S0-BAB-893

Progress in Pain Research and Management
Volume 17

Sex, Gender, and Pain

Mission Statement of IASP Press®

The International Association for the Study of Pain (IASP) is a nonprofit, interdisciplinary organization devoted to understanding the mechanisms of pain and improving the care of patients with pain through research, education, and communication. The organization includes scientists and health care professionals dedicated to these goals. The IASP sponsors scientific meetings and publishes newsletters, technical bulletins, the journal *Pain,* and books.

The goal of IASP Press is to provide the IASP membership with timely, high-quality, attractive, low-cost publications relevant to the problem of pain. These publications are also intended to appeal to a wider audience of scientists and clinicians interested in the problem of pain.

Previous volumes in the series
Progress in Pain Research and Management

Pharmacological Approaches to the Treatment of Chronic Pain: New Concepts and Critical Issues, edited by Howard L. Fields and John C. Liebeskind

Proceedings of the 7th World Congress on Pain, edited by Gerald F. Gebhart, Donna L. Hammond, and Troels S. Jensen

Touch, Temperature, and Pain in Health and Disease: Mechanisms and Assessments, edited by Jörgen Boivie, Per Hansson, and Ulf Lindblom

Temporomandibular Disorders and Related Pain Conditions, edited by Barry J. Sessle, Patricia S. Bryant, and Raymond A. Dionne

Visceral Pain, edited by Gerald F. Gebhart

Reflex Sympathetic Dystrophy: A Reappraisal, edited by Wilfrid Jänig and Michael Stanton-Hicks

Pain Treatment Centers at a Crossroads: A Practical and Conceptual Reappraisal, edited by Mitchell J.M. Cohen and James N. Campbell

Proceedings of the 8th World Congress on Pain, edited by Troels S. Jensen, Judith A. Turner, and Zsuzsanna Wiesenfeld-Hallin

Molecular Neurobiology of Pain, edited by David Borsook

Measurement of Pain in Infants and Children, edited by G. Allen Finley and Patrick J. McGrath

Sickle Cell Pain, by Samir K. Ballas

Assessment and Treatment of Cancer Pain, edited by Richard Payne, Richard B. Patt, and C. Stratton Hill

Chronic and Recurrent Pain in Children and Adolescents, edited by Patrick J. McGrath and G. Allen Finley

Opioid Sensitivity of Chronic Noncancer Pain, edited by Eija Kalso, Henry J. McQuay, and Zsuzsanna Wiesenfeld-Hallin

Psychological Mechanisms of Pain and Analgesia, by Donald D. Price

Proceedings of the 9th World Congress on Pain, edited by Marshall Devor, Michael C. Rowbotham, and Zsuzsanna Wiesenfeld-Hallin

Progress in Pain Research and Management
Volume 17

Sex, Gender, and Pain

Editor

Roger B. Fillingim, PhD

Departments of Psychology and Orthodontics,
University of Alabama, Birmingham, Alabama, USA

IASP PRESS® • SEATTLE

Timely topics in pain research and treatment have been selected for publication, but the information provided and opinions expressed have not involved any verification of the findings, conclusions, and opinions by IASP®. Thus, opinions expressed in *Sex, Gender, and Pain* do not necessarily reflect those of IASP or of the Officers and Councillors.

No responsibility is assumed by IASP for any injury and/or damage to persons or property as a matter of product liability, negligence, or from any use of any methods, products, instruction, or ideas contained in the material herein. Because of the rapid advances in the medical sciences, the publisher recommends that there should be independent verification of diagnoses and drug dosages.

Library of Congress Cataloging-in-Publication Data

Sex, gender, and pain / editor, Roger B. Fillingim.
p. ; cm. -- (Progress in pain research and management ; v. 17)
Includes bibliographical references and index.
ISBN 0-931092-35-3 (hard cover : alk. paper)
1. Pain--Sex factors. I. Fillingim, Roger B., 1962- II. Series.
[DNLM: 1. Pain. 2. Sex Characteristics. 3. Sex Factors. WL 704 S518 2000]
RB127.S44 2000
616'.0472--dc21

00-033589

Published by:

IASP Press
International Association for the Study of Pain
909 NE 43rd St., Suite 306
Seattle, WA 98105 USA
Fax: 206-547-1703
www.halcyon.com/iasp
www.painbooks.org

Printed in the United States of America

Contents

Part III Sex-Related Factors in Clinical Pain Conditions

Part IV Conclusions

Contributing Authors

Graciela S. Alarcón, MD, MPH *Division of Clinical Immunology and Rheumatology, University of Alabama at Birmingham, Birmingham, Alabama, USA*

Anna Maria Aloisi, MD, PhD *Institute of Human Physiology, University of Siena, Siena, Italy*

Karen J. Berkley, PhD *Program in Neuroscience, Florida State University, Tallahassee, Florida, USA*

Laurence A. Bradley, PhD *Division of Clinical Immunology and Rheumatology, University of Alabama at Birmingham, Birmingham, Alabama, USA*

Lin Chang, MD *CURE Digestive Diseases Research Center, Neuroenteric Disease Program, Department of Medicine, School of Medicine, University of California, Los Angeles, California, USA*

Roger B. Fillingim, PhD *Departments of Psychology and Orthodontics, University of Alabama at Birmingham, Birmingham, Alabama, USA; currently Department of Operative Dentistry, Public Health Services and Research, University of Florida, Gainesville, Florida, USA*

Robert W. Gear, DDS, PhD *Department of Oral and Maxillofacial Surgery, University of California, San Francisco, California, USA*

Maria Adele Giamberardino, MD *Pathophysiology of Pain Laboratory, Department of Medicine and Science of Aging, "G. D'Annunzio" University of Chieti, Chieti, Italy*

Alan R. Gintzler, PhD *Department of Biochemistry, Downstate Medical Center, Brooklyn, New York, USA*

Margaret M. Heitkemper, PhD, FAAN *Department of Biobehavioral Nursing and Health Systems, University of Washington, Seattle, Washington, USA*

Kenneth A. Holroyd, PhD *Department of Psychology, Ohio University, Athens, Ohio, USA*

Kevin S. Jones, MA *Department of Psychology, University of Western Ontario, London, Ontario, Canada*

Barry R. Komisaruk, PhD *Department of Psychology, Rutgers, The State University of New Jersey, Newark, New Jersey, USA*

Stefan Lautenbacher, PhD *Department of Psychiatry and Psychotherapy, University of Marburg, Marburg, Germany; and Department of Physiological Psychology, University of Bamberg, Bamberg, Germany*

Linda LeResche, ScD *Department of Oral Medicine, University of Washington, Seattle, Washington, USA*

Jon D. Levine, MD, PhD *Division of Neuroscience, NIH Pain Center, University of California, San Francisco, California, USA*

Gay L. Lipchik, PhD *Department of Psychology, Ohio University, Athens, Ohio, USA; currently Department of Physical Medicine and Rehabilitation, Saint Vincent Health Center, Erie, Pennsylvania, USA*

Nai-Jiang Liu, PhD *Department of Biochemistry, Downstate Medical Center, Brooklyn, New York, USA*

William Maixner, DDS, PhD *Dental Research Center, University of North Carolina, Chapel Hill, North Carolina, USA*

Emeran A. Mayer, MD *CURE Digestive Diseases Research Center, Neuroenteric Disease Program, Departments of Medicine and Physiology, School of Medicine, University of California, Los Angeles, California, USA*

Christine Miaskowski, RN, PhD, FAAN *Department of Physiological Nursing, University of California, San Francisco, California, USA*

Jeffrey S. Mogil, PhD *Department of Psychology and Program in Neuroscience, University of Illinois at Urbana-Champaign, Champaign, Illinois, USA*

Cynthia D. Myers, PhD *Department of Operative Dentistry, University of Florida, Gainesville, Florida, USA*

Bruce D. Naliboff, PhD *CURE Digestive Diseases Research Center, Neuroenteric Disease Program, Department of Psychiatry and Biobehavioral Sciences, University of California, Los Angeles, California, USA; and Department of Psychophysiology Research, VA Medical Center, Los Angeles, California, USA*

Timothy J. Ness, MD, PhD *Department of Anesthesiology, University of Alabama at Birmingham, Birmingham, Alabama, USA*

Joseph L. Riley III, PhD *Departments of Clinical and Health Psychology and Operative Dentistry, University of Florida, Gainesville, Florida, USA*

Michael E. Robinson, PhD *Department of Clinical and Health Psychology, University of Florida, Gainesville, Florida, USA*

Gary B. Rollman, PhD *Department of Psychology, University of Western Ontario, London, Ontario, Canada*

Wendy F. Sternberg, PhD *Department of Psychology, Haverford College, Haverford, Pennsylvania, USA*

R. William Stones, MD *Department of Obstetrics and Gynaecology, University of Southampton, Princess Anne Hospital, Southampton, United Kingdom*

Melissa W. Wachterman, BS *Department of Psychology, Haverford College, Haverford, Pennsylvania, USA*

Beverly Whipple, PhD, RN, FAAN *College of Nursing, Rutgers, The State University of New Jersey, Newark, New Jersey, USA*

Foreword

This book is a very welcome and thorough account of relationships between sex, gender, and pain. During the past decade, this topic has become much better understood due to extensive laboratory and clinical research. While much remains to be explored, the various chapters of this volume address the main issues of the biological and psychological influences of sex and gender on the many facets of pain experience and behavior.

In the first chapter, Roger Fillingim creates a context for the book by introducing three important issues—the magnitude of sex differences in pain, the mechanisms underlying these differences, and their clinical relevance. The remaining chapters continue to address these issues.

This book brings together experimental and clinical knowledge regarding the complex influences of sex and gender on pain. The literature reviewed in this book is rich yet raises numerous questions. Clinicians will appreciate the detail and thoroughness with which practical clinical questions are explored. At the same time, both clinicians and experimentalists will develop a deeper understanding of the world of those who treat pain.

Two unfortunate assumptions are often made by those wishing to provide simple, unifying explanations for sex and gender differences in pain—first, that these differences primarily result from "first-order" biological mechanisms, and second, that they reflect psychological differences. This book shows that the answer is more complex for it demonstrates that biological and psychological mechanisms are interdependent. We see how the transmission of pain-related information at all levels of the nervous system is subject to numerous psychological and biological influences—even dorsal horn neurons are directly influenced by psychological context.

Many chapters begin to fill the missing gaps in knowledge concerning interactions between biological and psychological effects of sex and gender, and some guide us toward future research areas. For example, Linda LeResche points out that the prevalence ratio of women to men with temporomandibular pain is about 2:1 in the general community, yet the ratio of women to men seeking health care for this type of condition is between 5:1 and 9:1. Thus, although greater prevalence is a contributing factor to greater health care utilization among women, it is not likely to be the exclusive factor; additional psychological and biological differences between men and women are likely to have critical influences. Chapters discussing experimental pain convincingly demonstrate sex and gender differences in subjects' responses and perceptions, and they reveal some implications of sex differences for development of persistent clinical pain conditions. For example, temporal summation of second pain ("wind-up") is, on average, of greater magnitude in women than in men. This difference has potential clinical interest because wind-up reflects the beginning stages of central sensitization, hence its mechanisms may support the hyperalgesia and allodynia of some persistent pain states. This consideration raises an important question. If women generally show greater magnitudes or rates of wind-up than men, could this sex difference explain the greater prevalence among women of pain conditions such as fibromyalgia, TMD, or irritable bowel syndrome? After all, these pain conditions are likely to be at least partly supported by mechanisms of central sensitization.

In reading these discussions of possible mechanisms underlying sex differences in pain, one cannot help being struck by the diversity of contributing factors, whether hormonal, psychological, neurophysiological, or neuropharmacological. The range of factors is almost overwhelming. Nevertheless, these multidimensional studies of sex and gender differences in pain produce an added and unexpected benefit by revealing the biological and psychological predisposing factors that produce common persistent pain conditions. As several chapters make clear, sex is only one of many interacting demographic factors that influence the magnitude and prevalence of different types of pain states.

In the last chapter Karen Berkley reflects on the important issues and questions raised in the previous chapters. She endorses a developmental lifespan perspective in which sex/gender is only one of several factors influencing the development of pain in individuals. This perspective emerges naturally from the varied topics presented and represents perhaps the book's most notable accomplishment.

Experienced scientists, clinicians, and students will find much to value within these pages. I am pleased to have this opportunity to introduce such an excellent book.

Donald D. Price, PhD
Departments of Oral and Maxillofacial Surgery and Neuroscience
University of Florida

Preface

Pain is a complex and personal experience sculpted by a multitude of forces both internal and external to the organism. Over the past 30 years, recognition of the multidimensional nature of pain has fostered an increased interest in understanding individual differences that can influence nociceptive processing. Even more recently, appreciation has grown for the potential role of sex- and gender-related factors in determining an individual's experience of pain. Indeed, the uncompromised pursuit of the equality of the sexes that characterized previous decades has given way to a constructive discourse regarding potentially important differences between women and men. Dramatic advances in pain research, together with sweeping changes in cultural attitudes, have revolutionized the field of research on sex-related differences in pain responses. Substantial evidence now indicates that females and males differ greatly in their nociceptive processing, in their responses to analgesic manipulations, and in their experience of clinical pain. Indeed, a recent Gallup survey on pain in America found that women are more likely than men to experience daily pain (46% of women vs. 37% of men) and that women are 50% more likely than men to have missed work in the past year because of pain.

This book provides a single resource summarizing many of the most important findings regarding sex, gender, and pain. Its contributors are leading international experts in this field whose perspectives include basic neuroscience, human laboratory research, clinical investigation, and epidemiological studies. This book provides information on multiple sex-related factors that can influence pain—factors such as genetic, hormonal, and psychosocial influences.

Part I is devoted to a discussion of several basic processes that may contribute to sex-related influences on pain. Chapter 1 provides the biopsychosocial framework for sex differences in pain. In Chapter 2, Anna Maria Aloisi reviews the wide-ranging somatosensory effects of gonadal hormones in both the peripheral and central nervous systems. She discusses the effects of such hormones on non-nociceptive systems as well as their influence on nociceptive processing. In the following chapter, Jeffrey Mogil discusses genetic influences on nociceptive sensitivity and their potential interactions with sex. He emphasizes the need to examine qualitative rather than simply quantitative sex differences in nociceptive processing. In Chapter 4, Michael Robinson and colleagues provide a very thorough review of the multiple psychosocial factors that may contribute to the sex-related differences in pain responses observed in human studies. This chapter discusses the importance of sex roles, social learning, and cognitive variables, and it describes sex differences in both clinical and experimental pain responses.

Part II focuses on the results of experimental research examining sex-related influences on pain. In Chapter 5, Wendy Sternberg and Melissa Wachterman review the complex nonhuman animal literature exploring sex differences and hormonal influences on nociceptive processing. This discussion covers not only the influence of sex and gonadal hormones on basal nociceptive responses, but also their effects on endogenous analgesic responses (e.g., stress-induced analgesia). Chapters 6 and 7 are devoted to two female-specific forms of analgesia. In Chapter 6, Alan Gintzler and Nai-Jiang Liu review Dr. Gintzler's pioneering exploration of how the hormonal events accompanying pregnancy alter nociceptive responses. The authors provide a logical analysis of research findings that have clarified the opioid and non-opioid neurochemistry underlying these effects. In Chapter 7, Barry Komisaruk and Beverly Whipple describe their impressive body of research demonstrating the analgesic effects of vaginocervical stimulation. The authors present both human and nonhuman animal data documenting these effects, and they discuss the neural mechanisms supporting this form of analgesia. In Chapter 8, Maria Adele Giamberardino discusses sex-related effects on visceral pain, which differs in important ways from the more typically studied pain arising in cutaneous and somatic structures. This comprehensive chapter reviews both the mechanisms underlying these effects and their clinical implications.

Gary Rollman and colleagues review human research on sex differences in experimental pain (Chapter 9). Rather than simply focusing on empirical findings, these authors provide an insightful discussion of multiple biopsychosocial mechanisms that may contribute to such differences. In Chapter 10, Tim Ness and I review the findings from prior research regarding the effects of the menstrual cycle and other hormonal events on pain responses in humans. This chapter discusses the clinical implications of these hormonal effects and analyzes their potential mechanisms. In Chapter 11, Christine Miaskowski and colleagues discuss sex-related differences in responses to analgesic medications. The authors include a review of their very interesting recent work on opioids and also consider other human and nonhuman animal research in order to better characterize the role that sex plays in analgesic responses.

Part III of the book considers sex-related contributions to various clinical pain conditions. In Chapter 12, Linda LeResche provides an overview of epidemiological perspectives and data relevant to sex differences in pain. She examines sex differences in the prevalence of several different pain conditions and highlights changes in prevalence across the life cycle, which may have important mechanistic implications. Chapter 13, by Kenneth Holroyd and Gay Lipchik, reviews sex-based mechanisms influencing recurrent headache disorders. The authors discuss sex differences in headache epidemiology, hormonal influences on headache symptoms, and clinical implications of these sex-related differences. In Chapter 14, Laurence Bradley and Graciela Alarcón discuss fibromyalgia, highlighting the reasons for its far greater prevalence among females. The authors present a model of heightened pain sensitivity in this disorder and incorporate sex-related factors that may contribute to the abnormal pain processing that is frequently observed in patients. In Chapter 15, William Maixner and I review sex-related contributions in temporomandibular disorders. We propose various neurobiological and psychophysiological mechanisms that may help explain the increased occurrence of this painful condition in females relative to males. Chapter 16, by Bruce Naliboff and colleagues, presents an overview of sex and gender as important contributors to irritable bowel syndrome and discusses mechanisms underlying sex-related influences in this disorder, including neuroanatomical, neuroendocrine, and gonadal hormonal factors. Chapter 17, by R. William Stones, reviews pelvic pain syndromes, a group of female-specific pain conditions. Dr. Stones presents diagnostic and treatment considerations in several different disorders and places these syndromes in a sociocultural context.

In the final chapter, Karen Berkley, clearly a pioneer in this field, distills and synthesizes the information presented by the authors of the other chapters. She discusses the limitations of our current knowledge and highlights the need for further research in several important areas.

I hope this volume will heighten the awareness of basic and clinical scientists and providers of pain treatment as it alerts them to the potential importance of sex-related factors in the experience of pain. This book should encourage us to discuss what we all believe: *women and men really are different!* A better understanding of the differences between the sexes will ultimately enhance our ability to diagnose and treat pain disorders of all types.

ROGER B. FILLINGIM, PHD

Part I

Basic Considerations for Sex, Gender, and Pain Research

Sex, Gender, and Pain, Progress in Pain Research and Management, Vol. 17, edited by R.B. Fillingim, IASP Press, Seattle, © 2000.

1

Sex, Gender and Pain: A Biopsychosocial Framework

Roger B. Fillingim

Departments of Psychology and Orthodontics, University of Alabama at Birmingham, Birmingham, Alabama, USA

The experience of being female or male depends on complex interactions among multiple endogenous and exogenous variables. These include obvious anatomical differences such as body size, genital organs, and muscle mass; differing levels and temporal patterns of gonadal hormones; psychosocial factors such as emotional experience and sex role expectancies; and multiple environmental and cultural influences. These and other variables are responsible for creating substantial differences between the sexes. However, investigators face the difficult task of determining when these differences are robust enough to overcome the tremendous variability *within* each sex and to merit scientific attention in and of themselves. The publication of this volume suggests that the topic of sex-related differences in pain has crossed that threshold. In this introductory chapter, I will outline recent events that have influenced research in this area, culminating in the publication of this book. I will then highlight several important issues regarding sex, gender, and pain, many of which will be addressed in detail in subsequent chapters.

RECENT DEVELOPMENTS

Important contributions to the literature on sex-related differences in the experience of pain have been made over many decades; however, I wish to focus on several recent events that provided important impetus and direction to this field. In pain research, as in all other areas of biomedical research, women have traditionally been eschewed as research subjects, partly because of the assumption that results derived from men were generalizable to women. When this assumption proved invalid, the vagaries of controlling for the pesky female menstrual cycle (or rodent estrous cycle) were used as an excuse to exclude women (and female rodents). Several years ago, Karen Berkley (1992) addressed this issue in a brief yet thought-provoking article emphasizing the importance of sex-related issues in neuroscience research. Her survey of 100 articles in reputable neuroscience journals indicated that 45% of the articles failed to report the sex of their subjects. The author also noted that the estrous cycle and other naturally occurring hormonal events in the female rat represent "experimental opportunities" rather than obstacles. In conclusion, Berkley stated that "the differences between females and males, which we all know to be important, can and should be exploited in scientific research." Shortly thereafter, M.A. Ruda wrote an editorial in the journal *Pain,* in which she discussed the importance of studying the differences between women and men, a topic that had been out of favor given the emphasis in the 1980s on equality of the sexes. These two publications both reflected and promoted renewed interest in the issue of sex-related differences in pain.

In 1995, we (Fillingim and Maixner 1995) wrote a review article in *Pain Forum* summarizing the literature on sex differences in experimental pain and providing a model for conceptualizing the mechanisms whereby sex differences could emerge. At about the same time, Karen Berkley (1997) prepared a review article for *Behavioral and Brain Sciences,* which received extensive commentary from many prominent pain scientists. Anita Unruh (1996) also published a comprehensive review article in *Pain* on sex differences in clinical pain. These and other publications indicated increasing interest in the topic in the 1990s, culminating in two National Institutes of Health (NIH) initiatives. First, in 1997, NIH issued a request for applications entitled "Sex and Gender-Related Differences in Pain and Analgesic Responses," which was sponsored by multiple institutes including the Office for Research on Women's Health. Then, in April 1998, the NIH Pain Research Consortium hosted a scientific conference entitled "Gender and Pain: A Focus on How Pain Impacts Women Differently Than Men," organized by M.A. Ruda. This well-attended conference featured presentations by many prominent basic and clinical scientists and received considerable attention in the popular media. Another important development began in August 1996 at the 8th World Congress on Pain in Vancouver, where Will Stones and Karen Berkley organized a meeting of researchers interested in sex, gender, and pain. This meeting led to the establishment of an International Association for the Study of Pain (IASP) Special Interest Group (SIG) on Sex, Gender and Pain, which held its first formal meeting in 1999 at the 9th World Congress on Pain in Vienna.

The objectives of this SIG are (1) to encourage basic and clinical research on how sex and gender affect pain mechanisms and all realms of its management, (2) to provide a central information resource on these issues, and (3) to develop multidisciplinary discussion groups on subtopics of these issues.

This group continues to thrive, and many of the authors in this volume are members. In summary, the 1990s witnessed several influential publications in the scientific press, strong support from the NIH for research in this area, and the organization of an international special interest group related to sex, gender, and pain. These events laid the groundwork for the publication of this book.

SEX DIFFERENCES IN PAIN

Many important issues are related to sex, gender, and pain. There is little doubt that female and male organisms of many species differ in their responses to pain. However, these differences can be complex and variable, and their exact nature is not always clear. Three important issues related to sex, gender, and pain are addressed in the chapters that follow: (1) the magnitude of sex differences in pain, (2) the mechanisms underlying these differences, and (3) their clinical relevance

THE MAGNITUDE OF SEX DIFFERENCES IN PAIN

Some authors have suggested that sex differences are relatively small (Berkley 1997), while others have reported moderate effects (Riley et al. 1998), and we have previously proposed that sex differences in pain responses are robust (Fillingim and Maixner 1995). Interestingly, all three opinions may be correct. The magnitude and direction of sex differences can be influenced by the type of pain being studied (i.e., experimental, acute clinical, or chronic), by the population under investigation (clinical vs. community-based), and by the specific empirical questions addressed in the study. For example, sex differences in experimental pain perception are well documented, but the consistency and magnitude of the effects vary across pain induction techniques (Riley et al. 1998). Also, sex differences in the epidemiology of certain pain disorders have been demonstrated, while other pain conditions appear to be equally common in women and men (LeResche 1999; see Chapter 12, this volume). However, in clinical samples of chronic pain populations, sex differences in pain reports have been difficult to detect (see Chapter 4). Thus, attempts to draw a general conclusion regarding the magnitude of sex differences in pain would be inadequate. A much more productive approach would emphasize better characterization of sex differences in specific settings and populations, with the ultimate goal of understanding the mechanisms and clinical importance of these effects.

MECHANISMS UNDERLYING SEX DIFFERENCES

We (Fillingim and Maixner 1995; Fillingim 2000; Fillingim and Ness 2000) and others (Unruh 1996; Berkley 1997) have proposed various explanations for the sex differences that have emerged in studies of both clinical and experimental pain. These explanations are often classified as either psychosocial or neurophysiological. Examples of the former include sex role expectancies (i.e., femininity vs. masculinity), cognitive/affective factors (e.g., anxiety, coping, self-efficacy), and social learning. Examples of the latter include gonadal hormones, genetic factors, blood pressure, and differences in endogenous pain inhibition. This distinction between psychosocial and neurophysiological mechanisms, while convenient, is artificial, because psychosocial factors inevitably produce their effects via neurophysiological mechanisms, and because neurophysiological influences also affect psychosocial processes. The evidence related to many of these mechanisms is thoroughly reviewed in several chapters of this volume. However, it is important to resist the temptation to decide which factor is the real culprit in producing sex-related differences in pain response. I prefer to adopt a biopsychosocial approach, which recognizes that the experience of pain is inevitably sculpted by complex and dynamic interactions among biological, psychological, and sociocultural factors (see Fig. 1). Thus, our task is not to decide

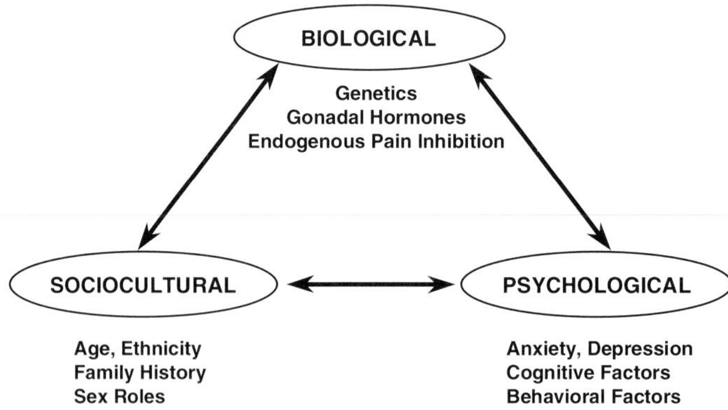

Fig. 1. Schematic diagram of the biopsychosocial model as it relates to sex differences in pain. Examples of biological, psychological, and sociocultural factors that may contribute to sex and gender effects on pain responses are included. The arrows indicate the important bidirectional interactions among the three sets of factors.

which factor is most important, but instead to determine the relative contributions of each of several factors from the three different but interdependent domains.

CLINICAL RELEVANCE

An inevitable question regarding sex-related differences in the experience of pain is, "How do sex differences influence diagnosis and treatment of patients in pain?" Of course, sex-related factors represent only one set of variables that may affect pain responses, and other variables such as age, psychosocial status, and disease activity may be more important in guiding clinical decisions. Nonetheless, sex-related factors may have important clinical ramifications. For example, data showing that certain analgesics appear to be more effective for women than for men (see Chapter 11) indicate that the patient's sex should influence the clinician's choice of analgesic agents. In addition, epidemiologic data clearly indicate that women are at greater risk for developing certain pain disorders, and hormonal factors are implicated in some of these (see Chapter 12). Thus, theories of the pathophysiology of these clinical conditions must account for the preponderance of female patients, which has implications for both diagnosis and treatment. Indeed, in a recent investigation of the influence of sex on the different phenotype of rheumatoid arthritis (RA), the authors state "Data ... are compatible with the interpretation that female and male RA follow different rules and represent distinguishable forms of the disease" (Weyand et al. 1998). Given their consistent and far-reaching effects on pain, it must be concluded that sex-related factors have tremendous clinical relevance. The task ahead is to understand the nature of these effects in order to incorporate them into clinical care as a way of enhancing the management of pain in women and men.

ACKNOWLEDGMENT

Preparation of this chapter was supported in part by NIH grant DE12261.

REFERENCES

Berkley KJ. Vive la difference. *Trends Neurosci* 1992; 15:331–332.
Berkley KJ. Sex differences in pain. *Behav Brain Sci* 1997; 20:371–380.
Fillingim RB. Sex, gender and pain: women and men really are different. *Curr Rev Pain* 2000; 4:24–30.

Fillingim RB, Maixner W. Gender differences in the responses to noxious stimuli. *Pain Forum* 1995; 4:209–221.

Fillingim RB, Ness TJ. Sex-related hormonal influences on pain and analgesic responses. *Neurosci Biobehav Rev* 2000; 24:485–501.

LeResche L. Gender considerations in the epidemiology of chronic pain. In: Crombie IK, Croft PR, Linton SJ, LeResche L, Von Korff M (Eds). *Epidemiology of Pain.* Seattle: IASP Press, 1999, pp 43–52.

Riley JL, Robinson ME, Wise EA, Myers CD, Fillingim RB. Sex differences in the perception of noxious experimental stimuli: a meta-analysis. *Pain* 1998; 74:181–187.

Unruh AM. Gender variations in clinical pain experience. *Pain* 1996; 65:123–167.

Weyand CM, Schmidt D, Wagner U, Goronzy JJ. The influence of sex on the phenotype of rheumatoid arthritis. *Arthritis Rheum* 1998; 41:817–822.

Correspondence to: Roger B. Fillingim, PhD, Department of Operative Dentistry, Public Health Services and Research, University of Florida, P.O. Box 100404, 1600 SW Archer Road, D8-37, Gainesville, FL 32610-0404, USA. Email: RFillingim@ufl.edu.

Sex, Gender, and Pain, Progress in Pain Research and Management, Vol. 17, edited by R.B. Fillingim, IASP Press, Seattle, © 2000.

2

Sensory Effects of Gonadal Hormones

Anna Maria Aloisi

Institute of Human Physiology, University of Siena, Siena, Italy

The 1990s saw the introduction of sex as a parameter in pain research. Although pioneering work was carried out at the beginning of the 20th century, general scientific knowledge about this topic has appeared only in recent years. Behavioral studies had approached the question of sex differences in pain responses, but there were few efforts to thoroughly explore the underlying neuronal circuits.

There is an impressive amount of information about the different circuits of the central nervous system (CNS) involved in collecting and processing information from the different sensory modalities—touch, smell, sight, hearing, and taste. Wonderful books have been written on their anatomy and physiology, so I will avoid summarizing these topics. Instead, I will concentrate on the influence of sex and gonadal hormones on sensory processing. I will include data not directly related to pain, but of potential interest for a better understanding of pain processes.

GONADAL HORMONES

In humans and experimental animals such as rats, the gonadal hormones are androgen and estrogen. Their effects on the CNS and many other tissues can be direct or may be mediated by numerous steroids. In this chapter, I will focus on testosterone and estradiol. Most of the information about the effects of gonadal hormones on the sensory system refers to estradiol-induced effects, and few data are available for testosterone. However, most of the testosterone-mediated actions in the male CNS are produced by estradiol obtained by the aromatization of testosterone (Naftolin et al. 1975; Horvath and Wikler 1999).

The sex differences in the CNS are produced by gonadal hormones during certain pre- and perinatal periods, which cause permanent changes in the hormone-sensitive neural substrate (Pilgrim and Hutchison 1994). These effects have been defined as "organizational" and are related to both reproductive and nonreproductive functions. In addition, gonadal hormones can modulate CNS functions throughout an individual's life by means of "activational" effects mostly related to their plasma concentrations (Arnold and Breedlove 1985). The adult mammalian brain shows remarkable plasticity in response to gonadal steroid manipulations (Kawata 1995).

In adulthood, blood levels of gonadal hormones differ by sex: testosterone is higher in males, while estradiol is higher in females. However, male and female rats have both hormones, and have receptors for both at very similar levels in the same brain regions, irrespective of sex (Kawata 1995; McEwen and Alves 1999). Gonadal hormones have a low molecular mass (270–379 kDa) and are sufficiently lipophilic to cross the blood-brain barrier by simple diffusion. Cholesterol is the precursor of both androgen and estrogen (Fig. 1). Some steroid hormones are synthesized within the nervous system, either de novo from cholesterol or via the metabolism of precursors originating in the circulation; these have been termed "neurosteroids" (Mensah-Nyagan et al. 1999).

In nonpregnant women, the ovaries secrete large amounts of estradiol, while during pregnancy the placenta secretes substantial amounts of estrogens. Estradiol has two types of receptors (ERα and ERβ), whose distribution differs in various tissues (Shughrue et al. 1996; Paech et al. 1997; Enmark and Gustafsson 1999). In the rat, the highest expression of ERα is in the uterus, testes, pituitary, ovaries, kidneys, epididymis, and adrenals,

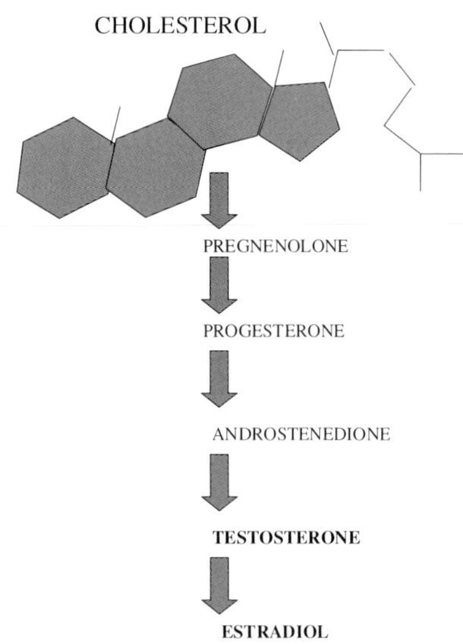

Fig. 1. Synthesis of gonadal hormones. Some of these metabolic pathways are present in the CNS.

whereas ERβ is the major estrogen receptor in the brain and is also present in the prostate, ovaries, lung, bladder, and epididymis (Kuiper et al. 1996).

Testosterone is synthesized in Leydig interstitial cells of the testis under the influence of the pituitary gonadotropic hormone. Only one kind of androgen receptor (AR) is known. In addition to being present in most peripheral structures, it is also present in the mammalian nervous system (Sar and Stumpf 1977), including the anterior and posterior horns of the spinal cord (Simerly et al. 1990). The AR regulates gene expression in both transactivation and transrepression modes and uses various strategies involving regions outside its DNA-binding domain to achieve its multiple functions (Turgeon and Waring 1999). For instance, Yang-Yen et al. (1990) demonstrated that AR in wild-type mice can have a marked dominant negative activity on transcription mediated by glucocorticoid and progesterone receptors.

Estradiol and testosterone act on neurons in which their receptors are present through two main pathways (Fig. 2). First, there is a classical pathway in which steroid hormones regulate genomic activity. After binding to its receptor, the hormone reaches the DNA and induces transcription of specific genes. These genes act on the neuronal substrate to cause permanent structural alterations. For instance, *c-Fos* gene expression can rapidly be induced by estradiol in several brain regions (Cattaneo and Maggi 1990; Insel 1990). Second, there is a nongenomic pathway of rapid gonadal hormone action, which appears not to involve effects on transcription (Schumacher 1990; Kawata 1995).

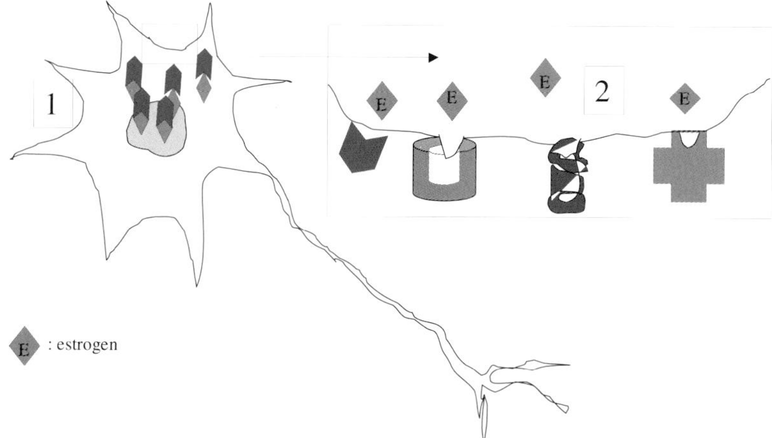

Fig. 2. Schematic representation of the action of gonadal hormones in neurons: (1) Through the classical genomic pathway, the hormone binds with its receptor, reaches the DNA and initiates the cascade of protein synthesis. (2) The rapid nongenomic pathway includes membrane receptors that are directly modulated by gonadal hormones without genomic effects.

Nongenomic effects are likely to be important supplementary mechanisms that fine-tune and modulate the actions that are set up by longer-lasting genomic effects. The nongenomic actions of estradiol on the firing of hypothalamic, hippocampal, cerebellar, and cortical neurons are believed to involve the chloride channel of the $GABA_A$ receptors (Weiland et al. 1997). Moreover, estrogen inhibits the entry of calcium through L-type channels (Nakajima et al. 1995; Mermelstein et al. 1996) and modulates protein kinase C activity and growth-associated protein 43 mRNA (Shughrue and Dorsa 1994; Sohrabji et al. 1994; Murphy and Segal 1996). Interestingly, some of these effects are implicated in neuronal mechanisms of learning and memory (Routtenberg 1985; McEwen and Alves 1999) and in the effects of stress on learning (Shors et al. 1997).

THE SEX-DEPENDENT SENSORY SYSTEMS

Discussion of the sensory modalities may seem a strange approach to enhancing our understanding of pain. However, the modulatory effects of pain on the perception of different stimuli have been confirmed by experimental evidence (Clark et al. 1986). Sex-related differences in the ability to detect sensory stimuli have repeatedly been shown by various approaches (Velle 1987). Women have lower sensory detection thresholds than men for most modalities. For taste, the sex differences increase with age; at around 40 years of age, women have a higher sensitivity than men for all substances tested. For smell, a number of well-planned and convincing investigations strongly support marked sex differences, with higher sensitivity in women. Estrogen has long been known to increase olfactory sensitivity, while androgens have the opposite effect (Le Magnen 1949). The threshold of sound perception is lower for women than for men, regardless of age (Corso 1959; Lopez-Escamez et al. 1999). Sex differences in the perception of auditory stimuli are most marked at higher frequencies. For touch, the general picture is the same for the skin senses as for taste and olfaction, since evidence strongly supports the contention that women show greater sensitivity than men to various stimuli.

Marked sex differences have been reported in physiological responses to the several categories included in the visual system. For instance, static and dynamic acuity is greater in men than in women (McGuinness 1976). However, women show more rapid scotopic adaptation than men. Interestingly, split visual field studies have revealed that males recognize pictures of faces faster when the stimulus is received by the right cerebral hemisphere (i.e., presented in the left visual field) than when received by the left hemisphere. For females, no difference between the two hemispheres was observed (Rizzolatti and Buchtel 1977).

GONADAL HORMONES AND PAIN

PERIPHERAL TISSUE

As early as 1894, Galton showed that women are more sensitive than men in the two-point discrimination test. Later, using an esthesiometer, Weinstein and Sersen (1961) showed that women are significantly more sensitive than men on the sole of the foot and the palm of the hand. Procacci and colleagues (1970a,b) found a lower pain threshold in women than men and also demonstrated that the pain threshold increases with advancing age in both sexes. Robinson and Short (1977) tested the skin of the nipples, areolae, and breast and found no sex differences in sensitivity *prepubertally*, while *postpubertally* sensitivity increases dramatically in women but not in men. This finding strongly supports the hypothesis that the differences are due to increasing levels of gonadal hormones. However, in neonates the electrical conductivity of the skin is considerably higher in females than in males (Weller and Bell 1965).

Several hypotheses have been advanced to explain these differences in sensitivity. For instance, sex differences in skin conductivity may be relevant to the measurement of skin sensitivity to electrical stimulation. The effects of gonadal hormones on skin characteristics are well known; puberty, estrous cycle phases, and menopause are all related to important skin variations. Estrogens enhanced dermal contents of water and collagen in a human study (Brincat et al. 1987). Larkin and colleagues (1986) reported that women are much more sensitive than men to electrocutaneous stimulation, particularly on the skin of the forearm. The sexes differed by at least 30% in all subgroups, although when the data were normalized with measures of body size (weight or surface area), no statistically significant male-female differences remained. In rodents, estrogen injection increased the size of the receptive area of trigeminal mechanoreceptors (Bereiter et al. 1980). In humans, Tan (1991) found a negative linear relationship between serum testosterone levels and the amplitude of the H-reflexes from thenar muscles of the right thumb. He also demonstrated that testosterone decreases the conduction time from the foot to the cerebral cortex; high testosterone levels were associated with short conduction times. These sensory experiments complement other studies looking at sex differences in pain in both animals and humans, which are reported throughout this volume.

In humans, the data that I consider of particular interest in understanding the involvement of gonadal hormones in pain processes are those related to the vascular system. The protective effect of estrogen in the cardiovascular system has prompted a number of studies whose focus includes molecules known to participate in nociception.

Estrogen exerts direct effects on blood vessels, promoting vasodilation by stimulating the synthesis of prostacyclin and nitric oxide (NO) (Hayashi et al. 1997). The vascular walls contain specific high-affinity receptors for estrogen (ER), and changes in the plasma estrogen concentration regulate the levels of ER in vascular tissue (Farhat et al. 1996). In particular, there are receptors in vascular smooth muscle, and specific binding sites have been demonstrated in the endothelium. The endothelium produces various vasoactive mediators such as prostacyclin and endothelium-derived NO. The vascular endothelium synthesizes NO from its natural precursor L-arginine via activity of the nitric oxide synthase (NOS) enzyme. These products are subject to regulation by estrogen. Moreover, estrogen stimulates the vessel wall to synthesize prostaglandin (Chang et al. 1980). These rapid vascular effects of estrogen are mediated by a mechanism independent of the classical genomic pathway of steroid action.

These findings implicate estrogen in pain-related effects through its vasodilatory action. However, in some instances estrogen appears to be involved in pain processes through potentiation of the spasmogenic response of vascular smooth muscle. This action may contribute to several pain syndromes with a recognized vascular component. For instance, migraine headache appears to be influenced by gender and by menstrual status (see Chapter 13). Moreover, the vasoconstriction observed in Raynaud's phenomenon, a disease most prominent in premenopausal women, may have the same estrogen-related mechanism (Levine and Taiwo 1989). This hypothesis is founded on the estrogen-induced enhanced sensitivity of small arterioles to norepinephrine and the increased number of α-adrenergic receptors in the myometrium (Altura 1975; Roberts et al. 1977). In rats (as in humans), these modifications could explain the decrease in the pressure nociceptive threshold observed 48 hours after β-estradiol administration. The decrease in the nociceptive threshold produced by norepinephrine in estradiol-treated rats was completely antagonized by sympathectomy (Levine and Taiwo 1989). The basis for the qualitative differences in the vasomotor responses to estrogen among different blood vessels is unclear.

DORSAL ROOT GANGLIA

The presence of estrogen receptors in the dorsal root ganglia (DRG) has repeatedly been reported, raising the possibility that estrogen modulates cutaneous sensation by acting directly on primary afferent cell body neurons. ERα is expressed in small DRG neurons (Sohrabji et al. 1994), while ERβ is abundantly expressed in large, medium, and small DRG neurons (Taleghany et al. 1999). Interestingly, in intact cycling female rats, ERα and ERβ mRNA levels in the DRG were both higher during proestrus than metestrus. The presence of ERα mRNA and protein in nerve growth factor (NGF)-dependent DRG neurons of adult female rats was related to the increased survival of DRG neurons (Patrone et al. 1999). In particular, estrogen regulates trkA mRNA levels even in the absence of NGF, which suggests that if estrogen collaborates with NGF in the maintenance of normal adult DRG gene expression and functions, the loss of estrogen (such as that associated with menopause) may contribute to a decline in DRG neuronal function and exacerbate ongoing neuropathic processes (Liuzzi et al. 1999). A reduction of estrogen in women has been associated with various pain syndromes in which no overt pathological condition can be identified (Heitkemper et al. 1993; Drexler and Schroeder 1994; Rosano et al. 1995).

SPINAL CORD

In the spinal cord, the interaction between pain and gonadal hormones has been studied mostly with reference to pregnancy-related events. In rodents, changes in pain perception during pregnancy revealed an opioid-mediated increase in the pain threshold, activated by sex hormones (Marcus 1995; Dawson-Basoa and Gintzler 1996); this phenomenon occurred in response to somatic as well as visceral noxious stimuli.

In rats, elevated response thresholds to aversive stimuli are most apparent during late pregnancy and around parturition. In women, antinociception appears during a similar period, i.e., 18 days before parturition (Cogan and Spinnato 1986). Moreover, it appears that the exposure of nonpregnant animals to the blood concentrations of estradiol and progesterone shown by pregnant females activates a κ-opioid receptor analgesic system in the spinal cord (see Chapter 6). The ability of spinal κ-opioid receptors to mediate sex-steroid-induced antinociception is consistent with their location within the spinal cord. Kappa-opioid receptors are present in high densities in the lumbosacral area of both rats and humans. In the rat spinal cord, κ-opioid binding sites are dense in superficial layers of the dorsal horn and in lamina X around the central canal, regions that are involved in the processing of nociceptive stimuli (Gouarderes et al. 1985). A progressive increase in the circulating levels of estradiol and progesterone, such as occurs during pregnancy, modulates a spinal dynorphin/κ-opioid analgesic system both presynaptically and postsynaptically. The μ-opioid-receptor analgesic system in the spinal cord does not appear to be sensitive to the blood profile of estradiol and progesterone during pregnancy, or to participate in the antinociception associated with gestation.

We have recently found (Aloisi and Ceccarelli 2000) that in intact male rats, intracerebroventricular administration of estrogen decreases the formalin-induced paw jerk (the repetitive phasic flexion of the injected limb), an effect counteracted by pretreatment with naloxone (Fig. 3). This finding suggests that estrogen can also influence pain transmission in the male spinal cord. Interestingly, in female rats Amandusson et al. (1999) demonstrated that estrogen receptors are present in large numbers of neurons in the spinal dorsal horn in the same location as the enkephalin-expressing neurons. The same authors showed that estrogen administration rapidly increases spinal cord enkephalin mRNA levels in ovariectomized rats.

THALAMUS

The thalamus is a supraspinal center in which external stimuli could be greatly affected by different endogenous conditions. Thus, it is interesting that thalamic circuits are also sensitive to circulating levels of gonadal

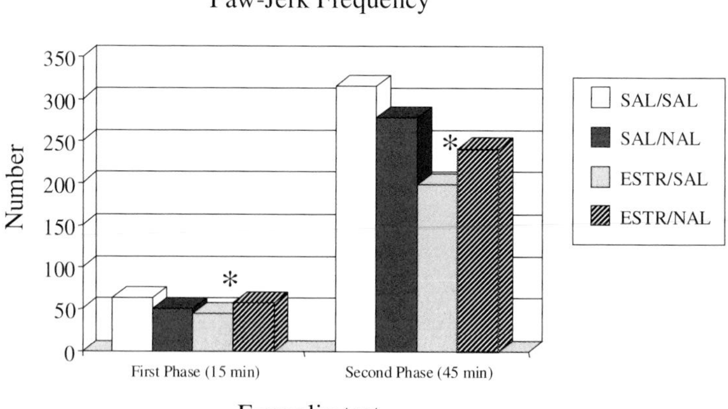

Fig. 3. In intact animals, estrogen treatment decreases paw-jerk frequency during both the first and the second phase of the formalin test; this effect is counteracted by pretreatment with naloxone. ESTR = estradiol; NAL = naloxone; SAL = saline. Asterisks (*) denote $P < 0.005$ versus SAL/SAL. Data are from Aloisi and Ceccarelli (2000).

steroids. Wardlaw and colleagues (1982) reported that castrated female rats exposed for 3 weeks to estrogens exhibited a decrease of thalamic endorphin, with important effects on somatosensory transmission. More recently, in a study of dyskinesia, Bosse and DiPaolo (1996) suggested that GABAergic output to the thalamus decreases after ovariectomy (as a model of menopause); the thalamus is thus less inhibited and becomes overactive, sending excessive glutamatergic signals. Therefore, it appears that gonadal hormones can significantly affect thalamic transmission through different neural circuits. We are not aware of any studies aimed at understanding the importance of gonadal hormones in nociceptive transmission through the thalamus.

BRAIN

Many morphological and functional sex differences have been described throughout the brain. For instance, Levy (1980) reported marked sex differences in cerebral organization. Estrogen has been associated with enhanced verbal fluency, and testosterone with better visual-spatial abilities (Kimura 1992; Van Goozen et al. 1995). Ho et al. (1986) used signal detection analyses to demonstrate that men and women use different strategies to complete experimental tasks. In particular, women gave more false alarms and responded more rapidly depending on the stage of their cycle, although the number of their correct answers remained relatively stable. McGaughy and Sarter (1999) reported that the attentional performance of intact female rats was better in diestrus than in proestrus.

Estrogens affect cognitive functions through their actions on the cholinergic system (Luine 1997; Miller et al. 1999). In addition, estrogen enhances mood and subjective well-being in the perimenopausal and postmenopausal periods (Schneider et al. 1977; Gerdes et al. 1982). Interestingly, estrogen receptors and cholinergic muscarinic or nicotinic sites coexist on many cortical and hippocampal neurons (Hosli and Hosli 1999). Affective disorders, such as postnatal depression, premenstrual syndrome, and postmenopausal depression, are associated with a large decrease in serum estrogen levels. However, estradiol and testosterone were affected differently by painful stimuli in animal experiments. Testosterone was unaffected or increased by painful stimuli (pinching or formalin treatment) (Tsuchiya 1994; Aloisi and Ceccarelli 2000), whereas estrogens were greatly decreased after formalin-induced pain (Aloisi and Ceccarelli 2000). This finding suggests that females exhibit a kind of vicious circle in which the decrease of estrogen can contribute to the further increase of pain, and so on. On the other hand, estrogen replacement increases the incidence of temporomandibular joint disorders (LeResche et al. 1997).

Pain has both sensory and affective components. A selective modulation of the affective component is strongly correlated with changes in activity within the anterior cingulate cortex, but not in the primary somatosensory cortex (Rainville et al. 1997). The cingulate cortex is part of an affective pain response system and contributes to the perception of pain and to the learning process associated with predicting and avoiding noxious stimuli. Studies on humans and animals have consistently shown that cingulate neurons respond to noxious stimuli and can undergo plastic changes during persistent pain (Zhuo et al. 1998).

Becerra et al. (1999) showed distinct differences in CNS activation in the anterior cingulate, insula, and frontal lobes in women at the mid-follicular and mid-luteal menstrual cycle phases following either 41°C or 46°C stimulation. The pain ratings were the same for the two phases, and activation during the mid-follicular phase closely approximated activation in men given the same thermal stimuli. Moreover, painful stimuli applied to the forearm induced similar reflex responses in males and females, but significantly greater activation of the contralateral prefrontal cortex, insula, and thalamus in females, which suggests a different supraspinal processing of similar input (Casey 1999). This finding agrees with data obtained in rats; with different techniques, neuronal activity was higher after painful stimuli in females than in males (Brown et al. 1996; Aloisi et al. 1997).

GONADAL HORMONES AND NEUROTRANSMITTERS

MONOAMINES

The differences observed between males and females cannot be explained by gender-related anatomical variations alone. Thus, functional differences have been hypothesized. In 1968, Bowerman and colleagues (1968) proposed that gonadal hormones play an active role in modulating the balance between norepinephrine- and acetylcholine-mediated action. These two neurotransmitters belong to the autonomic system and also act as chemical transmitters in the CNS. The authors suggested that the sex differences could reflect the balance between the activating effect of central adrenergic processes and the inhibitory effect of central cholinergic processes. This balance can be influenced by sex hormones, since estrogens appear to be stronger activators of the adrenergic system than androgens. Other studies, in particular those of Frankenhaeuser and colleagues (1978), confirmed this hypothesis in humans. They showed that although basal adrenergic metabolism does not differ between the sexes, the levels of adrenalin excretion after stress are much higher in males than in females. Heritage and colleagues (1980) found in rodents that estradiol target sites are present in the nuclei of many catecholamine bodies in the brainstem, which primarily contain norepinephrine. In the locus ceruleus, 25% of the catecholamine neurons contain estradiol target sites.

Estrogen influences the serotonergic system (Bethea et al. 1998). In addition to influencing serotonin plasma levels, female sex hormones alter both the number and binding capabilities of serotonin receptors. Peak estrogen levels in the rat are associated with decreased numbers of available serotonin receptors (Marcus 1995) and thus with a greater availability of serotonin. However, during the withdrawal phase following an estrogen peak, estrogen receptor affinity decreases and the number of available serotonin receptors increases (Biegon and McEwen 1982; Uphouse et al. 1986). Interestingly, Stratz et al. (1993) found a significant correlation between the number of tender points and serotonin levels in fibromyalgia patients, and reported a significantly lower level of plasma serotonin in patients than in controls. Cyclic variations of plasma estrogen levels may thus influence serotonin levels, which in turn may modulate the soreness of tender points (Klein et al. 1992; Russell et al. 1992; Yunus 1992).

OPIOIDS

Gonadal hormones also influence the endogenous opioid system (Shoupe et al. 1985; Hammer and Bridges 1987; Aloisi and Ceccarelli 2000). The endogenous opioid peptides belong to three families: endorphins (EP), enkephalins (ENK), and dynorphins. All the β-EP in the limbic-hypothalamic circuit originates in the cell bodies of the hypothalamic arcuate nucleus (Mansour et al. 1988). In contrast, ENK cells are extensively distributed throughout all the nuclei of the limbic-hypothalamic circuit. The expression of both β-EP and ENK is sensitive to sex steroids. For instance, Thornton et al. (1994) showed that estrogen treatment significantly increases the number of β-EP-immunoreactive cells in ovariectomized (OVX) guinea pigs with respect to OVX vehicle-treated animals. This was true for all areas of the arcuate nucleus of the hypothalamus. In OVX rats, 2 or 3 weeks of treatment with estradiol benzoate significantly decreased hypothalamic proopiomelanocortin mRNA levels and β-EP content (Thornton et al. 1994). The treatment led to increased expression of the ENK gene (Romano et al. 1988; Priest et al. 1995), an effect that is probably mediated by intracellular estrogen receptors (Pfaff et al. 1994). The estrogen receptor can bind directly to the ENK gene and thereby influence its transcriptional activity (Zhu and Pfaff 1995).

In the brain of the female rat, the number of μ-type opioid receptors fluctuates during the different phases of the estrous cycle, which may explain the different magnitude of the effects exerted by opioid agonists and antagonists in the different phases of the ovulatory cycle. Piva and colleagues (1995) reported that treatment with estradiol benzoate alone increased the number of binding sites of dihydromorphine (a specific μ-receptor ligand) in the hippocampus and thalamus, without modifying the receptor status of the other brain regions. In primates, Wehrenberg et al. (1982) reported significant reductions of hypothalamic β-EP following ovariectomy; in intact animals, plasma β-EP levels rose during times of increased estrogen and were undetectable at menstruation, when serum levels of ovarian steroids were minimal.

In summary, the effects of estrogen on β-EP neurons are complex. Numerous factors, primarily the neuronal population considered but also the time of day and the time after estrogen treatment, may affect the response of β-EP neurons to estrogen (Genazzani et al. 1990; Wise et al. 1990).

MENSTRUAL CYCLE CHANGES

The human menstrual cycle is characterized by increasing levels of estrogen in the blood during the follicular phase, with a peak near the time of ovulation. Diurnal variations in pain thresholds and cyclic changes covering longer periods have been detected in both sexes (Procacci et al. 1970b, 1974). In women, the pain threshold varies with the stage of the estrous cycle. As early as 1944, Haman advanced the hypothesis of a general lowering of the sensory threshold in correspondence to menses; this was substantiated by a number of studies that found the pain threshold to be highest in the follicular phase and lowest in the luteal phase. However, this finding does not hold true for all kinds of painful stimulation. While the pain threshold is higher in the follicular phase for almost all natural stimuli, the opposite occurs for electrical stimuli, i.e., there is a lower threshold in the follicular phase (see Chapter 10 for a detailed review).

Migraine is prevalently a female disorder and is significantly related to reproductive life events. The menstrual period represents a phase of maximal vulnerability to migraine attacks. Baseline sex hormone levels are altered in some women with migraine. Epstein et al. (1975) reported higher mean estrogen and progesterone levels in migraine patients than in headache-free controls throughout most of the menstrual cycle. Indeed, migraine tended to improve with physiological menopause.

An earlier hypothesis to explain pain threshold variation during the menstrual cycle stated that variations in the extracellular fluid at the receptor site or increased skin impedance may change the conductance into deeper tissues and thus alter the aversiveness of the electrical stimulation (Tedford et al. 1977). Indeed, Morton et al. (1953) noted that women's average weight increase due to premenstrual water retention was 1.36 kg. Interestingly, a somewhat regular cyclic variation in pain threshold has also been reported for males (Velle 1987).

CONCLUSIONS

Gonadal hormones are substances that induce the development of primary and secondary sexual characteristics. Among their effects are several important modulatory actions on the CNS, including pain circuits. Data concerning sex differences in the sensory system are scarce and have not yet been consolidated, as is apparent from the absence of such information in physiology textbooks.

The clinical approach to many illnesses has always been sex-dependent. However, for pain syndromes, information on sex differences is still mostly limited to epidemiologic data indicating that women are more susceptible than men to the development of chronic pain syndromes. Thus, basic and clinical studies of the sexual differentiation of the nervous system and of the structural basis of sex differences in physiological functions and behavioral patterns would help in understanding why females are more at risk for chronic pain.

Delving deeper into the sex differences in each body region would certainly disclose some secrets. The information provided in this chapter about gonadal hormones and the somatosensory system is certainly not exhaustive; it is intended only to provide an overview of the widespread action of these substances.

Gonadal hormones are necessary for reproduction, but it appears that no body region, no neuronal circuit, and virtually no cell is unaffected by them. Thus, in pain research, increased attention toward these molecules would appear to be obligatory.

ACKNOWLEDGMENT

The author thanks the University of Siena and is grateful to Dr. Ilaria Ceccarelli for her indispensable help.

REFERENCES

Aloisi AM, Ceccarelli I. Role of gonadal hormones in formalin-induced pain responses of male rats: modulation by estradiol and naloxone administration. *Neuroscience* 2000; 95:559–566.

Aloisi AM, Zimmermann M, Herdegen T. Sex-dependent effects of formalin and restraint on c-Fos expression in the septum and hippocampus of the rat. *Neuroscience* 1997; 81:951–958.

Altura BM. Sex and estrogens and responsiveness of terminal arterioles to neurohypophyseal hormones and catecholamines. *J Pharmacol Exp Ther* 1975; 193:403–412.

Amandusson A, Hallbeck M, Hallbeck A, Hermanson O, Blomqvist A. Estrogen-induced alterations of spinal cord enkephalin gene expression. *Pain* 1999; 83:243–248.

Arnold AP, Breedlove SM. Organizational and activational effects of sex steroids on brain and behavior: a reanalysis. *Horm Behav* 1985; 19:469–498.

Becerra LR, Breiter HC, Stojanovic M, et al. Human brain activation under controlled thermal stimulation and habituation in noxious heat: an fMRI study. *Magn Reson Med* 1999; 41:1044–1057.

Bereiter DA, Stanford LR, Barker DJ. Hormone-induced enlargement of receptive fields in trigeminal mechanoreceptive neurons. II. Possible mechanisms. *Brain Res* 1980; 184:411–423.

Bethea CL, Pecins-Thompson M, Schutzer WE, Gundlah C, Lu ZN. Ovarian steroids and serotonin neural function. *Mol Neurobiol* 1998; 18:87–123.

Biegon A, McEwen BS. Modulation by estradiol of serotonin receptors in brain. *J Neurosci* 1982; 2:199–205.

Bosse R, DiPaolo T. The modulation of brain dopamine and GABAA receptors by estradiol: a clue for CNS changes occurring at menopause. *Cell Mol Neurobiol* 1996; 16:199–212.

Bowerman DM, Klaiber EL, Kobayashi Y, Vogel W. Roles of activation and inhibition in sex differences in cognitive abilities. *Psychol Rev* 1968; 75:23–50.

Brincat M, Moniz CF, Kabalan S, et al. Decline in skin collagen content and metacarpal index after the menopause and its prevention with sex hormone replacement. *Br J Obstet Gynaecol* 1987; 94:126–129.

Brown LL, Siegel H, Etgen AM. Global sex differences in stress-induced activation of cerebral metabolism revealed by 2-deoxyglucose autoradiography. *Horm Behav* 1996; 30:611–617.

Casey KL. Forebrain mechanisms of nociception and pain: analysis through imaging. *Proc Natl Acad Sci USA* 1999; 96:7668–7674.

Cattaneo E, Maggi A. c-fos induction by estrogen in specific rat brain areas. *Eur J Pharmacol* 1990; 188:153–159.

Chang WC, Nakao J, Orimo H, Murota SI. Stimulation of prostaglandin cyclooxygenase and prostacyclin synthetase activities by estradiol in rat aortic smooth muscle cells. *Biochim Biophys Acta* 1980; 620:472–482.

Clark WC, Yang JC, Janal MN. Altered pain and visual sensitivity in humans: the effects of acute and chronic stress. *Ann NY Acad Sci* 1986; 467:116–129.

Cogan R, Spinnato JA. Pain and discomfort thresholds in late pregnancy. *Pain* 1986; 27:63–68.

Corso JF. Age and sex differences in thresholds. *J Acoust Soc Am* 1959; 31:489–507.

Dawson-Basoa ME, Gintzler AR. Estrogen and progesterone activate spinal kappa-opiate receptor analgesic mechanisms. *Pain* 1996; 64:608–615.

Drexler H, Schroeder JS. Unusual forms of ischemic heart disease. *Curr Opin Cardiol* 1994; 9:457–464.

Enmark E, Gustafsson J. Oestrogen receptors—an overview. *J Intern Med* 1999; 246:133–138.

Epstein MT, Hockaday JM, Hockaday TD. Migraine and reproductive hormones throughout the menstrual cycle. *Lancet* 1975; 1:543–548.

Farhat MY, Lavigne MC, Ramwell PW. The vascular protective effects of estrogen. *FASEB J* 1996; 10:615–624.

Frankenhaeuser M, von Wright MR, Collins A, et al. Sex differences in psychoneuroendocrine reactions to examination stress. *Psychosom Med* 1978; 40:334–343.

Galton F. The relative sensitivity of men and women at the nape of the neck by Webster's test. *Nature* 1894; 50:40–42.

Genazzani AR, Trentini GP, Petraglia F, et al. Estrogens modulate the circadian rhythm of hypothalamic beta-endorphin contents in female rats. *Neuroendocrinology* 1990; 52:221–224.

Gerdes LC, Sonnendecker EWW, Polakow ES. Psychological change effected by estrogen-progesterone and clonidine treatment in climacteric women. *Am J Obstet Gynaecol* 1982; 142:98–104.

Gouarderes C, Cros J, Quirion R. Autoradiographic localization of mu, delta and kappa opioid receptor binding sites in rat and guinea pig spinal cord. *Neuropeptides* 1985; 6:331–342.

Haman JO. Pain threshold and dysmenorrhea. *Am J Obstet Gynaecol* 1944; 47:686–691.

Hammer RP Jr, Bridges RS. Preoptic area opioids and opiate receptors increase during pregnancy and decrease during lactation. *Brain Res* 1987; 420:48–56.

Hayashi T, Yamada K, Esaki T, Mutoh E, Iguchi A. Effect of estrogen on isoforms of nitric oxide synthase: possible mechanism of anti-atherosclerotic effect of estrogen. *Gerontology* 1997; 43:24–34.

Heitkemper MM, Jarrett M, Caudell KA, Bond E. Women with gastrointestinal symptoms: implications for nursing research and practice. *Gastroenterol Nurs* 1993; 15:226–232.

Heritage AS, Stumpf WE, Sar M, Grant LD. Brainstem catecholamine neurons are target sites for sex steroid hormones. *Science* 1980; 207:1377–1379.

Ho HZ, Gilger JW, Brink TM. Effects of menstrual cycle on spatial information-processes. *Percept Mot Skills* 1986; 63:743–751.

Horvath TL, Wikler KC. Aromatase in developing sensory systems of the rat brain. *J Neuroendocrinol* 1999; 11:77–84.

Hosli E, Hosli L. Cellular localization of estrogen receptors on neurones in various regions of cultured rat CNS: coexistence with cholinergic and galanin receptors. *Int J Dev Neurosci* 1999; 17:317–330.

Insel TR. Regional induction of c-fos-like protein in rat brain after estradiol administration. *Endocrinology* 1990; 126:1849–1853.

Kawata M. Roles of steroid hormones and their receptors in structural organization in the nervous system. *Neurosci Res* 1995; 24:1–46.

Kimura D. Sex differences in the brain. *Sci Am* 1992; 267:118–125.

Klein R, Bansch M, Berg PA. Clinical relevance of antibodies against serotonin and gangliosides in patients with primary fibromyalgia syndrome. *Psychoneuroendocrinology* 1992; 17:593–598.

Kuiper GG, Enmark E, Pelto-Huikko M, Nilsson S, Gustafsson JA. Cloning of a novel receptor expressed in rat prostate and ovary. *Proc Natl Acad Sci USA* 1996; 93:5925–5930.

Larkin WD, Reilly JP, Kittler LB. Individual differences in sensitivity to transient electrocutaneous stimulation. *IEEE Trans Biomed Eng* 1986; 33:495–504.

Le Magnen J. Physiologie des sensations—variation spécifique des séniles olfactifs chez l'homme sous actions androgène et oestrogène. *C R Hebd Seances Acad Sci* 1949; 228:947–948.

LeResche L, Saunders K, Von Korff MR, Barlow W, Dworkin SF. Use of exogenous hormones and risk of temporomandibular disorder pain. *Pain* 1997; 69:153–160.

Levine JD, Taiwo YO. Beta-estradiol induced catecholamine-sensitive hyperalgesia: a contribution to pain in Raynaud's phenomenon. *Brain Res* 1989; 487:143–147.

Levy J. Cerebral asymmetry and the psychology of man. In: Wittrock MC (Ed). *The Brain and the Psychology*. New York: Academic Press, 1980.

Liuzzi FJ, Scoville SA, Bufton SM. Effects of short-term estrogen replacement on trkA mRNA levels in axotomized dorsal root ganglion neurons. *Exp Neurol* 1999; 159:433–440.

Lopez-Escamez JA, Salguero G, Salinero J. Age and sex differences in latencies of waves I, III and V in auditory brainstem response of normal hearing subjects. *Acta Otorhinolaryngol Belg* 1999; 53:109–115.

Luine VN. Steroid hormone modulation of hippocampal dependent spatial memory. *Stress* 1997; 2:21–36.

Mansour A, Khachaturian H, Lewis ME, Akil H, Watson SJ. Anatomy of CNS opioid receptors. *Trends Neurosci* 1988; 11:308–314.

Marcus DA. Interrelationships of neurochemicals, estrogen, and recurring headache. *Pain* 1995; 62:129–139.

McEwen BS, Alves SE. Estrogen actions in the central nervous system. *Endocr Rev* 1999; 20:279–307.

McGaughy J, Sarter M. Effects of ovariectomy, 192 IgG-saporin-induced cortical cholinergic deafferentation, and administration of estradiol on sustained attention performance in rats. *Behav Neurosci* 1999; 113:1216–1232.

McGuinness D. Sex differences in the organisation of perception and cognition. In: Lloyd B, Archer J (Eds). *Exploring Sex Differences*. London: Academic Press, 1976, pp 123–155.

Mensah-Nyagan AG, Do-Rego JL, Beaujean D, et al. Neurosteroids: expression of steroidogenic enzymes and regulation of steroid biosynthesis in the central nervous system. *Pharmacol Rev* 1999; 51:63–81.

Mermelstein PG, Becker JB, Surmeier DJ. Estradiol reduces calcium currents in rat neostriatal neurons via a membrane receptor. *J Neurosci* 1996; 16:595–604.

Miller MM, Hyder SM, Assayag R, et al. Estrogen modulates spontaneous alternation and the cholinergic phenotype in the basal forebrain. *Neuroscience* 1999; 91:1143–1153.

Morton JH, Additon H, Addison RG, Hunt L, Sullivan JJ. A clinical study of premenstrual tension. *Am J Obstet Gynaecol* 1953; 65:1182–1191.

Murphy DD, Segal M. Regulation of dendritic spine density in cultured rat hippocampal neurons by steroid hormones. *J Neurosci* 1996; 16:4059–4068.

Naftolin F, Ryan KJ, Davies IJ, et al. The formation of estrogens by central neuroendocrine tissues. *Recent Prog Horm Res* 1975; 31:295–319.

Nakajima T, Kitazawa T, Hamada E, et al. 17beta-Estradiol inhibits the voltage-dependent L-type Ca^{2+} currents in aortic smooth muscle cells. *Eur J Pharmacol* 1995; 294:625–635.

Paech K, Webb P, Kuiper GG, et al. Differential ligand activation of estrogen receptors ER-alpha and ER-beta at AP1 sites. *Science* 1997; 277:1508–1510.

Patrone C, Andersson S, Korhonen L, Lindholm D. Estrogen receptor-dependent regulation of sensory neuron survival in developing dorsal root ganglion. *Proc Natl Acad Sci USA* 1999; 96:10905–10910.

Pfaff DW, Schwartz-Giblin S, McCarthy MM, Kow L. Cellular and molecular mechanisms of female reproductive behaviors. In: Knobil E, Neill JD (Eds). *The Physiology of Reproduction*. New York: Raven Press, 1994, pp 107–220.

Pilgrim C, Hutchison JB. Developmental regulation of sex differences in the brain: can the role of gonadal steroids be redefined? *Neuroscience* 1994; 60:843–855.

Piva F, Limonta P, Dondi D, et al. Effects of steroids on the brain opioid system. *J Steroid Biochem Mol Biol* 1995; 53:343–348.

Priest CA, Eckersell CB, Micevych PE. Estrogen regulates preproenkephalin-A mRNA levels in the rat ventromedial nucleus: temporal and cellular aspects. *Brain Res Mol Brain Res* 1995; 28:251–262.

Procacci P, Bozza G, Buzzelli G, Della CM. The cutaneous pricking pain threshold in old age. *Gerontol Clin (Basel)* 1970a; 12:213–218.

Procacci P, Buzzelli G, Passeri I, et al. Studies on the cutaneous pricking pain threshold in man. Circadian and circatrigintan changes. *Res Clin Stud Headache* 1970b; 3:260–276.

Procacci P, Della CM, Zoppi M, et al. Pain threshold measurements in man. In: Bonica JJ, Pagni CA (Eds). *Recent Advances on Pain*. Springfield: Thomas, 1974.

Rainville P, Duncan GH, Price DD, Carrier B, Bushnell MC. Pain affect encoded in human anterior cingulate but not somatosensory cortex. *Science* 1997; 277:968–971.

Rizzolatti G, Buchtel HA. Hemispheric superiority in reaction time to faces: a sex differences. *Cortex* 1977; 13:300–305.

Roberts JM, Insel PA, Goldfien RD, Goldfien A. alpha Adrenoreceptors but not beta adrenoreceptors increase in rabbit uterus with oestrogen. *Nature* 1977; 270:624–625.

Robinson E, Short RV. Changes in breast sensitivity at puberty, during the menstrual cycle, and at parturition. *BMJ* 1977; 7:1188–1191.

Romano GJ, Harlan RE, Shivers BD, Howells RD, Pfaff DW. Estrogen increases proenkephalin messenger ribonucleic acid levels in the ventromedial hypothalamus of the rat. *Mol Endocrinol* 1988; 2:1320–1328.

Rosano GM, Collins P, Kaski JC, et al. Syndrome X in women is associated with oestrogen deficiency. *Eur Heart J* 1995; 16:610–614.

Routtenberg A. Protein kinase C activation leading to protein F1 phosphorylation may regulate synaptic plasticity by presynaptic terminal growth. *Behav Neural Biol* 1985; 44:186–200.

Russell IJ, Michalek JE, Vipraio GA, et al. Platelet 3H-imipramine uptake receptor density and serum serotonin levels in patients with fibromyalgia/fibrositis syndrome. *J Rheumatol* 1992; 19:104–109.

Sar M, Stumpf WE. Androgen concentration in motor neurons of cranial nerves and spinal cord. *Science* 1977; 197:77–79.

Schneider MA, Brotherton PL, Hailes J. The effect of exogenous oestrogens on depression in menopausal women. *Med J Aust* 1977; 2:162–163.

Schumacher M. Rapid membrane effects of steroid hormones: an emerging concept in neuroendocrinology. *Trends Neurosci* 1990; 13:359–362.

Shors TJ, Elkabes S, Selcher JC, Black IB. Stress persistently increases NMDA receptor-mediated binding of [^{3}H]PDBu (a marker for protein kinase C) in the amygdala, and re-exposure to the stressful context reactivates the increase. *Brain Res* 1997; 750:293–300.

Shoupe D, Montz FJ, Lobo RA. The effects of estrogen and progestin on endogenous opioid activity in oophorectomized women. *J Clin Endocrinol Metab* 1985; 60:178–183.

Shughrue PJ, Dorsa DM. Estrogen and androgen differentially modulate the growth-associated protein GAP-43 (neuromodulin) messenger ribonucleic acid in postnatal rat brain. *Endocrinology* 1994; 134:1321–1328.

Shughrue PJ, Komm B, Merchenthaler I. The distribution of estrogen receptor-beta mRNA in the rat hypothalamus. *Steroids* 1996; 61:678–681.

Simerly RB, Chang C, Muramatsu M, Swanson LW. Distribution of androgen and estrogen receptor mRNA-containing cells in the rat brain: an in situ hybridization study. *J Comp Neurol* 1990; 294:76–95.

Sohrabji F, Miranda RC, Toran-Allerand CD. Estrogen differentially regulates estrogen and nerve growth factor receptor mRNAs in adult sensory neurons. *J Neurosci* 1994; 14:459–471.

Stratz T, Samborski W, Hrycaj P, et al. Serotonin concentration in serum of patients with generalized tendomyopathy (fibromyalgia) and chronic polyarthritis. *Med Klin* 1993; 88:458–462.

Taleghany N, Sarajari S, DonCarlos LL, Gollapudi L, Oblinger MM. Differential expression of estrogen receptor alpha and beta in rat dorsal root ganglion neurons. *J Neurosci Res* 1999; 57:603–615.

Tan U. Association of serum testosterone levels with latencies of somatosensory evoked potentials from right and left posterior tibial nerves in right-handed young male and female subjects. *Int J Neurosci* 1991; 60:249–277.

Tedford WHJ, Warren DE, Flynn WE. Alteration of shock aversion thresholds during the menstrual cycle. *Percept Psychophys* 1977; 21:193–196.

Thornton JE, Loose MD, Kelly MJ, Ronnekleiv OK. Effects of estrogen on the number of neurons expressing beta-endorphin in the medial basal hypothalamus of the female guinea pig. *J Comp Neurol* 1994; 341:68–77.

Tsuchiya T. Effects of cutaneous mechanical stimulation on plasma corticosterone, luteinizing hormone (LH), and testosterone levels in anesthetized male rats. *Hokkaido Igaku Zasshi* 1994; 69:217–235.

Turgeon JL, Waring DW. Androgen modulation of luteinizing hormone secretion by female rat gonadotropes. *Endocrinology* 1999; 140:1767–1774.

Uphouse L, Williams J, Eckols K, Sierra V. Variations in binding of [3H]5-HT to cortical membranes during the female rat estrous cycle. *Brain Res* 1986; 381:376–381.

Van Goozen SH, Cohen-Kettenis PT, Gooren LJ, Frijda NH, Van de Poll NE. Gender differences in behaviour: activating effects of cross-sex hormones. *Psychoneuroendocrinology* 1995; 20:343–363.

Velle W. Sex differences in sensory functions. *Perspect Biol Med* 1987; 30:490–522.

Wardlaw SL, Thoron L, Frantz AG. Effects of sex steroids on brain beta-endorphin. *Brain Res* 1982; 245:327–331.

Wehrenberg WB, Wardlaw SL, Frantz AG, Ferin M. beta-Endorphin in hypophyseal portal blood: variations throughout the menstrual cycle. *Endocrinology* 1982; 111:879–881.

Weiland NG, Orikasa C, Hayashi S, McEwen BS. Distribution and hormone regulation of estrogen receptor immunoreactive cells in the hippocampus of male and female rats. *J Comp Neurol* 1997; 388:603–612.

Weinstein S, Sersen E. Tactile sensitivity as a function of handedness and laterality. *J Comp Physiol Psychol* 1961; 54:665–669.

Weller GM, Bell RQ. Basal skin conductance and neonate state. *Child Dev* 1965; 36:647–657.

Wise PM, Scarbrough K, Weiland NG, Larson GH. Diurnal pattern of proopiomelanocortin gene expression in the arcuate nucleus of proestrous, ovariectomized, and steroid-treated rats: a possible role in cyclic luteinizing hormone secretion. *Mol Endocrinol* 1990; 4:886–892.

Yang-Yen HF, Chambard JC, Sun YL, et al. Transcriptional interference between c-Jun and the glucocorticoid receptor: mutual inhibition of DNA binding due to direct protein-protein interaction. *Cell* 1990; 62:1205–1215.

Yunus MB. Towards a model of pathophysiology of fibromyalgia: aberrant central pain mechanisms with peripheral modulation. *J Rheumatol* 1992; 19:846–850.

Zhu YS, Pfaff DW. DNA binding of hypothalamic nuclear proteins on estrogen response element and preproenkephalin promoter: modification by estrogen. *Neuroendocrinology* 1995; 62:454–466.

Zhuo M, Lee DE, Li P, Calejesan AA. The cingulate cortex biphasically regulate spinal nociception. *Soc Neurosci Abstracts* 1998; 24:1135.

Correspondence to: Anna Maria Aloisi, MD, PhD, Institute of Human Physiology, University of Siena, Via Aldo Moro, 53100 Siena, Italy. Email: aloisi@unisi.it.

Sex, Gender, and Pain, Progress in Pain Research and Management, Vol. 17, edited by R.B. Fillingim, IASP Press, Seattle, © 2000.

3

Interactions between Sex and Genotype in the Mediation and Modulation of Nociception in Rodents

Jeffrey S. Mogil

Department of Psychology and Neuroscience Program, University of Illinois at Urbana-Champaign, Champaign, Illinois, USA

INDIVIDUAL DIFFERENCES IN PAIN AND PAIN INHIBITION

Experimental data are most often, and most appropriately, presented as group means accompanied by some index of variance (e.g., standard deviations or standard errors). It is, of course, the first priority of the experimenter to account for the means. Although much can also be learned from a consideration of the variance among randomly sampled individuals, this aspect is routinely ignored. Some proportion of observed variance is attributable to experimental error, but much derives from intrinsic differences among the subjects. For example, it is well known that 10 mg morphine, *on average,* will effectively inhibit a wide range of clinical and experimental pain in humans. We now understand a great deal about how morphine works on a molecular, cellular, and systems level (see Basbaum and Fields 1984; Pasternak 1993; Kieffer 1999). What we do not yet know is why morphine works well in some individuals, but more poorly in others.

Many factors have been proposed to contribute to such variability. For example, it is thought that some types of pain (e.g., neuropathic pain) are relatively insensitive to opiate inhibition (Arnér and Meyerson 1988), whereas other types (e.g., inflammatory pain) are relatively sensitive (Kayser and Guilbaud 1983). Both nociceptive sensitivity and response to analgesics vary with photoperiod, suggesting the involvement of circadian rhythmicity (Morris and Lutsch 1967; Folkard 1976). A number of ontogenetic and adult environmental factors can affect pain sensitivity in rats, including prenatal and postnatal stress (Kinsley et al. 1988; Pieretti et al. 1991), perinatal lead exposure (Jackson and Kitchen 1989), diet (Frye et al. 1993; Shir et al. 1998), and housing (group vs. isolation) (Adler et al. 1975; Puglisi-Allegra and Oliverio 1983).

In addition, factors intrinsic to the subjects can account for considerable variability. The most studied of these "organismic" variables are age (see Hamm and Knisely 1988; Chung et al. 1995; Fitzgerald 1995), genetic background (see Mogil 1999), and sex. Within a particular sex, physiological/hormonal status (e.g., menstrual/estrous cycle phase, pregnancy) is a well-known if not particularly well understood modifying factor. This chapter describes the influence of both genetic variation and sex on nociception and antinociception in laboratory rodents, especially in terms of how these variables interact. Recent findings in my laboratory strongly suggest that the modulatory effect of either of these organismic variables on pain-related traits can only be understood in the context of the other. That is, sex differences vary with, and are specific to, the particular genetic background in question, and genetic differences (between strains) can sometimes be observed in one sex but not the other. This chapter will focus both on quantitative sex differences (i.e., *more* or *less* pain) and on qualitative sex differences indicating the recruitment of neurochemically distinct neural circuitry.

GENETICS OF PAIN AND PAIN INHIBITION: A MINIREVIEW

Genetic background (or "genotype") may be the organismic factor of greatest relevance to explaining variance in studies of pain, because of all the factors described above, genotype is the least likely to be controlled for within an experiment. This is because all studies in humans and most studies in animals are performed in genetically heterogeneous populations. Although all members of a mammalian species have virtually identical genomes—in that they possess and express the same 50,000–150,000 genes (excluding catastrophic mutations)—genetic diversity results from DNA sequence variants (or "alleles") in or near these genes. These allelic variants, called "mutations" if rare and "polymorphisms" if more common, are inherited in a Mendelian fashion, and occur with a frequency of approximately 1 per 350 base pairs in humans (Cargill et al. 1999). Since most pain-related traits (or "phenotypes") are polygenic, i.e., mediated by multiple genes, each gene contributes only partially to the expression of the phenotype.

Pain-related traits, like virtually all others, are influenced by both genetic and environmental factors ("nature and nurture"). Therefore, inheritance of particular alleles at pain-relevant genes accounts only for a proportion of overall phenotypic variance; that proportion is known as "heritability." Heritability estimates for pain, established largely via twin studies in humans, have ranged from 10% for experimental pressure pain (MacGregor et al. 1997) to 21% for sciatica (Heikkila et al. 1989) to >50% for migraine (e.g., Honkasalo et al. 1995; Larsson et al. 1995; Ziegler et al. 1998) and menstrual pain (Treloar et al. 1998). For some of these pain syndromes, heritability appears to be considerably higher in females than males. For instance, estimated heritability of sciatica in females was 26.2% compared to 14.0% in males (Heikkila et al. 1989), and that of migraine was 49–58% in females compared to 39–44% in males (Larsson et al. 1995). Finally, one study revealed a sex difference in the proportion of variance in migraine occurrence due to genetic dominance (Honkasalo et al. 1995). Heritability estimates for a variety of nociception and antinociception traits in rodents also span a wide range, but they average approximately 50% (e.g., Mogil et al. 1999).

Once the heritability of a pain-related trait has been established, the arduous but important task of genetic dissection can begin. Three pain traits have thus far yielded to genetic explanation. Indo and colleagues (1996) demonstrated that mutations of the *NTRK1* gene, encoding the high-affinity nerve growth factor receptor, are the cause of congenital insensitivity to pain with anhidrosis (CIPA; hereditary sensory neuropathy, type IV). Ophoff and colleagues (1996) showed that mutations of the *CACNL1A4* gene, encoding a subunit of a P/Q-type voltage-gated calcium channel, can produce familial hemiplegic migraine. The relevance of this gene to idiopathic migraine remains unclear. Finally, it is well established that various polymorphisms of the *CYP2D6* gene, encoding a neuronal cytochrome P450 enzyme, are relevant to (among other things) the analgesic efficacy of codeine (see Meyer 1994). Individuals rendered "poor metabolizers" by virtue of inheriting one of these polymorphisms (7–10% of the Caucasian population) are unable to convert codeine to morphine, and thus receive no therapeutic benefit from this opiate.

The three successful genetic dissections described above were greatly facilitated by the "all-or-none" nature of the pain traits in question, indicative of their mediation by single genes. The situation is more complicated for the vast majority of pain-related phenotypes in which multiple genes contribute. The extra burden imposed by having to isolate the effects of individual genes from all other genetic and environmental factors is mitigated somewhat by the extra statistical power realized by the use of experimental crosses in laboratory mice. My laboratory has used quantitative trait locus (QTL) mapping in several studies relevant to pain, the results of which will be discussed below. Such efforts typically involve a sequence of steps (see Lander and Schork 1994; Belknap et al. 1996). First, an inbred strain survey is performed to define the heritability of the trait and identify extreme-responding strains. Inbred strains are particularly useful genetically, since they represent genomes (and thus, particular alleles of pain-relevant genes) that have been fixed in a homozygous state (i.e., identical-by-descent) by repeated brother-sister matings. Each individual member of an inbred strain is essentially a clone of all other members, irrespective of time or geography. Thus, any observed variability within a strain must by definition be due to environmental factors, whereas a comparison of between-strain means reflects genetic contributions. Once extreme-responding (say, nociception-sensitive and nociception-resistant) inbred strains are identified, a test cross (e.g., backcross, F_2 intercross, recombinant inbred [RI] strains) can be produced as a genetically segregating mapping population. All members of the mapping population are "phenotyped" for the trait at hand, and then "genotyped" for their inheritance of DNA markers spanning the genome. We and many others use "microsatellite" markers (i.e., simple sequence repeat/length polymorphisms), which are common throughout the mammalian genome, of known location, easily typed by size, and especially polymorphic in their repeat length, even between closely related inbred strains. The genetic "linkage" (i.e., partial coinheritance) of the phenotype and genotype of a particular microsatellite suggests a QTL at the approximate chromosomal location of the linked microsatellite; an inference is made in turn that a gene contributing to the phenotype also resides nearby. Following the identification of QTLs, a consultation of existing linkage maps may identify "candidate genes," which can be evaluated using conventional methods. Alternately, positional cloning efforts may begin in an attempt to clone the gene based on its location.

QUANTITATIVE SEX DIFFERENCES IN RODENTS: INTERACTIONS WITH GENOTYPE

As described in Chapter 5, sex differences in nociception and opioid antinociception are somewhat less controversial in the rodent literature than in the analogous human literature. We recently reviewed the existing rodent data (Mogil et al. 2000), and made the following broad conclusions: (1) female rats are more sensitive than males to electric shock and chemical nociception; (2) this sex difference is abolished or even *reversed* in rats when noxious heat is used as a stimulus (although species differences may exist here); and (3) male rodents are universally more sensitive to morphine antinociception than females (although the situation is more complicated for other opioid and non-opioid analgesics). When compiling this review, we were struck by the realization that virtually the entire literature used one of the following subject populations: Sprague Dawley rats, Swiss-derived mice, and deer mice (*Peromyscus maniculatus*).

This discovery was unsettling because of a recent finding we had made using inbred mouse strains. In that experiment, male and female mice of 11 inbred strains were tested for their nociceptive sensitivity on the 49°C tail-withdrawal test, and also for their antinociceptive sensitivity to supraspinally administered morphine (Kest et al. 1999). Of the 11 strains considered, three (AKR/J, C3H/HeJ, and C57BL/6J) displayed significant sex differences in basal nociceptive sensitivity, with females proving more sensitive than males in each case. With respect to morphine antinociception, significant sex differences were observed in four strains. Male AKR/J, C57BL/6J, and SWR/J mice were 6.9-, 3.6-, and 3.5-fold more sensitive than their female counterparts, respectively, whereas CBA/J females were 5.5-fold more sensitive than males of that strain (Kest et al. 1999). Another intriguing finding was that the variability of cumulative half-maximal antinociceptive doses (AD_{50}s) among female strain means greatly exceeded that of males. The highest and lowest female mean AD_{50} differed by 41-fold (CBA/J females, 0.12 μg; SWR/J females, 4.95 μg), whereas the analogous range for males was only 14-fold (C3H/HeJ males, 0.11 μg; SJL/J male, 1.64 μg). Since within-strain variance was equivalent between the sexes (even though we did not control for estrous phase in females), this differential between-strain variability corresponds to far higher heritability estimates for supraspinal morphine antinociception in females compared to males.

Although we identified sex differences in both basal nociception and morphine antinociception in some strains in this study, most strains showed no evidence of sex differences. Despite using small samples (n = 8 mice of each sex per strain), we might at least have expected to see a *trend* toward sex differences (Kest et al. 1999), but most strains showed no such trend. Thus, a major conclusion of this study was that the presence of sex differences depends on the genetic background under consideration. We believe that this conclusion is generalizable to other nociceptive assays (e.g., the hot-plate test) and analgesics (the κ-opioid receptor agonist U50,488 and the synthetic cannabinoid WIN55,212-2) (see Table I).

While intriguing, these findings are not immediately relevant to the existing literature, since nongeneticists do not widely use inbred strains because of their poor fecundity and (resultant) high purchase price. Therefore, we attempted to determine whether the presence of sex differences would depend on the outbred subject population chosen. Outbred strains (more correctly, randomly bred stocks) of rodents represent the vast majority

Table I
Which rodent strains show sex differences in nociception and antinociception?

Male > Female	Male = Female[a]	Female > Male
Basal Thermal Nociceptive Sensitivity (Kest et al. 1999; Mogil et al. 1999a)		
Sprague Dawley rats	Wistar Kyoto rats Swiss Webster mice[b] CD-1 (ICR) mice[b] 8 inbred strains (129/J, A/J , BALB/cJ, CBA/J, DBA/2J, LP/J, SJL/J, SWR/J)	Long Evans rats Swiss Webster mice[b] AKR/J mice C3H/HeJ mice C57BL/6J mice
Morphine Antinociception (Kest et al. 1999; Mogil et al. 1999a)		
Long Evans rats Sprague Dawley rats CD-1 (ICR) mice AKR/J mice[c] C57BL/6J mice[c] SWR/J mice[c]	Wistar Kyoto rats Swiss Webster mice 7 inbred strains[c] (129/J, A/J, BALB/cJ, C3H/HeJ, DBA/2J, LP/J, SJL/J)	CBA/J mice[c]
WIN55,212-2 Antinociception[d] (Wilson et al. 1999)		
129/J mice BALB/cJ mice	9 inbred strains (A/J, AKR/J, C3H/HeJ, C57BL/6J, C57BL/10J, C58/J, CBA/J, DBA/2J, RIIIS/J)	
U50,488 Antinociception[e] (J.S. Mogil, unpublished observations)		
129/J mice C3H/HeJ mice	8 inbred strains (A/J, AKR/J, C57BL/6J, C57BL/10J, C58/J, DBA/2J, RIIIS/J, SM/J)	BALB/cJ mice

Note: All tests used the 49°C tail-withdrawal assay.
[a] With conventional sample sizes of $n < 25$ individuals/sex.
[b] Depending on vendor (see text). Note, though, that with sufficiently high sample sizes ($n > 40$ individuals/sex), all outbred mouse lines tested showed female > male sex differences, but with varying magnitude.
[c] In this study (Kest et al. 1999), sensitivity to supraspinal (intracerebroventricular) administration of morphine was assessed.
[d] Sensitivity based on a single dose of systemic WIN55,212-2 (6.0 mg/kg), near the half-maximal antinociceptive dose (AD_{50}) of outbred mice.
[e] Sensitivity based on a single dose of systemic U50,488 (25 mg/kg), near the AD_{50} of outbred mice.

of subjects in biobehavioral research, and can be obtained inexpensively from a number of large commercial suppliers. Although such suppliers attempt to minimize inbreeding in order to maintain heterozygosity, which in turn maintains fecundity, partial inbreeding is nonetheless unavoidable in finite populations (Falconer and Mackay 1996). Many researchers assume that by using outbred mice or rats they are testing a "mixed" or "average" sample of the species. In fact, although much genetic heterogeneity still exists among individual members of an outbred strain, allele frequencies of pain-relevant genes may be highly divergent (and even fixed) in one strain compared to another.

To test this hypothesis, we obtained males and females of some of the most popular rodent strains: Long Evans rats, Sprague Dawley rats, Wistar Kyoto rats, CD-1 (ICR) mice, and Swiss Webster mice (from two different suppliers, Harlan Sprague Dawley, Inc., and Simonsen Laboratories, Inc.). We tested the animals for nociceptive sensitivity on the 49°C tail-withdrawal test, and subsequently for systemic morphine antinociception (Mogil et al. 2000). Again, we found strong evidence for a fundamental interaction between strain and sex (see Table I). In rats, Long Evans females were more sensitive to thermal nociception than males, but the direction of the sex difference was reversed in Sprague Dawleys (in accordance with most of the existing literature). In mice, all three populations displayed a trend in the same direction, with females proving more sensitive to thermal nociception than males. However, the sex difference differed by strain in its robustness; with a sample of about 25 rats of each sex per strain, the sex difference was highly significant ($P < 0.001$) in Swiss Webster mice from Simonsen, almost significant in Swiss Webster mice from Harlan ($P = 0.08$), and clearly nonsignificant in CD-1 mice ($P = 0.44$). After sample sizes were doubled, the sex difference was rendered significant in all three mouse populations. At standard biobehavioral experiment group sizes ($n \approx 5$–15), it is likely that a significant sex difference would be obtained only when using Swiss Webster (Simonsen) mice. Similar findings were obtained with respect to morphine antinociception. Significant sex differences in morphine AD_{50}—with males proving more sensitive to morphine than females in each case—were obtained in Sprague Dawley rats and CD-1 mice, and strong trends toward significance were observed in Long Evans rats and Swiss Webster (Harlan) mice, but the morphine dose-response curves obtained in male and female Wistar Kyoto rats and Swiss Webster (Simonsen) mice were superimposable (Mogil et al. 2000). Again, although it is entirely possible that sex differences would eventually emerge in all populations given sufficient statistical power, with commonly used sample sizes only Sprague Dawley rats and CD-1 mice are likely to exhibit significant sex differences.

These findings are sobering because they suggest that the overall conclusions derived from the rodent sex difference in pain literature are not readily generalizable, even within a given species. Had the bulk of these data been collected using a rat strain other than Sprague Dawley, for example, a wholly different consensus might have emerged regarding the presence and even direction of sex differences. These findings have considerable practical utility, however, for future investigations. Investigators who wish to study sex differences in morphine antinociception are advised to use Sprague Dawley rats or CD-1 mice, in which such differences are robust. Those conducting morphine experiments with both sexes (as is, of course, recommended), but where sex differences are not a focus, would be better off using Wistar rats or Swiss Webster (Simonsen) mice in which sex differences are less likely to emerge as a confounding variable.

The demonstration of sex/genetic interactions in rodents has implications for humans as well. If this interaction applies to our species, then the following prediction would be made: "Some women (i.e., those with certain alleles of relevant genes) will be more sensitive to pain and less sensitive to morphine analgesia than some men, and vice versa." The virtually tautological nature of this statement begs the question as to why so much research focuses on demonstrating overall quantitative differences between the sexes. As I have argued previously, it is the qualitative differences between the sexes in their processing of pain that are truly of interest, and most likely to lead to scientific and clinical advances.

QUALITATIVE SEX DIFFERENCES IN RODENTS: INTERACTIONS WITH GENOTYPE

The clearest evidence for qualitative sex differences in pain processing comes from studies of stress-induced antinociception (SIA) in rodents. Although less frequently studied in recent years, SIA is thought to represent the endogenous substrate for exogenous analgesics such as morphine. Pain-modulatory mechanisms did not evolve so that animals would respond to the opium poppy, but rather so that exposure to life-threatening environmental stressors might temporarily inhibit pain perception. One might argue, therefore, that if fundamental differences exist between the sexes with respect to pain modulation, the study of SIA is more likely to uncover such differences than the study of responses to drugs like morphine. One very early discovery about SIA (e.g., Hayes et al. 1976) was that multiple, neurochemically distinct types exist. The most replicated distinction is between opioid SIA (involving the release of one or more endogenous opioid peptides, acting on one or more opioid receptor types) and non-opioid SIA (see Watkins and Mayer 1986). Much work has gone into defining the neurochemical identity of the latter, with conflicting results (Gogas et al. 1986; Rodgers and Shepherd 1989; Rodgers et al. 1990; Marek et al. 1992; Watkins et al. 1992). Thus, as a practical matter, non-opioid SIA is considered that which is insensitive to blockade by high doses of the prototypic opioid receptor antagonists, naloxone or naltrexone. It has become clear, however, that adjustment of stressor parameters can elicit either "pure" opioid or non-opioid SIA, or a mixed SIA with both opioid and non-opioid components (Lewis et al. 1980; Terman et al. 1986; Mogil et al. 1996). In general, milder stressors (e.g., short swims in warm water) produce opioid SIA, and more severe stressors (e.g., long swims in cold water) produce non-opioid SIA, although an important interaction with genotype has been demonstrated here (Urca et al. 1985a; Tierney et al. 1991; Mogil and Belknap 1997).

The first suggestion that the neurochemical nature of SIA might interact with sex was made by Romero and colleagues (1988), who observed that the SIA produced by intermittent cold-water swims (18 10-second swims in 2°C water, each separated by a 10-second recovery period) was sensitive to antagonism by 14 mg/kg naloxone in males but not females. This sexual dimorphism in naloxone sensitivity persisted whether there was a sex difference in SIA magnitude (as was the case when electric shock jump thresholds were used as the dependent measure) or not (as was the case when using radiant heat tail-flick latencies). The exact opposite sex difference in the naloxone sensitivity of SIA was observed by Wong, who reported that the SIA produced in mice by 60 minutes of restraint (Wong 1992) or by 30-second swims in 30°C water (Wong 1987) was dose-dependently reversed by 1–4 mg/kg naloxone in females but not males. Finally, Lipa and Kavaliers (1990) noted that the opioid (i.e., naloxone-sensitive) antinociception produced either by morphine or restraint stress was completely reversed as well by a high dose (0.25 mg/kg) of the *N*-methyl-D-aspartate (NMDA) receptor blocker, MK-801 (dizocilpine), in male deer mice. This dose of MK-801 produced significant antagonism in female deer mice as well, but in this sex the reversal was far from complete.

This latter finding was intriguing to our group in the early 1990s because we were performing experiments evaluating the role of NMDA receptors in *non*-opioid SIA. We found that a far lower dose of MK-801, 0.075 mg/kg, produced a specific blockade of non-opioid SIA produced by cold-water swims (3 minutes in 15°C water), but not by opioid SIA produced by warm-water swims (3 minutes in 32°C water) (Marek et al. 1992). A reanalysis of these data by sex revealed, intriguingly, that MK-801 was only efficacious in blocking non-opioid SIA in male subjects. As follow-up studies demonstrated, female mice were completely insensitive to MK-801 antagonism of SIA produced by 3-minute swims in 15°C water, even though the SIA was indeed non-opioid in females, and, importantly, of equal magnitude to the MK-801-sensitive SIA displayed by males (Mogil et al. 1993). We hypothesized that females must possess another mechanism to account for the SIA they were clearly exhibiting, a mechanism that was neither opioid nor NMDAergic. The existence of such a mechanism, which we showed to be dependent on the presence of estrogen (Mogil et al. 1993) but *not* modulated by estrous-cycle-related changes in estrogen levels (Sternberg et al. 1994), has been confirmed and our results have been replicated and extended, largely through the efforts of Sternberg (Sternberg et al. 1996) and Kavaliers (Kavaliers and Galea 1995; Kavaliers and Choleris 1997; Kavaliers et al. 1998).

The findings of Kavaliers and Choleris (1997) deserve special mention. These investigators showed that the same sexual dimorphism observed in multiple SIA paradigms can also be seen for the selective κ-opioid agonist, U-69,593. That is, U-69,593 antinociception in males is completely blocked by NMDA antagonism using the competitive antagonist, NPC 12626, whereas equipotent U-69,593 antinociception in females is completely resistant to such antagonism. Indeed, several previous studies have suggested the paradoxically "non-opioid" character of κ-opioid antinociception (Kest et al. 1992; Saucier and Kavaliers 1994). Thus, it is intriguing that Gear and colleagues (1996a,b) have demonstrated a sex difference in clinical analgesic response to κ-opioid-preferring drugs in humans, with women enjoying more analgesia than men. Our findings and those of Kavaliers and Choleris (1997) suggest that this apparent quantitative sex difference may really represent the differential output of largely distinct analgesic circuitries in each sex.

As mentioned above, compelling evidence indicates that the activation of opioid versus non-opioid SIA mechanisms following exposure to a stressor depends on the genotype of the test subject. Urca and colleagues (1985a) have shown, for example, that identical parameters of footshock stress (30 minutes of intermittent footshock; 3 mA, 1 second on, 5 seconds off) produced opioid SIA in Sabra strain rats and in Sprague Dawley rats from a local Israeli supplier, but non-opioid SIA in six other rat populations tested. Further experiments revealed an interaction between strain and age in determining what form of SIA would be produced (Urca et al. 1985b,c). None of these reports, however, made any mention of the sex of the subjects tested. Since our demonstration of the existence of a female-specific SIA mechanism was based on results from a single mouse strain (Swiss Webster mice obtained from Bantin & Kingman, Inc.), we attempted to replicate the phenomenon in three different strains: Swiss Webster (obtained from Simonsen), C57BL/6J, and DBA/2J (Mogil and Belknap 1997). Results from the former two strains paralleled our previous findings: the equipotent, non-opioid SIA produced by 3-minute, 15°C swims in male and female mice was antagonized by MK-801 in male mice only. Although DBA/2 females also displayed equipotent non-opioid and non-NMDAergic SIA, the SIA in male mice of this strain was sensitive to naloxone rather than MK-801. Thus, this study demonstrated that neurochemical mediation of SIA interacts not only with sex, but also with genetic background (in males) (Mogil and Belknap 1997). In an ongoing study of swim SIA involving the C3HeB/FeJ strain (J.S. Mogil et al., unpublished observations), we have noted that 3-minute,

15°C swims produce a mixed opioid/NMDAergic SIA in males, whereas females exhibit a mixed opioid/non-NMDAergic SIA. For endogenous antinociception too, then, sex and genotype interact with stress severity to determine the neurochemical nature, if not the magnitude, of antinociception.

SEX-SPECIFIC QUANTITATIVE TRAIT LOCI

My laboratory is primarily concerned at the present time with identifying pain-related QTLs. QTLs, as mentioned above, are chromosomal regions showing statistically significant linkage, or co-inheritance, with continuously varying traits. It is presumed that one or more genes affecting the trait—and more importantly, affecting individual differences in the expression of the trait—lie within the fairly broad region defined by a QTL. When conducting QTL-mapping experiments, we collect data from male and female mice as a matter of course. What we have consistently noted in these efforts is the existence (and perhaps even preponderance) of sex-specific QTLs, in which linkage is obtained in one sex but not the other. Such sex-specific QTLs have consistently been found on autosomes,

not on the X or Y chromosomes. Of course, the identification of a sex-specific QTL does *not* imply that males and females have different genes (they do not, except for those few genes found on the Y chromosome), or even that males and females necessarily express different subsets of those genes. The identification of a sex-specific QTL *does* imply that the gene(s) representing the QTL are only relevant to trait variation in that sex. This in turn implies that the sexes possess at least partially distinct physiological mechanisms mediating the trait in question.

Our first discovery of a sex-specific QTL (and only the second such discovery after Melo et al. 1996, although there have been several since) was obtained in a mapping study of basal thermal nociceptive sensitivity on the 54°C hot-plate test (Mogil et al. 1997a). Using C57BL/6J (sensitive) and DBA/2J (resistant) progenitor strains, the study used a two-phase approach in which putative QTLs identified in BXD/Ty RI strains (26 re-inbred strains from a [C57BL/6J × DBA/2J] F_2 intercross) were verified using a new F_2 intercross (see Gora-Maslak et al. 1991; Belknap et al. 1996). A QTL was identified on mouse chromosome 4 (50–80 cM from the centromere), which was statistically associated with hot-plate latencies at $P = 0.0026$, close to or exceeding the threshold for "suggestive linkage" proposed by Lander and Kruglyak (1995). When male and female data were analyzed separately, the equivalent P values were 0.005 and 0.085 for males and females, respectively. Although owing to the restricted sample size, both the existence of the QTL and its sex-specificity should be regarded as provisional, a simple pharmacological experiment inspired by this finding lends support to both contentions. We noted that within the QTL region lies the murine *Oprd1* gene at 65 cM from the centromere. If this gene represents the QTL for basal hot-plate sensitivity on chromosome 4, we should be able to show strain-dependent (and in this case, sex-dependent) effects of pharmacological blockade of its gene product, the δ-opioid receptor. We pretreated male and female mice of both progenitor strains, C57BL/6J and DBA/2J, with either saline or one of the following opioid receptor type antagonists: high-dose naloxone (10 mg/kg; to block all opioid receptors), low-dose naloxone (0.1 mg/kg; to block μ receptors only), nor-binaltorphimine (5 mg/kg; to block κ receptors only), or naltrindole (5 mg/kg; to block δ receptors only). Although high-dose naloxone was able to reduce hot-plate latencies in DBA/2J mice down to the level of C57BL/6J mice, low-dose naloxone and nor-binaltorphimine had no effect in any group, arguing against the involvement of μ or κ receptors in setting basal nociceptive thresholds. However, pretreatment with naltrindole resulted in differential effects among the groups, causing a 41% decrease in threshold latencies in DBA/2J males, a 26% decrease in C57BL/6J males, a nonsignificant 16% decrease in DBA/2J females, and a nonsignificant 2% decrease in C57BL/6J females (Mogil et al. 1997a). That is, as would be predicted if *Oprd1* truly was a sex-specific QTL for thermal nociception in these strains, blockade of δ receptors caused a sex- and strain-dependent effect on this trait. We also demonstrated in this study that pretreatment with the δ_2-receptor antagonist naltriben produced virtually identical decreases to naltrindole, whereas the δ_1-receptor blocker 7-benzylidenenaltrexone was ineffective in all groups, suggesting the relevance of the δ_2-receptor subtype in this phenomenon.

An even clearer demonstration of a sex-specific QTL followed our mapping of non-opioid swim SIA (Mogil et al. 1997b). Again, we used a two-phase approach, subjecting putative QTLs identified using BXD/Ty RI strains to confirmation in (C57BL/6J × DBA/2J) F_2 hybrids. Two QTLs were found, one on chromosome 6 at 20–40 cM ($P = 0.002$, close to or exceeding the threshold for "suggestive linkage") and one on distal chromosome 8 (> 50 cM). This latter QTL is unambiguously sex-specific, with a significance level of $P = 0.00000012$ in females (corresponding to a LOD, or logarithm of the odds, value of 6.1) but only $P = 0.038$ in males (LOD = 0.9). In females, this P value far exceeds Lander and Kruglyak's (1995) threshold for "significant linkage." This QTL accounts for between 53–85% of the genetic variance in 15°C swim SIA in female mice, or between 17–26% of the overall trait variance. Female F_2 hybrid mice inheriting one or both copies of the dominant DBA/2J allele at marker loci in this region of chromosome 8 exhibit threefold more SIA than those inheriting two copies of the C57BL/6J allele; whereas in males inheritance of any genotype does not affect SIA (Mogil et al. 1997b). Unfortunately, unlike with the chromosome 4 hot-plate QTL, no immediately obvious candidate gene(s) for non-opioid SIA are known to reside in the distal portion of chromosome 8. We are currently attempting to further refine the location of this female-specific QTL to facilitate the identification of the responsible gene. Concurrently, we are testing for the sex-specific involvement in SIA of the protein products of some less obvious candidate genes in the region. Achieving this goal should give the first glimpse into the nature of the female-specific antinociceptive mechanism. However, the very fact that an obvious sex-specific QTL was uncovered for this trait supports the notion that a female-specific mechanism exists.

CONCLUSIONS

The results of our studies of the interaction of sex and genotype suggest that the efforts of talented investigators in the sex differences in pain field are being directed toward a question of limited significance, namely: are women more sensitive to pain than men? As Berkley (1997) recently concluded, "the most striking feature of sex differences in reported pain experience is the apparent overall lack of them" (p. 371). Our data in rodents show that sex differences will be larger if males and females of certain subpopulations of a species are compared, and smaller (or reversed) if other subpopulations are used instead. Knowing this, the demonstration of sex differences in the species *overall* becomes less meaningful. At the same time, the rodent data are very compelling in their suggestion that males and females may be modulating pain by the activation of dissociable neural circuitry. If this is actually true, whether the output of this differential circuitry is quantitatively equivalent or not is of comparably little interest. The elucidation of sex-specific physiology, perhaps aided by the identification of sex-specific genes, presages the development of sex-specific therapy for pain. I submit that it is far less important to explain why women may experience more pain than men (if this is even true), than to be able to tailor parameters/doses and even *classes* of analgesic manipulations to most effectively manage the pain of individual members of either sex.

ACKNOWLEDGMENTS

The author is supported by PHS grants DA11394 (NIDA) and DE12735 (NIDCR).

REFERENCES

Adler MW, Mauron C, Samanin R, Valzelli L. Morphine analgesia in grouped and isolated rats. *Psychopharmacologia (Berlin)* 1975; 41:11–14.

Arnér S, Meyerson BA. Lack of analgesic effect of opioids on neuropathic and idiopathic forms of pain. *Pain* 1988; 33:11–23.

Basbaum AI, Fields HL. Endogenous pain control systems: brainstem spinal pathways and endorphin circuitry. *Annu Rev Neurosci* 1984; 7:309–338.

Belknap JK, Dubay C, Crabbe JC, Buck KJ. Mapping quantitative trait loci for behavioral traits in the mouse. In: Blum K, Noble EP (Eds). *Handbook of Psychiatric Genetics.* New York: CRC Press, 1996, pp 435–453.

Berkley KJ. Sex differences in pain. *Behav Brain Sci* 1997; 20:371–380.

Cargill M, Altshuler D, Ireland J, et al. Characterization of single-nucleotide polymorphisms in coding regions of human genes. *Nat Genet* 1999; 22:231–238.

Chung JM, Choi Y, Yoon YW, Na HS. Effects of age on behavioral signs of neuropathic pain in an experimental rat model. *Neurosci Lett* 1995; 183:54–57.

Falconer DS, Mackay TFC. *Introduction to Quantitative Genetics.* Essex, UK: Longman, 1996.

Fitzgerald M. Developmental biology of inflammatory pain. *Br J Anaesth* 1995; 75:177–185.

Folkard S. Diurnal variation and individual differences in the perception of intractable pain. *J Psychosom Res* 1976; 20:289–301.

Frye CA, Cuevas CA, Kanarek RB. Diet and estrous cycle influence pain sensitivity in rats. *Pharmacol Biochem Behav* 1993; 45:255–260.

Gear RW, Gordon NC, Heller PH, et al. Gender difference in analgesic response to the kappa-opioid pentazocine. *Neurosci Lett* 1996a; 205:207–209.

Gear RW, Miaskowski C, Gordon NC, et al. Kappa-opioids produce significantly greater analgesia in women than in men. *Nat Med* 1996b; 2:1248–1250.

Gogas KR, Hough LB, Glickl SD, Su K. Opposing actions of cimetidine on naloxone-sensitive and naloxone-insensitive forms of footshock-induced analgesia. *Brain Res* 1986; 370:370–374.

Gora-Maslak G, McClearn GE, Crabbe JC, et al. Use of recombinant inbred strains to identify quantitative trait loci in psychopharmacology. *Psychopharmacology* 1991; 104:413–424.

Hamm RJ, Knisely JS. Developmental aspects of nociception. *Brain Res Bull* 1988; 21:933–946.

Hayes RL, Bennett GJ, Newlon P, Mayer DJ. Analgesic effects of certain noxious and stressful manipulations in the rat. *Soc Neurosci Abstracts* 1976; 2:1350.

Heikkila JK, Koskenvuo M, Heliovaara M, et al. Genetic and environmental factors in sciatica: evidence from a nationwide panel of 9365 adult twin pairs. *Ann Med* 1989; 21:393–398.

Honkasalo M-L, Kaprio J, Winter T, et al. Migraine and concomitant symptoms among 8167 adult twin pairs. *Headache* 1995; 35:70–78.

Indo Y, Tsurata Y, Karim MA, et al. Mutations in the TRKA/NGF receptor gene in patients with congenital insensitivity to pain with anhidrosis. *Nat Genet* 1996; 13:485–488.

Jackson HC, Kitchen I. Perinatal lead exposure impairs opioid but not non-opioid stress-induced antinociception in developing rats. *Br J Pharmacol* 1989; 97:1338–1342.

Kavaliers M, Choleris E. Sex differences in *N*-methyl-D-aspartate involvement in κ opioid and non-opioid predator-induced analgesia in mice. *Brain Res* 1997; 768:30–36.

Kavaliers M, Galea LAM. Sex differences in the expression and antagonism of swim stress-induced analgesia in deer mice vary with the breeding season. *Pain* 1995; 63:327–334.

Kavaliers M, Colwell DD, Choleris E. Sex differences in opioid and *N*-methyl-D-aspartate mediated non-opioid biting fly exposure induced analgesia in deer mice. *Pain* 1998; 77:163–177.

Kayser V, Guilbaud G. The analgesic effects of morphine, but not those of the enkephalinase inhibitor thiorphan, are enhanced in arthritic rats. *Brain Res* 1983; 267:131–138.

Kest B, Marek P, Liebeskind JC. The specific *N*-methyl-D-aspartate (NMDA) receptor antagonist blocks U50,488, but not morphine antinociception. *Brain Res* 1992; 589:139–142.

Kest B, Wilson SG, Mogil JS. Sex differences in supraspinal morphine analgesia are dependent on genotype. *J Pharmacol Exp Ther* 1999; 289:1370–1375.

Kieffer BL. Opioids: first lessons from knockout mice. *Trends Pharmacol Sci* 1999; 20:19–26.

Kinsley CH, Mann PE, Bridges RS. Prenatal stress alters morphine and stress-induced analgesia in male and female rats. *Pharmacol Biochem Behav* 1988; 30:123–128.

Lander ES, Kruglyak L. Genetic dissection of complex traits: guidelines for interpreting and reporting linkage results. *Nat Genet* 1995; 11:241–247.

Lander ES, Schork NJ. Genetic dissection of complex traits. *Science* 1994; 265:2037–2048.

Larsson B, Bille B, Pedersen NL. Genetic influence in headaches: a Swedish twin study. *Headache* 1995; 35:513–519.

Lewis JW, Cannon JT, Liebeskind JC. Opioid and non-opioid mechanisms of stress analgesia. *Science* 1980; 208:623–625.

Lipa SM, Kavaliers M. Sex differences in the inhibitory effects of the NMDA antagonist, MK-801, on morphine and stress-induced analgesia. *Brain Res Bull* 1990; 24:627–630.

MacGregor AJ, Griffiths GO, Baker J, Spector TD. Determinants of pressure pain threshold in adult twins: evidence that shared environmental influences predominate. *Pain* 1997; 73:253–257.

Marek P, Mogil JS, Sternberg WF, et al. *N*-methyl-D-aspartic acid (NMDA) receptor antagonist MK-801 blocks non-opioid stress-induced analgesia. II. Comparison across three swim stress paradigms in selectively bred mice. *Brain Res* 1992; 578:197–203.

Melo JA, Shendure J, Pociask K, Silver LM. Identification of sex-specific quantitative trait loci controlling alcohol preference in C57BL/6 mice. *Nat Genet* 1996; 13:147–153.

Meyer UA. The molecular basis of genetic polymorphisms of drug metabolism. *J Pharm Pharmacol* 1994; 46:409–415.

Mogil JS. The genetic mediation of individual differences in sensitivity to pain and its inhibition. *Proc Natl Acad Sci USA* 1999; 96:7744–7751.

Mogil JS, Belknap JK. Sex and genotype determine the selective activation of neurochemically-distinct mechanisms of swim stress-induced analgesia. *Pharmacol Biochem Behav* 1997; 56:61–66.

Mogil JS, Sternberg WF, Kest B, et al. Sex differences in the antagonism of swim stress-induced analgesia: effects of gonadectomy and estrogen replacement. *Pain* 1993; 253:17–25.

Mogil JS, Sternberg WF, Balian H, et al. Opioid and non-opioid swim stress-induced analgesia: a parametric analysis in mice. *Physiol Behav* 1996; 59:123–132.

Mogil JS, Richards SP, O'Toole LA, et al. Genetic sensitivity to hot-plate nociception in DBA/2J and C57BL/6J inbred mouse strains: possible sex-specific mediation by δ_2-opioid receptors. *Pain* 1997a; 70:267–277.

Mogil JS, Richards SP, O'Toole LA, et al. Identification of a sex-specific quantitative trait locus mediating nonopioid stress-induced analgesia in female mice. *J Neurosci* 1997b; 17:7995–8002.

Mogil JS, Wilson SG, Bon K, et al. Heritability of nociception. I. Responses of eleven inbred mouse strains on twelve measures of nociception. *Pain* 1999; 80:67–82.

Mogil JS, Chesler EJ, Wilson SG, et al. Sex differences in thermal nociception and morphine antinociception in rodents depend on genotype. *Neurosci Biobehav Rev* 2000; 24:375–389.

Morris RW, Lutsch EF. Susceptibility to morphine-induced analgesia in mice. *Nature* 1967; 216:494–495.

Ophoff RA, Terwindt GM, Vergouwe MN, et al. Familial hemiplegic migraine and episodic ataxia type-2 are caused by mutations in the Ca^{2+} channel gene CACNL1A4. *Cell* 1996; 87:543–552.

Pasternak GW. Pharmacological mechanisms of opioid analgesics. *Clin Neuropharmacol* 1993; 16:1–18.

Pieretti S, d'Amore A, Loizzo A. Long-term changes induced by developmental handling on pain threshold: effects of morphine and naloxone. *Behav Neurosci* 1991; 105:215–218.

Puglisi-Allegra S, Oliverio A. Social isolation: effects on pain threshold and stress-induced analgesia. *Pharmacol Biochem Behav* 1983; 19:6479–681.

Rodgers RJ, Shepherd JK. 5-HT_{1A} agonist, 8-hydroxy-2-(DI-n-propylamino)tetralin (8-OH-DPAT), inhibits non-opioid analgesia in defeated mice: influence of route of administration. *Psychopharmacology* 1989; 97:163–165.

Rodgers RJ, Shepherd JK, Randall JI. Highly potent inhibitory effects of 5-HT3 receptor antagonist, GR38032F, on non-opioid defeat analgesia in male mice. *Neuropharmacology* 1990; 29:17–23.

Romero M-T, Kepler KL, Bodnar RJ. Gender determinants of opioid mediation of swim analgesia in rats. *Pharmacol Biochem Behav* 1988; 29:705–709.

Saucier DM, Kavaliers M. Antagonistic effects of the selective, competitive *N*-methyl-D-aspartate (NMDA) receptor antagonist, NPC12626, on kappa opiate-induced analgesia in male deer mice. *Brain Res* 1994; 637:292–296.

Shir Y, Ratner A, Raja SN, et al. Neuropathic pain following partial nerve injury in rats is suppressed by dietary soy. *Neurosci Lett* 1998; 240:73–76.

Sternberg WF, Mogil JS, Pilati ML, et al. Neurochemical quality of nonopioid stress-induced analgesia is not altered by estrous phase in female mice. *Proc West Pharmacol Soc* 1994; 37:141–143.

Sternberg WF, Mogil JS, Kest B, et al. Neonatal testosterone exposure influences neurochemistry of swim stress-induced analgesia in adult mice. *Pain* 1996; 63:321–326.

Terman GW, Morgan MJ, Liebeskind JC. Opioid and non-opioid stress analgesia from cold water swim: importance of stress severity. *Brain Res* 1986; 372:167–171.

Tierney G, Carmody JJ, Jamieson D. Stress analgesia: the opioid analgesia of long swims suppresses the non-opioid analgesia induced by short swims in mice. *Pain* 1991; 46:89–95.

Treloar SA, Martin NG, Heath AC. Longitudinal genetic analysis of menstrual flow, pain, and limitation in a sample of Australian twins. *Behav Genet* 1998; 28:107–116.

Urca G, Segev S, Sarne Y. Footshock-induced analgesia: its opioid nature depends on the strain of rat. *Brain Res* 1985a; 329:109–116.

Urca G, Segev S, Sarne Y. Footshock-induced analgesia: neurochemical correlates and pharmacological profile. *Eur J Pharmacol* 1985b; 114:283–290.

Urca G, Segev S, Sarne Y. Stress-induced analgesia: its opioid nature depends on the strain of rat but not on the mode of induction. *Brain Res* 1985c; 343:216–222.

Watkins LR, Mayer DJ. Multiple endogenous opiate and non-opiate analgesia systems: evidence of their existence and clinical implications. *Ann NY Acad Sci* 1986; 467:273–299.

Watkins LR, Wiertelak EP, Grisel JE, et al. Parallel activation of multiple spinal opiate systems appears to mediate 'non-opiate' stress-induced analgesias. *Brain Res* 1992; 594:99–108.

Wilson SG, Melton KA, Wickesburg RE, Mogil JS. Strain-dependent antinociception from the cannabinoid receptor agonist, WIN 55,212-2. *Soc Neurosci Abstracts* 1999; 25:924.

Wong C-L. Sex difference in naloxone antagonism of swim stress induced antinociception in mice. *Methods Find Exp Clin Pharmacol* 1987; 9:275–278.

Wong C-L. The effect of naloxone on restraint-induced antinociception in mice. *Methods Find Exp Clin Pharmacol* 1992; 14:695–700.

Ziegler DK, Hur YM, Bouchard TJ Jr, et al. Migraine in twins raised together and apart. *Headache* 1998; 38:417–422.

Correspondence to: Jeffrey S. Mogil, PhD, Dept. of Psychology, University of Illinois at Urbana-Champaign, 603 E. Daniel St., Champaign, IL 61820, USA. Tel: 217-333-6546; Fax: 217-244-5876; email: jmogil@s.psych.uiuc.edu.

Sex, Gender, and Pain, Progress in Pain Research and Management, Vol. 17, edited by R.B. Fillingim, IASP Press, Seattle, © 2000.

4

Psychosocial Contributions to Sex-Related Differences in Pain Responses

Michael E. Robinson,[a] Joseph L. Riley III,[a,b] and Cynthia D. Myers[b]

Departments of [a]Clinical and Health Psychology and [b]Operative Dentistry, University of Florida, Gainesville, Florida, USA

Approximately one out of every six adults living in the United States is in pain at any given moment (Wall and Jones 1991). Epidemiologic and experimental pain studies suggest that women may be over-represented among those reporting pain. According to a recent review of the epidemiologic literature (Unruh 1996), women more often report multiple pain sites, intense pain, and frequent pain. Fillingim and Maixner (1995) reviewed a representative sample of experimental pain studies and concluded that females have lower pain thresholds and exhibit less pain tolerance than males. A subsequent meta-analysis (Riley et al. 1998b) provided quantitative confirmation of this finding and revealed moderate effect sizes for sex-related differences in experimental pain report.

Results of clinical pain research comparing female and male patients have been less consistent. Some studies have found significant sex-related differences in pain report among patients diagnosed with the same medical condition (Lawlis et al. 1984). Other researchers have reported either small or no sex-related differences in clinical samples (Buckelew et al. 1990; Lander et al. 1990; Bush et al. 1993). Robinson and colleagues (1998) calculated small effect sizes (ranging from 0.015 to 0.34, Cohen's d) associated with sex-related differences in pain report in five large groups of patients with chronic pain conditions.

Several possible mechanisms have recently been proposed to explain sex-related differences in pain. Investigators have focused on biological differences, including genetic, hormonal, anatomical, and physiological differences between the sexes (Berkley 1997). Fillingim and Maixner (1995) provided a review and heuristic organization of potential mechanisms underlying sex differences in pain perception. They proposed four interactive components that include: (1) primary afferent systems, (2) central nervous system processing of nociceptive input, (3) peripheral physiological responses to noxious stimuli, and (4) differences in activation of pain modulatory systems by physiological responses. Sex differences in any of these systems, according to Fillingim and Maixner, offer at least a partial explanation of observed sex differences in pain response.

In most of the recent efforts, researchers have placed far more emphasis on first-order biological factors than on psychosocial factors that may also account for sex-related differences in pain response. By contrast, other investigators have emphasized psychosocial inputs such as sex-differentiated learning history, socialization, behavior, and risk factors relating to pain. For example, Riley et al. (1998a) found that among female patients presenting for treatment in a facial pain clinic, those who reported a history of sexual or physical abuse reported greater pain severity than other patients. Fillingim and colleagues (1999b) recently reported similar findings in a nonclinical sample of young adults, and concluded that a self-reported history of abuse was associated with increased pain complaints and higher pain severity for both females and males. Given national statistics on the prevalence of abuse (Potter et al. 1999), these studies have important implications and illustrate learning and history effects that may contribute to sex-related differences in pain responding.

A consensus is building that there are important sex-related differences in pain, and that these differences are poorly understood. The relative contributions of biological, psychological, and sociocultural factors to sex-related differences in the pain experience and in pain reporting behaviors have yet to be adequately examined. However, prevailing models conceptualize pain as a multidimensional perceptual phenomenon comprising a complex interaction of biological and psychosocial factors (Melzack and Wall 1965). Sex-correlated differences in psychosocial and behavioral variables related to pain are therefore critically important to investigate. In this chapter, we selectively review theoretical and empirical literature addressing psychological and sociocultural factors of particular relevance to sex-related differences in pain. We review three topic areas: sex-related differences in gender stereotypes, sex-correlated differences in cognitive factors related to the pain experience, and sex-correlated differences in affective factors related to the pain experience.

SEX-RELATED DIFFERENCES IN GENDER STEREOTYPES

In discussions of male-female differences in pain behavior, the influences of gender role stereotypes are often inferred, but rarely directly examined. Conceptual problems appear to complicate this task. The common practice of using the terms "sex" and "gender" interchangeably in the pain literature illustrates these problems. A useful distinction can be made between the two terms (Unger 1979). In our discussion, we will use the term "sex" when referring to biologically determined aspects of femaleness and maleness, and the term "gender" when referring to modifiable, socioculturally shaped behavior and traits such as femininity and masculinity. We will use the terms "sex-related differences" and "sex-correlated differences" interchangeably, rather than the term "sex differences," in order to signal that the term "sex" is being used as a marker, rather than to connote biologically deterministic assumptions (Deaux 1993).

PSYCHOSOCIAL THEORIES OF GENDER

Social-cognitive learning theory (Mischel 1966; Bandura 1986) and cognitive-developmental theory (Kohlberg 1966) propose that young children develop a sense of themselves as male or female, termed gender identity, and acquire knowledge of their appropriate gender role through the same processes that are involved in all learning. These processes include modeling, imitation, reinforcement, and punishment. Gender schema theory (Bem 1981, 1985) integrates elements of both social learning theory and cognitive-developmental theory in explaining the means by which males and females become masculine and feminine by conforming to cultural stereotypes of these traits. Bem does not specifically reference pain in her research program, but the hypothesis that men and women would respond differently to painful stimuli based on adherence to cultural norms for the sexes is consistent with her theory. To the extent that the masculine gender role norm emphasizes tolerance of pain in order to avoid appearing unmasculine, gender schema theory would predict that males who conformed to the masculine stereotype would be motivated to appear invulnerable to pain.

Social cognitive learning theory, cognitive-developmental theory, and gender schema theory construe gender in terms of personality constructs that, while culturally instilled and not inherent, develop early in life and endure as stable traits across situations through the lifespan. Social psychologists Deaux and Major (1987, 1990, 1998) propose a behavioral, interactive model of gender that shifts the focus of attention away from distal processes involved in the early acquisition of gender traits, and toward proximal, situational factors that govern the display of gender-linked behaviors within specific interpersonal interactions. Expectancy confirmation and self-presentation strategies are two important constructs in their model. Deaux and Major have not specifically referenced pain in their work, but their model could be used to examine gender-related displays of pain behavior in specific research contexts such as the pain laboratory.

PSYCHOSOCIAL THEORIES OF PAIN BEHAVIOR

Psychosocial theories of pain behavior have focused on the effects of contingencies on the emergence and persistence of pain behaviors (Fordyce 1986), and on the significance of learning acquired through observing pain models and through the reinforcing or punishing consequences of others' pain behaviors (Craig 1986). Empirical examinations of the influences of pain modeling demonstrate strong effects. Craig and Weiss (1971) demonstrated a threefold increase in pain threshold when subjects were given a pain-tolerant model. Craig and Prkachin (1978) demonstrated that high and low tolerance models of pain responding were effective in altering subjects' responses to similar painful stimulation. The demonstration of bidirectional influences of modeling provides particularly strong evidence of the effects of social modeling on pain responsivity. Turkat and Guise (1983) and Turkat et al. (1983) also demonstrated bidirectional influences of high and low pain-tolerance models on subjects' pain responsivity. Craig et al.'s studies included only male subjects, while Turkat and colleagues included only female subjects, so no direct sex comparisons can be made. Importantly, the sizes of the effects of these social modeling manipulations are as large as or larger than those obtained in a meta-analysis of sex differences in experimental pain (Riley et al. 1998b); this finding emphasizes the importance of investigating these influences as they relate to sex-correlated differences in pain responsivity.

EMPIRICAL LINKS AMONG SEX, GENDER, AND PAIN BEHAVIOR

Gender role expectations and social role modeling of pain may interact early in life. Mechanic (1964) examined the relationship between age, sex, and children's attitudes toward risk and denial of pain in order to detect conformity with societal expectations that boys will have a greater "ability to take it" (p. 448). Both younger and older boys (fourth and eighth graders) were significantly more likely than their female peers to indicate that they had no fear of getting hurt and that they did not pay attention to pain. In a group of hospitalized children, Savedra et al. (1982) found that girls conformed to the feminine stereotype of emotional expressivity by using more affective descriptors of pain than did boys.

Several authors have investigated the influence of a family history of pain. Edwards and colleagues (1985) reported that the number of family members with pain was positively associated with the frequency of recent pain complaints among young adults. Interestingly, the relationship between family history and pain complaints was stronger for females than males. Relatedly, Lester and colleagues (1994) found that a family history of pain was associated with increased pain reports among college students. Koutantji et al. (1998) recently demonstrated that subjects' sex and family history of pain are related to report of current pain and awareness of others' pain. Women from a nonclinic student population had more pain models than did men, had a greater awareness of pain in others, and appeared to be more susceptible to pain models as a result of this heightened awareness. In explanation, the authors suggested that social roles for women are more supportive of pain expression and pain awareness. For both sexes, there was a significant relationship between the number of pain models reported and the number of pain symptoms. Men and women did not differ in the frequency of pain symptoms after menstrual pain was controlled. Fillingim and colleagues (2000) recently found that a reported familial pain history was associated with greater recent pain complaints and with enhanced experimental pain sensitivity among females, but not males.

In an analogue study of imagined pain in several body locations, Klonoff et al. (1993) found that men indicated they would respond to pain with embarrassment and would be reluctant to disclose their pain. Women, by contrast, indicated that they would respond to pain with anxiety and a high likelihood of disclosing their pain. Levine and De Simone (1991) found that males reported less pain during a cold-pressor task when the experimenter was an attractive 28-year-old female dressed in a manner intended to accentuate her femininity than when the experimenter was male. No such interaction was found in the absence of deliberate accentuation of gender cues in the experimenters' appearance (Feine et al. 1991). The studies reviewed suggest that gender role stereotypes are exerting an effect on behavior; however, they did not directly measure the construct of gender.

In a study of male college students, using the Masculine Gender Role Stress Scale as a measure of masculinity, Lash et al. (1990) found that "high-masculine" males showed greater systolic blood pressure changes during a painful cold-pressor task than did "low-masculine" males, but only when the task was presented as a masculine achievement challenge. When the cold pressor was presented as a neutral task, the high-masculine and low-masculine males did not differ from one another in pain response. Lash and colleagues reasoned that cardiovascular reactivity was, in part, a function of men's cognitive appraisal of, and stress response to, the experimental instructions. They concluded that the masculine challenge was particularly stressful for men with more stereotypically masculine self-images. The challenge instructions emphasized successful performance and physical adequacy, both of which had been appraised in previous research as more stressful domains for men than women (Eisler and Skidmore 1987). In two later studies, Lash and colleagues (1991, 1995) included females in their samples in order to examine the gender relevance of stressors as mediators of sex-related differences in cardiovascular reactivity. These authors manipulated masculine, feminine, and neutral challenge instructions for the cold-pressor task, and found that males showed greater systolic reactivity in the masculine challenge condition, that females showed greater reactivity in the feminine challenge condition, and that the sexes did not differ in the neutral condition. These results are consistent with gender schema theory, which would predict that instructions to withstand pain should be less salient and pose less of a challenge to women than to men, according to conventional gender stereotypes.

One study directly investigated the interaction of biological sex, conformity to dominant societal gender role norms, and pain responsivity in a sample of healthy undergraduates (Otto and Dougher 1985). Using the Bem Sex Role Inventory (Bem 1974) as a measure of gender-related personality traits, and mechanical pressure as the noxious stimulus, the researchers found a significant interaction between masculinity-femininity scores and subjects' sex when testing pain threshold. Males who scored highest on the masculinity scale reported the highest pain thresholds, consistent with a masculine gender stereotype. Females reported more pain, irrespective of their gender role scale scores. The investigators interpreted their results as reflecting a masculinity-enhancing reporting bias among stereotypically masculine males; however, sex-related differences in pain threshold and tolerance remained significant even after controlling for masculinity-femininity scores. A more recent experimental pain study using the Bem Sex Role Inventory as a measure of gender and the cold pressor as the noxious stimulus found no effects of gender when controlling for sex and blood pressure reactivity (Myers et al. 1998).

GENDER AND EXPECTATIONS OF PAIN RESPONSIVITY

Our own work suggests that women and men have very different expectations of pain (Robinson et al. 1999). These expectations tend to be gender stereotyped. Pilot data on our newly developed Gender Role Expectations of Pain (GREP) questionnaire also suggest that socialization regarding pain differs between men and women. The GREP comprises 12 visual analogue scales that assess a subject's view of the typical man and woman with respect to pain sensitivity, pain endurance, and willingness to report pain. The questionnaire also assesses the subject's personal attribution of his or her pain sensitivity, pain endurance, and willingness to report pain relative to the typical man and woman. Initial psychometrics from a sample of 390 undergraduate men and women are encouraging. The instrument showed good internal consistency, with high negative correlations between items that theoretically should have been reciprocal. For example, the correlation between the rating of the typical man's versus the typical woman's sensitivity to pain was –0.70. Similar correlations were obtained for the correlations between ratings of the typical pain endurance of men and women ($r = -0.71$) and the typical man's versus the typical woman's willingness to report pain ($r = -0.81$). A smaller sample of subjects ($n = 21$) resulted in test-retest correlations ranging from 0.44 to 0.87 for individual items.

A factor analysis of the original sample of 390 subjects resulted in a five-factor solution accounting for 75% of the variance in item scores. The five factors closely resemble the theoretical structure intended in the construction of the questionnaire: (1) stereotypic willingness to report pain, (2) stereotypic sensitivity to pain, (3) personal sensitivity and willingness to report pain, (4) personal endurance of pain, and (5) stereotypic endurance of pain. Additional analyses indicated that both men and women thought that the typical man was less willing to report pain than the typical woman ($F_{1,389} = 336$, $P < 0.001$). Sex accounted for 46% of the variance in subjects' perceptions of gender-stereotyped willingness to report pain. Evidence also indicated what might be termed a "male enhancement bias" for the endurance measures, with men reporting that the typical man has higher endurance of pain than the typical woman ($F_{1,389} = 65.7$, $P < 0.001$). Sex accounted for approximately 15% of the variance of gender-stereotyped pain endurance. Men felt that they had higher endurance than the typical man or woman ($F_{1,389} = 40.9$, $P < 0.001$); sex accounted for 9.5% of the variance in this relationship.

Results of our own studies to date indicate a large discrepancy between sex differences observed in experimental pain studies (moderate to large effect sizes) and clinical pain studies (quite small effect sizes). The distinct possibility exists that a significant number of the sex differences observed in experimental pain studies are situation specific and do not reflect physiological or anatomical differences between the sexes. One mechanism that has been understudied in the pain literature is that of gender role. The gender role construct is very likely to be multidimensional (reviewed in Ashmore and Sewell 1998), and is itself a special case of a broader rubric of social learning influences on a wide variety of behavior, including pain responding.

SOCIAL LEARNING FACTORS IN SEX-RELATED DIFFERENCES IN HEALTH CARE UTILIZATION

Sex-differentiated learning histories about symptom reporting and illness behavior in general may contribute to epidemiologic findings of sex-related differences in pain and in the use of clinical services specializing in pain assessment and treatment (reviewed in Unruh 1996). Several studies have documented higher per capita use of health care services by women compared to men for all types of morbidity (Verbrugge 1979; Cleary et al. 1982; Gijsbers et al. 1992; Verbrugge and Patrick 1995). Unruh concluded that this pattern was also true for pain-related health care use.

Observed sex differences in health care use have been explained as a function of differences in health status, health-seeking behavior, biases in health care provision, and differences in mortality (Mustard et al. 1998). Other studies have shown that illness orientation, symptom perception, caregiving responsibilities, social acceptability of admitting to illness, and willingness to seek care are likely candidates for explaining sex differences in health care use (Hibbard and Pope 1983). Hibbard and Pope found that illness orientation variables were related to medical care utilization for both men and women, although women showed greater concern for health and greater perception of symptom severity. These results were most pronounced in the middle range of symptom frequency, with no sex differences when either high or low rates of symptoms were compared between men and women. Meininger (1986) reported that men and women also have different rates of seeking lay health consultants, and that this sex difference interacted with socioeconomic status. Other authors have indicated that men and women have different belief systems with respect to their causal attributions about illness. For example, Klonoff and Landrine (1994) found that women were more likely than men to view illness as a form of punishment.

Sex-related differences in interactions between health care providers and patients are also potential factors in the observed sex differences in health care use. Safran and colleagues (1997) reported that women were 3.6 times more likely to be prescribed activity restriction, even though the level of symptoms was equivalent for men and women. The investigators suggested that there is an interaction between the sex of the practitioner and the patient that highlights the social biases evident in the practice of medicine.

Clear evidence shows that, on average, women and men differ in their use of health care, and that sex-related differences in health beliefs, health concerns, symptom perception, patient-practitioner relationships, and willingness to seek care all contribute significantly to this outcome. These findings point directly to the important contribution of sex-differentiated social learning histories to sex-correlated differences in health care use in general. The results of research on health care utilization in general are likely to apply to pain symptoms because pain is such a common complaint of most illness; this is a rich area to investigate further. Medical sociologist David Mechanic (1986) wrote: "Illness behavior involves a complex interaction between the quality of bodily dysfunction, the sociocultural and psychological orientations brought by individuals to their situation, and the unique demands of the immediate social context" (p. 6). Paraphrasing Mechanic to apply to the current topic, pain behavior is a complex interaction between nociception, sex-differentiated learning histories brought by individual women and men to their situations, and the unique demands of the social context.

PLACING SEX AND GENDER INTO CONTEXT

Obviously, biological sex is only one of several important dimensions on which individuals differ. Individuals also vary with respect to cultural background, ethnicity, socioeconomic status, education level, and age, and in other important ways. Cultural and ethnic norms, beliefs, and attitudes regarding pain reporting have been examined in non-sex-differentiated groups in both clinical and experimental settings through use of qualitative, descriptive, and experimental, quantitative methodologies (e.g., Zborowski 1952; Zola 1966; Lawlis et al. 1984; Lipton and Marbach 1984; Zatzick and Dimsdale 1990; van den Akker et al. 1995; Bates 1996). Results have been very mixed, with interpretation made difficult by the tremendous heterogeneity of populations studied and pain methodologies employed. Sex-related differences have not typically been central to these investigations, but within-sex cross-cultural comparisons suggest that this is an important area for further investigation (reviewed in Rollman 1998).

SEX-CORRELATED DIFFERENCES IN COGNITIVE FACTORS RELATED TO THE PAIN EXPERIENCE

The gate control theory of pain postulates the physiological process through which psychosocial and behavioral factors are integrated into the subjective experience of pain (Melzack and Wall 1965). The subjectivity of the experience of pain implies that an individual's beliefs, appraisals, and coping strategies are likely to contribute to the maintenance, exacerbation, or attenuation of pain perception or pain behavior. Furthermore, these forces are likely to interact through reciprocal feedback loops, so that effects can also be causes.

Numerous important individual differences have been demonstrated in beliefs, appraisals, and coping strategies as they relate to pain and to emotional responses to pain (Turk and Rudy 1986; Jensen et al. 1991b). These psychosocial variables have been examined in non-sex-differentiated samples, with numerous studies demonstrating the importance of their influence. When males and females demonstrate different behavioral responses to pain (e.g., report of pain intensity or unpleasantness, or health care use), one possible explanation is that the influences of these psychosocial and behavioral factors interact with each other or with pain differently across the sexes.

MEN AND WOMEN COPE DIFFERENTLY WITH STRESS

If individuals develop their own strategies for coping with painful sensations, and if men and women experience pain differently (i.e., frequency, intensity, temporal pattern, location, and syndrome), men and women may develop different pain coping styles. Evidence indicates that men and women cope differently with stress generally. Pain can certainly be defined as a stressor, and coping with pain can be defined as a purposeful attempt to manage a stressful situation (Lazarus and Folkman 1984). The literature on sex differences in coping with stress is thus germane to our topic and will be reviewed briefly.

Vingerhoets and Van Heck (1990) studied sex-related differences in coping styles in response to psychological and somatic symptoms. Consistent with earlier coping research, men were more inclined to use active, problem-focused coping. In contrast, women tended to use emotion-focused coping, to express their emotions, to seek social support, and to blame themselves. Wallbott and Scherer (1991) examined the interaction effects of sex and coping style on two types of cognitive and emotional stressors. Sex was an important mediator, especially with regard to behavioral arousal in certain situations. Women consistently reacted negatively to cognitive stressors while showing less arousal in emotional situations, whereas men showed the opposite response pattern. Other studies show that compared to men, women make more use of social support in coping with stress. For example, in a study on sex differences in coping styles across the lifespan, Diehl and colleagues (1996) found that women were more likely than men to focus on the intra- and interpersonal aspects of conflict situations. A study of coping among gymnasts (Kolt et al. 1995) found that female gymnasts were more likely than their male counterparts to use social support to cope with performance problems. Hobfoll et al. (1994) developed a dual-axis model of coping on the dimensions of active versus passive and pro-social versus antisocial coping strategies. Their results showed that women and men did not differ on the active versus passive dimension, but that women were much more likely than men to use pro-social coping strategies. Additionally, men who were at the extremes on the social dimension (i.e., men who were either very pro-social or antisocial), suffered from greater emotional distress than women, suggesting that social coping strategies may be more limited for men in general than for women. Collectively, the coping studies reviewed here suggest that men and women cope with stress differently and in ways that are consistent with dominant cultural gender role stereotypes: women focus more on the interpersonal and emotional aspects of a situation, while men concentrate more on problem-solving strategies.

SEX-CORRELATED DIFFERENCES IN CHRONIC PAIN COPING

The literature on the effectiveness of various pain coping styles has been somewhat mixed. Jensen et al. (1991a) detected considerable variability in the efficacy of different coping strategies. Unruh (1996) suggested that social influences may predispose males and females to learn different coping strategies; however, few studies have directly tested for sex-related differences in pain coping. More commonly, researchers have controlled for sex as a demographic variable when testing for associations with measures of pain, mood, or functioning (i.e., Spinhoven et al. 1989; Keefe et al. 1991; Tota-Faucette et al. 1993; Lefebvre 1999). These studies typically show minimal or no effect of sex in their analysis. Most studies reporting sex-related differences in use of coping strategies appear to have analyzed sex post hoc, secondary to the testing of other primary hypotheses. For example, Harkapaa (1991) examined the relationships among control beliefs, psychological distress, and coping strategies in a sample of low back pain patients in Finland. Sex was initially used with other control variables and was forced into a logistic regression model in the first step. However, sex differences were reported as significantly and positively associated with preventive action, coping self-statements, hoping/praying, and diverting one's attention from pain. Williams and Keefe (1991) examined whether beliefs about pain were related to the use of specific coping strategies. Using multivariate cluster analysis, these authors identified three subgroups related to pain beliefs in a sample of 120 chronic pain patients. Males and females were equally represented among those patients who viewed their pain as mysterious and enduring and among others who viewed pain as understandable and of short duration. More males than females viewed pain as long-term and understandable, and this group also provided the lowest rating of their ability to decrease pain by using coping strategies. In a sample of 75 patients with rheumatoid arthritis, Affleck et al. (1992) found that compared to men, women implemented more daily coping activities, had recourse to a greater number of different coping methods, and were more likely to seek emotional support.

We found three studies that hypothesized and tested for sex differences in pain coping across patients grouped by sex. I. Jensen et al. (1994) assessed sex differences in coping with the consequences of long-term musculoskeletal pain among 121 consecutive referrals to a Swedish orthopedic clinic. The investigators controlled for differences in subjective health status, pain, and occupation status. Women engaged in significantly more behavioral activity as a coping strategy than did men. A trend was observed for men to report more frequent use of coping self-statements and a greater likelihood of reinterpreting or ignoring pain. Additionally, when data from males and females were separated, regression analysis indicated that coping self-statements and a tendency to ignore pain sensations were negatively related to a measure of pain for females, but not males.

Using a questionnaire survey, Weir et al. (1996) studied sex differences in a sample of 222 patients referred to a pain clinic to determine the relationship between health care needs and the use of health care services for pain. Based on scores from a measure of psychosocial changes resulting from illness, respondents were grouped by sex into three psychological adjustment categories. Females in the poorly adjusted group differed from females in the good or fair adjustment groups in terms of social support, having fewer confident relationships, and less caring or supportive relationships. Males in the poorly adjusted group differed from their respective good and fair groups only on perceived social support. In a stepwise regression, females' adjustment was accounted for by cognitive variables (impact of life role meaning of the condition), and males' adjustment was explained by loss of their life role.

Unruh (1999) performed a telephone survey to study 309 community-based adults experiencing troublesome pain in the previous 2 weeks. Consistent with past studies, women reported having more intense pain and using more coping strategies, relative to men. Of the commonly reported coping strategies, women used significantly more positive self-statements, palliative behaviors, and problem solving and sought more social support, but were not different on information seeking, distraction, or internalizing/catastrophizing.

Consistent with the broader coping literature, the authors of the three studies specifically examining sex-related differences in chronic pain coping found that women report using a broader array of coping strategies and in particular, they use more social/emotional support than men.

SEX-CORRELATED DIFFERENCES IN PAIN-RELATED APPRAISALS

A number of studies suggest that beliefs or appraisals about pain influence the experience of pain through mechanisms such as the type of coping strategies used to manage pain or the emotional response to pain (Turner and Clancy 1986; Crisson and Keefe 1988; Keefe and Williams 1990; Buescher et al. 1991; Jensen and Karoly 1991; Haythornthwaite 1998). Thus, cognitive evaluations, which include control appraisals and catastrophizing, may be important in mediating or moderating the sex differences observed in pain, pain coping, and adjustment.

SEX-RELATED DIFFERENCES IN CONTROL OF PAIN

Few studies in the chronic pain literature report sex differences in measures of control. Buckelew et al. (1990) studied adjustment to persistent pain among 160 subjects (67 males and 93 females) referred to a comprehensive pain rehabilitation program. Multivariate cluster analysis suggested that males and females fit different subgroup profiles on dimensions of health locus of control. For females more than males, cluster assignment was more related to the use of coping strategies. Strong et al. (1994) also used cluster analysis to develop a multidimensional assessment model for chronic low back pain patients and to classify patients into subgroups. More males than females were classified as being "in control," which was characterized by low levels of pain, a strong attitude that one can control pain, and low catastrophizing. More females than males were in the active coping group, which reported higher levels of pain and use of more cognitive coping strategies (reinterpreting pain, denial, or diverting attention) than the predominately male group. Males and females were equally represented in a high dysfunction group. Haythornthwaite et al. (1998) tested the association between perceptions of control, coping strategies, coping flexibility, and a number of outcomes in 195 pain patients with mixed pain etiology who were admitted to an inpatient pain clinic. Sex was not found to be related to perceived control, and so was not considered in subsequent analyses.

Two studies using community-based samples have reported sex differences in perceived control. Liddell and Locker (1997) studied the association between attitudes about dental pain and pain control in 2609 adults living in metropolitan Toronto. Women expressed a significantly greater need for control but were not different from men in perceived control. The authors concluded that women were at greater disadvantage in the dental situation because of their greater desire for control but lower perception of actual control. In her community-based telephone survey study, Unruh (1999) tested the hypothesis that sex would moderate the association between appraisals and coping for individuals experiencing troublesome pain in the previous 2 weeks. There were no sex differences in the overall magnitude of threat or challenge appraisals; however, women's threat appraisal increased sooner in relationship to interference from pain than did men's. Unruh also found a sex-by-appraisal interaction for indirect help seeking such as crying, moaning, or seeking comfort.

SEX-RELATED DIFFERENCES IN CATASTROPHIZING ABOUT PAIN

Catastrophizing has been identified as an important variable in the assessment and treatment of pain (Turk and Rudy 1986). Catastrophizing, which can be defined as perceived lack of control, excessive worry about the future, and a tendency to view life as overwhelming, is a key factor in the relationship between chronic pain and negative affect (Keefe et al. 1989; Sullivan and D'Eon 1990; Jensen et al. 1991b; Geisser et al. 1994). Few studies have investigated sex differences in catastrophizing or in the way catastrophizing could mediate between the various dimensions of chronic pain and negative affect. Sex-related differences in pain catastrophizing have been documented in undergraduates' responses to pain questionnaires (Osman et al. 1997; Fillingim et al. 1999b). I. Jensen et al. (1994) found that female chronic pain patients engaged in more catastrophizing than males, even though the study controlled for pain and subjective health status. Strong et al. (1994) also reported evidence that females catastrophize more than males, finding a predominately male subgroup with low catastrophizing in comparison with two other groups in which females and males were equally distributed. Harkapaa (1991), however, did not find sex differences in catastrophizing in their sample of Finnish chronic low back pain patients. In addition, Unruh (1999) did not find differences in the magnitude of catastrophizing between men and women, but reported a sex-related association between catastrophizing and threat appraisals.

COGNITIVE FACTORS CONTRIBUTING TO SEX-RELATED DIFFERENCES IN EXPERIMENTAL PAIN

Although sex-related differences are not universally found in experimental pain research, such differences are common, with women usually reporting more pain relative to men (Fillingim and Maixner 1995; Riley et al. 1998b). In experimental pain studies, cognitive and affective factors relate significantly to pain responsivity; however, sex differences or similarities in cognitive and affective factors relating to experimental pain are largely unstudied. To the extent that psychosocial factors differ in women and men who participate as subjects in laboratory pain studies, such factors may help to explain sex-related differences in experimental pain.

Catastrophizing has been related to decreased tolerance for cold-pressor pain (Geisser et al. 1992). An interesting finding is that catastrophizers seem to experience difficulty shifting attentional focus away from pain, with the result that they amplify the somatosensory information associated with noxious stimuli (Crombez et al. 1998). Although the evidence is mixed, some studies indicate that women catastrophize more than men with regard to pain (reviewed above), suggesting that a link between catastrophizing and attention may contribute to sex differences in experimental pain responsivity.

Self-efficacy expectancies for pain coping were significantly related to tolerance for cold-pressor pain and were superior to pain ratings in predicting pain tolerance in college students (Dolce et al. 1986; Baker and Kirsch 1991). Use of positive self-statements about pain coping was associated with increased exposure time in a cold-pressor paradigm relative to use of negative coping self-statements in a clinic sample of patients with chronic orofacial pain (N.M. Litwins et al., unpublished manuscript). Evidence for sex-related differences in the relationship between self-efficacy and pain response comes from a study in which higher pain-related efficacy and control beliefs were associated with lower thermal pain sensitivity in women, but not in men (Fillingim et al. 1996). Additional evidence was provided by a cold-pressor study involving 40 male and 40 female healthy adults (Weisenberg et al. 1995), in which men exhibited higher self-efficacy for pain control, lower anxiety ratings, and lower skin resistance response, greater pain tolerance, and higher estimation of the importance of keeping the arm immersed in the cold water.

Cultural variability in attitudes toward health, illness, pain, and gender stereotypes may influence pain-related cognitions and responsivity to laboratory-induced pain. Three recent reviews (Zatzick and Dimsdale 1990; Rollman 1998; Wise et al. 1999) of cross-cultural differences in responses to experimental pain emphasized the mixed results of these studies. The reviewers encountered difficulties in making comparisons across studies due to diversity in racial and ethnic groups involved, mixed socioeconomic status and education level of participants, and variability in method of pain induction. Sex-related differences within cultures have yet to be adequately addressed, and they add another layer of complexity to results that are already difficult to interpret in cross-cultural investigations.

SEX-CORRELATED DIFFERENCES IN AFFECTIVE FACTORS RELATED TO THE PAIN EXPERIENCE

SEX-RELATED DIFFERENCES IN AFFECTIVE RESPONSE TO CLINICAL PAIN

The association between pain and the affective response to pain is well documented. Pain and measures of negative affect have been positively correlated with comorbidity to a varying degree, depending on the specific pain condition, the clinical sample studied, and the dimension of negative emotion measured (for review, see Robinson and Riley 1999). Various theories about the nature of these relationships hold that negative emotion increases somatic sensitivity, that negative emotion causes some pain, or that negative emotion can result from the experience of chronic pain (Watson and Pennebaker 1989; Banks and Kerns 1996; Fishbain et al. 1997). The finding that women report more psychological distress in the general population than men (Nolen-Hoeksema 1990) may contribute to sex differences in the experience of pain, in that females with ongoing pain would continue to be more likely to experience negative affect.

SEX-CORRELATED DIFFERENCES IN PAIN-RELATED DEPRESSION AND ANXIETY

Community-based samples have provided limited evidence that women with pain experience more emotional distress then men. Magni et al. (1990) found that among 2324 participants in the National Health and Nutrition Examination Survey, pain and depressive symptoms tended to be more evident in women reporting chronic pain than in corresponding men, when compared to controls of the same sex. As with other constructs in the clinical pain literature, sex differences in emotional response to pain are infrequently reported as the primary analysis. We will review several studies that have found differences in measures of pain-related depression and anxiety.

Sex differences in emotional response to pain may influence an individual's report of clinical pain. In a study of back pain patients, Bolton

(1994) found that increased somatic awareness and depressive symptoms were associated for females but not males. She suggested that it may be "more socially acceptable for women to admit to distress than men, and that women have a greater perception of their symptoms and body awareness than do men" (p. 352). She noted that the correlation between somatic awareness and depression that is found in women but not men suggests fundamental differences in the psychosocial profile of each gender. Haley et al. (1985) reported sex-related patterns in pain and mood, with depression being significantly related to pain for females, whereas for males, depression was associated with activity but not with pain. More recently, Edwards and colleagues (2000) noted that women and men from a heterogeneous chronic pain population reported equivalent levels of pain-related anxiety. However, high pain-related anxiety was associated with greater pain severity, greater interference from pain, and low levels of daily activity among men but not women.

Two studies in the headache literature have reported sex differences in psychological distress. Lacriox and Barbaree (1990) found that among headache sufferers, females had a higher mean score than males on a psychosomatic symptom checklist and more frequent disruption in social and family life. Gilbar et al. (1998) also reported data consistent with the hypothesis that sex is a risk factor for psychological distress secondary to headache. Their study compared the psychological symptoms of 26 young men and 65 young women referred to a neurology clinic for medical advice regarding headache. Women demonstrated more psychological symptoms than the men on measures of somatization and depression. The authors suggested that women with multiple roles (housekeeper, parent, employee) were overwhelmed with role conflicts.

In studies of rheumatoid arthritis patients, women reported higher rates of depression (Fifield et al. 1994) and greater negative (but not positive) affect than did male patients (Fifield et al. 1996). Building on these two studies, Dowdy et al. (1996) directly tested whether psychological adjustment could be explained by differences in sex, over and above the variance associated with physical impairment, coping strategies, and emotional support. Using a stepwise regression model, the authors found that these control variables only partially accounted for the association between sex and negative affect. Sex-related differences were most marked for measures assessing negative affective symptoms associated with depression, and weakest with scores more closely associated with anxiety, suggesting that the emotional component on which the sexes differ most is depression.

Evers et al. (1997) studied rheumatoid arthritis patients over the course of the first year following diagnosis and examined the determinants of psychological distress. Females reported higher mean levels of anxiety and depression at initial diagnosis. Depression and anxiety immediately following the initial diagnosis were predicted by female sex, high levels of pain, negative life events, and low social support. One year after diagnosis, disease severity and female sex continued to be related to psychological distress. In addition, a decrease in depression was associated with a larger social network at initial diagnosis for all patients. This finding is consistent with several of the coping studies reviewed above, suggesting that the use of passive coping strategies may be more detrimental for females because of their need for social support. Furthermore, the use of passive coping is associated with increased symptoms in studies of depression (Nolen-Hoeksema 1990; Nolen-Hoeksema et al. 1993).

SEX-RELATED DIFFERENCES IN OTHER EMOTIONS ARE LESS WELL STUDIED

Although emotions such as anger (Wade et al. 1990; Fernandez and Turk 1995) and fear (Wade et al. 1990; Asmundson et al. 1999) are now recognized as prominent emotions experienced by chronic pain patients, few studies have tested for related sex differences. Burns et al. (1998) examined associations between anger management style and adjustment in 127 married chronic pain patients prior to entry into a multidisciplinary pain management program. These authors found a significant interaction of anger expression and sex. Among men, anger expression was negatively correlated with gains in physical therapy, and anger suppression was negatively associated with improvements in depression and general activities; these effects remained significant after controlling for trait anger. Furthermore, adjustment in highly anger-expressing men was negatively associated with critical responses from their spouses, whereas among women, no association was observed. The authors concluded that how anger is managed, at least among male pain patients, appears to have a unique influence on patient outcomes, suggesting that that optimal treatment approaches could differ for males and females.

Sex differences in fear of movement and behavioral performance have been reported (Vlaeyen 1995). Females reported higher scores on a measure of fear of re-injury from movement, although primary independent variables in the study were catastrophizing, depression, and pain coping. In a regression model, a block of control variables, including sex, accounted for 14% of the variance in fear of movement. The sex variable had a significant standardized beta of –0.18, when controlling for pain and compensation status. Liddel and Locker (1997) found that community-based women reported more problematic anxiety related to fear of dental pain than did men. The results suggested that compared to men, female respondents avoided pain more, accepted pain less and feared it more, and desired control more; however, the sexes did not differ on perceived control during a dental procedure.

We are aware of only one study that has systematically examined sex differences in dimensions of pain across multiple emotions (J.L. Riley et al., unpublished manuscript). This study used simultaneous regression to test for sex differences in dimensions of pain processing with data collected from a sample of 1647 chronic pain patients (680 males and 967 females). Male and female patients experienced different emotional responses to their chronic pain. Of the five negative emotions assessed (depression, anxiety, anger, fear, and frustration), frustration best characterized the emotional response to pain for females, and anxiety for males. Univariate analyses indicated that females experienced statistically higher fear and frustration than males, but the effects were small. The most interesting finding was that the associations between emotions and pain were not in the direction hypothesized. In contrast to studies reviewed above (Haley et al. 1985; Bolton 1994; Evers et al. 1997), males demonstrated an overall higher linear association between pain unpleasantness and emotions compared to females. The authors concluded that the most important sex differences in pain-related emotions may not manifest themselves as group differences, but as differences in linear relationships between immediate pain unpleasantness and discrete emotional feelings, such as frustration and fear.

As evidenced by Riley et al.'s study (unpublished manuscript), not all studies of clinical samples are consistent with respect to the direction of sex differences in emotional response to pain. Using a global instrument of psychological distress (Symptom Check List 90), Buckelew et al. (1990) found that males scored significantly higher on somatization, depression, and anxiety. In a recently reported null result, Turk and Okifuji (1999) examined sex differences in a number of variables representing adaptation to pain. This study used multiple samples, one consisting of 143 cancer patients and a second comprising 428 patients suffering nonmalignant pain. These researchers tested for sex-related differences on several measures of depression, disability, and impact from pain (interference). Women in the nonmalignant pain sample reported more depressive symptoms than men and were likely to qualify for a clinical diagnosis using the Center for Epidemiological Study Depression Scale cutoff. Other variables were not statistically different across sex in either sample. Turk and Okifuji emphasized the fact that the differences between the sexes were less notable than variability within sex.

SEX-CORRELATED DIFFERENCES IN AFFECTIVE FACTORS RELATED TO EXPERIMENTAL PAIN

Lautenbacher and Rollman (1993) suggested that stimulation-related anxiety level may be a critical variable in explaining sex differences as well as discrepancies among types of stimulation. Their argument is based on speculation that more sex differences were observed in studies using higher ramping slopes with thermal stimuli (i.e., Feine et al. 1991) or longer electrical pulse duration (Robin et al. 1987). Lautenbacher and Rollman suggested that anxiety generated by the stimuli itself influenced the response of females more than that of males. Earlier investigators (Malow 1981; Cornwall and Donderi 1988) have shown that induced anxiety affects pain perception, but these results are inconsistent with respect to the direction of influence and the pain measure affected. Unfortunately, neither of these two studies employed females as subjects, prohibiting assessment of sex or gender influences on pain. The Cornwall and Donderi (1988) study was consistent with the speculations of Lautenbacher and Rollman in that stimulus-specific anxiety increased pain responsivity.

The hypothesis that stimulation characteristics affect the anxiety-by-sex interaction is supported by findings of other studies. For example, Robin et al. (1987) tested the influence of sex and anxiety on pain perception in a sample of 50 volunteers (healthy dental students). Minimum perceptible threshold, pain threshold, and pain tolerance threshold were determined by delivering electrical stimulation at regular intervals. The results showed a lower pain threshold and tolerance in females than in males and a significant correlation between the score on Cattell's anxiety test and these pain measures. Weisenberg et al. (1995) also reported a sex-by-anxiety-by-trial interaction, with females showing reduced anxiety on the second trial. However, the results of a study performed by Fillingim et al. (1999a) fail to support Lautenbacher and Rollman's (1993) hypothesis. Their subjects underwent heat pain threshold assessment via the method of levels using fast (4.0°C/s) and slow (0.5°C/s) rates of rise. Fillingim et al. found that females demonstrated lower thresholds than males on both slow and fast rates of rise, inconsistent with the sex-by-rate interaction hypothesis.

Another hypothesis regarding sex differences in pain perception relates to the increased prevalence of depression in women. Depressed patients are thought to be more sensitive to pain (Watson and Pennebaker 1989), and a cognitive process has been suggested involving excessive somatic focus and overinterpretation of physical sensations (Barsky and Wyshak 1990). However, we were unable to find a single study testing this sex difference hypothesis using experimental pain.

CAUTIONS

The studies reviewed above must be interpreted with several caveats in mind. A bias toward overestimating sex-related differences in psychosocial response to pain may exist in the pain literature for several reasons. First, when sex-related differences are not found in secondary analyses of published studies, they are less likely to be reported, and studies finding a null result with a primary hypothesis for sex-related differences may not be accepted for publication at all. Second, given that painful sensations are frequently accompanied by emotional discomfort, psychosocial distress may influence health care use via symptom magnification or by triggering the decision to seek care. The prevalence of negative emotions in pain clinic patients is well documented (Engel et al. 1996). For example, Gatchel et al. (1995) showed that measures of negative affect predicted chronicity of an injury. Therefore, there may be a symptom-related bias across sex that triggers the decision to seek care, introducing a confounding variable into the sampling of individuals experiencing pain in studies using clinical samples. Consequently, this potential sex-related interaction between an individual's pain condition and his or her emotional response to pain, which appears to be predictive of health care use, may be either a cause or an effect of sex-correlated differences.

Furthermore, one can easily criticize the studies reviewed above as accounting for only a small proportion of the overall variance in the relationships studied. However, sex-correlated differences in human behavior of any kind are likely to be more complex than the models we are currently testing. Therefore, one of the problems in determining or understanding the true nature of these sex differences is the lack of larger multifactorial models that include pain, pain coping, emotions, and sociocultural influences including gender role socialization to guide our methodologies and related hypothesis testing.

SUMMARY

The evidence is clear that in laboratory settings, men and women differ on average with respect to pain report across a number of types of stimulation and psychophysical protocols. It seems equally clear that women report more pain symptoms in epidemiologic studies and also attend pain clinics in greater numbers. Scientific attention has increasingly turned to these issues. The focus of much, if not most of the research on sex differences in pain responding has been on discovering the physiological/anatomical determinants of sex differences in laboratory settings. The emerging data supporting first-order biological contributions to sex differences are compelling, but the relative contributions of biological and social learning influences have not been adequately studied. To a large degree, the social influences that come to bear in laboratory settings, and particularly the potential differences in those influences for men and women, have not been adequately explored. The social milieu of the laboratory may be significantly different for men and women, affecting how each sex behaves in that milieu. Expressing pain in a public arena is likely to be very different for men and women, and may be better explained by social factors rather than by biological factors. Countless behavioral differences between women and men, for example communication styles, attire, and vocational and avocational interests, seem most parsimoniously explained by differences in social learning and social customs rather than as a function of biology. It seems logical that sociocultural gender norms should also influence women and men when they report on a stimulus applied as part of a laboratory study of pain.

Findings from research into health care utilization suggest that, on average, men and women make different attributions about clinical symptoms, differ in their perceptions of symptom severity and significance, have different values associated with health and health care, and report different expectations about sex-typed responding to pain. Men and women employ coping strategies to different degrees with respect to clinical pain. Women and men also differ in their expression of negative emotion, which is a critical part of any clinical pain condition. However, the relationship of clinical pain to negative mood differs between the sexes, suggesting additional complexity from social factors.

We believe there is compelling evidence to suggest that anyone interested in studying sex-related pain responding needs to take into account psychosocial factors including gender socialization, learning history, cognitive factors, and affective factors in any pain measurement. The attribution of differences to men and women based on chromosomal sex alone appears to us to be overly simplistic and may, in fact, ignore the greater contribution to sex-related differences from the way in which men and women are socialized with respect to symptom perception and symptom reporting.

REFERENCES

Affleck G, Urrows S, Tennen H, Higgins P. Daily coping with pain from rheumatoid arthritis: patterns and correlates. *Pain* 1992; 51:221–229.

Ashmore RD, Sewell AD. Sex/gender and the individual. In: Barone DF, Hersen H, VanHasselt VB (Eds). *Advanced Personality*. New York: Plenum, 1998.

Asmundson GJ, Norton PJ, Norton GR. Beyond pain: the role of fear and avoidance in chronicity. *Clin Psychol Rev* 1999; 19(1):97–119.

Baker SL, Kirsch I. Cognitive mediators of pain perception and tolerance. *J Pers Soc Psychol* 1991; 61:504–510.

Bandura A. *Social Foundations of Thought and Action: A Social Cognitive Theory*. Englewood Cliffs, NJ: Prentice-Hall, 1986.

Banks SM, Kerns RD. Explaining high rates of depression in chronic pain: a diathesis-stress framework. *Psychol Bull* 1996; 119:95–110.

Barsky AJ, Wyshak G. Hypochondriasis and somatosensory amplification. *Br J Psychiatry* 1990; 140:273–283.

Bates MS. *Biocultural Dimensions of Chronic Pain: Implications for Treatment of Multi-Ethnic Populations*. Albany, NY: State University of New York Press, 1996.

Bem SL. The measurement of psychological androgyny. *J Consult Clin Psychol* 1974; 42(2):155–162.

Bem SL. Gender schema theory: a cognitive account of sex-typing. *Psychol Rev* 1981; 88:354–364.

Bem SL. Androgyny and gender schema theory. In: Sonderegger TB (Ed). *Psychology and Gender: Nebraska Symposium on Motivation, 1984*. Lincoln, NE: University of Nebraska Press, 1985.

Berkley KJ. Sex differences in pain. *Behav Brain Sci* 1997; 20:371–380.

Bolton JE. Psychological distress and disability in back pain patients: evidence of sex differences. *J Pychosom Res* 1994; 38(8):849–858.

Buckelew SP, Shutty MS, Hewett J, et al. Health locus of control, gender differences and adjustment to persistent pain. *Pain* 1990; 42:287–294.

Buescher KL, Johnston JA, Parker JC, et al. Relationship of self-efficacy to pain behavior. *J Rheumatol* 1991; 18(7):968–972.

Bush FM, Harkins SW, Harrington WG, Price DD. Analysis of gender effects on pain perception and symptom presentation in temporomandibular pain. *Pain* 1993; 53:73–80.

Burns JW, Johnson BJ, Devine J, Mahoney N, Pawl R. Anger management style and the prediction of treatment outcome among male and female chronic pain patients. *Behav Res Ther* 1998; 36(11):1051–1062.

Cleary PD, Mechanic D, Greenley JR. Sex differences in medical care utilization: an empirical investigation. *J Health Soc Behav* 1982; 23(2):106–119.

Cornwall A, Donderi D. The effect of experimentally induced anxiety on the experience of pressure pain. *Pain* 1988; 35:105–113.

Craig KD. Social modeling influences: pain in context. In: Sternbach RA (Ed). *The Psychology of Pain,* 2nd ed. New York: Raven Press, 1986.

Craig KD, Prkachin KM. Social modeling influences on sensory decision theory and psychophysiological indexes of pain. *J Pers Soc Psychol* 1978; 36:805–815.

Craig KD, Weiss SM. Vicarious influences on pain-threshold determinations. *J Pers Soc Psychol* 1971; 19:53–59.

Crisson JE, Keefe FJ. The relationship of locus of control to pain coping strategies and psychological distress in chronic pain patients. *Pain* 1988; 35(2):147–154.

Crombez G, Eccleston C, Baeyens F, Eelen P. When somatic information threatens, catastrophic thinking enhances attentional interference. *Pain* 1998; 75:187–198.

Deaux K. Commentary: Sorry, wrong number—a reply to Gentile's call. *Psychol Sci* 1993; 4(2):125–126.

Deaux K, LaFrance M. Gender. In: Gilbert DT, Fiske ST (Eds). *The Handbook of Social Psychology,* Vol. 2, 4th ed. Boston: McGraw-Hill, 1998, pp 788–827.

Deaux K, Major B. Putting gender into context: an interactive model of gender-related behavior. *Psychol Rev* 1987; 94 (3):369–389.

Deaux K, Major B. A social-psychological model of gender. In: Rhode DL (Ed). *Theoretical Perspectives on Sexual Difference*. New Haven: Yale University Press, 1990, pp 89–99.

Diehl M, Coyle N, Labouvie-Vief G. Age and sex differences in strategies of coping and defense across the life span. *Psychol Aging* 1996; 11(1):127–139.

Dolce JJ, Doleys DM, Raczynski JM, et al. The role of self-efficacy expectancies in the prediction of pain tolerance. *Pain* 1986; 27(2):261–272.

Dowdy SW, Dwyer KA, Smith CA, Wallston KA. Gender and psychological well-being of persons with rheumatoid arthritis. *Arthritis Care Res* 1996; 9(6):449–456.

Edwards PW, O'Neill GW, Zeichner A, Kuczmierczyk AR. Effects of familial pain models on pain complaints and coping strategies. *Percept Mot Skills* 1985; 61(3 Pt 2):1053–1054.

Edwards RR, Augustson E, Fillingim RB. Sex-specific effects of pain-related anxiety on adjustment to chronic pain. *Clin J Pain* 2000; 16:43–53.

Eisler RM, Skidmore JR. Masculine gender role stress: scale development and component factors in the appraisal of stressful situations. *Behav Modif* 1987; 11:123–136.

Engel CC, von Korff M, Katon WJ. Back pain in primary care: predictors of high health-care costs. *Pain* 1996; 65:197–204.

Evers AW, Kraaimaat FW, Geenen R, Bijlsma JW. Determinants of psychological distress and its course in the first year after diagnosis in rheumatoid arthritis patients. *J Behav Med* 1997; 20(5):489–504.

Feine JS, Bushnell MC, Miron D, Duncan GH. Sex differences in the perception of noxious heat stimuli. *Pain* 1991; 44:255–262.

Fernandez E, Turk DC. The scope and significance of anger in the experience of chronic pain. *Pain* 1995; 61:165–175.

Fifield J, Reisine S, Sheehan TJ. Gender differences in the expression of depressive symptoms in patients with rheumatoid arthritis. *Arthritis Rheum* 1994; 7(Suppl 9):S283.

Fifield J, Reisine S, Sheehan TJ, McQuillan J. Gender, paid work, and symptoms of emotional distress in rheumatoid arthritis patients. *Arthritis Rheum* 1996; 39(3):427–435.

Fillingim RB, Maixner W. Gender differences in the responses to noxious stimuli. *Pain Forum* 1995; 4(4):209–221.

Fillingim RB, Keefe FJ, Light, Booker, Maixner W. The influence of gender and psychological factors on pain perception. *J Gender Culture Health* 1996; 1:21–36.

Fillingim RB, Maddux V, Shackelford JA. Sex differences in heat pain thresholds as a function of assessment method and rate of rise. *Somatosens Mot Res* 1999a; 16(1):57–62.

Fillingim RB, Wilkinson CS, Powell T. Self-reported abuse history and pain complaints among young adults. *Clin J Pain* 1999b; 15:85–91.

Fillingim RB, Edwards RR, Powell T. Sex-dependent effects of reported familial pain history on clinical and experimental pain responses. *Pain* 2000; 86:87–94.

Fishbain DA, Cutler R, Rosomoff HL, Rosomoff RS. Chronic pain-associated depression: antecedent or consequence of chronic pain? A review. *Clin J Pain* 1997; 13:116–137.

Fordyce WE. Learning processes in pain. In: Sternbach RA (Ed). *The Psychology of Pain.* New York: Raven Press, 1986.

Gatchel RJ, Polatin PB, Kinney RK. Predicting outcome of chronic back pain using clinical predictors of psychopathology: a prospective analysis. *Health Psychol* 1995; 14:415–420.

Geisser ME, Robinson ME, Pickren W. Differences in cognitive coping strategies among pain-sensitive and pain-tolerant individuals on the cold-pressor test. *Behav Ther* 1992; 23:31–41.

Geisser ME, Robinson ME, Keefe FJ, Weiner ML. Catastrophizing, depression and the sensory, affective and evaluative aspects of chronic pain. *Pain* 1994; 58:79–83.

Gijsbers van Wijk CM, Kolk AM, van den Bosch WJ, van den Hoogen HJ. Male and female morbidity in general practice: the nature of sex differences. *Soc Sci Med* 1992; 35(5):665–678.

Gilbar O, Bazak Y, Harel Y. Gender, primary headache, and psychological distress. *Headache* 1998; 38(1):31–34.

Haley WE, Turner JA, Romano JM. Depression in chronic pain patients: relation to pain, activity, and sex differences. *Pain* 1985; 23(4):337–343.

Harkapaa K. Relationships of psychological distress and health locus of control beliefs with the use of cognitive and behavioral coping strategies in low back pain patients. *Clin J Pain* 1991; 7:275–282.

Haythornthwaite JA, Menefee LA, Heinberg IJ, Clark MR. Pain coping strategies predict perceived control over pain. *Pain* 1998; 77(1):33–39.

Hibbard JH, Pope CR. Gender roles, illness orientation and use of medical services. *Soc Sci Med* 1983; 17:129–137.

Hobfoll SE, Dunahoo CL, Ben-Porath Y, Monnier J. Gender and coping: the dual-axis model of coping. *Am J Community Psychol* 1994; 22(1):49–82.

Jensen I, Nygren A, Gamberale F, Goldie I, Westerholm P. Coping with long-term musculoskeletal pain and its consequences: is gender a factor? *Pain* 1994; 57:167–172.

Jensen MP, Karoly P. Control beliefs, coping efforts, and adjustment to chronic pain. *J Consult Clin Psychol* 1991; 59(3):431–438.

Jensen MP, Turner JA, Romano JM. Self-efficacy and outcome expectancies: relationship to chronic pain coping strategies and adjustment. *Pain* 1991a; 44(3):263–269.

Jensen MP, Turner JA, Romano JM, Karoly P. Coping with chronic pain: a critical review of the literature. *Pain* 1991b; 47:249–283.

Jensen MP, Turner JA, Romano JM, Lawler BK. Relationship of pain-specific beliefs to chronic pain adjustment. *Pain* 1994; 57(3):301–309.

Keefe FJ, Williams DA. A comparison of coping strategies in chronic pain patients in different age groups. *J Gerontol* 1990; 45(4):161–165.

Keefe FJ, Brown GK, Wallston KA, Caldwell DS. Coping with rheumatoid arthritis pain: catastrophizing as a maladaptive strategy. *Pain* 1989; 37:51–56.

Keefe FJ, Caldwell DS, Martinez S, et al. Analyzing pain in rheumatoid arthritis patients. Pain coping strategies in patients who have had knee replacement surgery. *Pain* 1991; 46(2):153–160.

Klonoff EA, Landrine H. Culture and gender diversity beliefs about the causes of six illnesses. *J Behav Med* 1994; 17(4):407–418.

Klonoff EA, Landrine H, Brown M. Appraisal and response to pain may be a function of its bodily location. *J Psychosom Res* 1993; 37(6):661–670.

Kohlberg LA. A cognitive-developmental analysis of children's sex-role concepts and attitudes. In: Maccoby EE (Ed). *The Development of Sex Differences.* Stanford, CA: Stanford University Press, 1966, pp 82–173.

Kolt G, Kirkby RJ, Lindner H. Coping processes in competitive gymnasts: gender differences. *Percept Mot Skills* 1995; Dec, 81(3 Pt 2):1139–1145.

Koutantji M, Pearce SA, Oakley DA. The relationship between gender and family history of pain with current pain experience and awareness of pain in others. *Pain* 1998; 77(1):25–31.

Lacroix R, Barbaree HE. The impact of recurrent headaches on behavior lifestyle and health. *Behav Res Ther* 1990; 28(3):235–242.

Lander J, Fowler-Kerry S, Hill A. Comparison of pain perception among males and females. *Can J Nurs Res* 1990; 22(1):39–49.

Lash SJ, Eisler RM, Schulman RS. Cardiovascular reactivity to stress in men: Effects of masculine gender role stress appraisal and masculine performance challenge. *Behav Modif* 1990; 14(1):3–20.

Lash SJ, Gillespie BL, Eisler RM, Stouthard DR. Sex differences in cardiovascular reactivity: effects of the gender relevance of the stressor. *Health Psychol* 1991; 10:392–398.

Lash SJ, Eisler RM, Stouthard DR. Sex differences in cardiovascular reactivity as a function of the appraised gender relevance of the stressor. *Behav Med* 1995; 21:86–94.

Lawlis GF, Achterberg J, Kenner L, Kopetz K. Ethnic and sex differences in response to clinical and induced pain in chronic spinal pain patients. *Spine* 1984; 9(7):751–754.

Lautenbacher S, Rollman G. Sex differences in pain responsiveness to painful and non-painful stimuli are dependent on the stimulation method. *Pain* 1993; 55:255–264.

Lazarus RA, Folkman S. *Stress, Appraisal, and Coping*. New York: Springer, 1984.

Lefebvre JC, Keefe FJ, Affleck G, et al. The relationship of arthritis self-efficacy to daily pain, daily mood, and daily pain coping in rheumatoid arthritis patients. *Pain* 1999; 80(1–2):425–435.

Lester N, Lefebvre JC, Keefe FJ. Pain in young adults: I. Relationship to gender and family pain history. *Clin J Pain* 1994; 10(4):282–289.

Levine FM, De Simone LL. The effects of experimenter gender on pain report in male and female subjects. *Pain* 1991; 44:69–72.

Liddell A, Locker D. Gender and age differences in attitudes to dental pain and dental control. *Community Dent Oral Epidemiol* 1997; 25(4):314–318.

Lipton JA, Marbach JJ. Ethnicity and the pain experience. *Soc Sci Med* 1984; 19:1279–1298.

Magni G, Moreschi C, Rigatti-Luchini S, Merkse H. Prospective study on the relationship between depressive symptoms and chronic musculoskeletal pain. *Pain* 1990; 56:289–297.

Malow R. The effects of induced anxiety on pain perception: a signal detection analysis. *Pain* 1981; 11:397–405.

Mechanic D. The influence of mothers on their children's health attitudes and behavior. *Pediatrics* 1964; 33:444–453.

Mechanic D. The concept of illness behavior: culture, situation, and personal predisposition. *Psychol Med* 1986; 16:1–7.

Melzack R, Wall PD. Pain mechanisms: a new theory. *Science* 1965; 150:971–979.

Meininger JC. Sex differences in factors associated with use of medical care and alternative illness behaviors. *Soc Sci Med* 1986; 22(3):289–292.

Mischel W. A social-learning view of sex differences in behavior. In: Maccoby EE (Ed). *The Development of Sex Differences*. Stanford, CA: Stanford University Press, 1966, pp 56–81.

Mustard CA, Kaufert P, Kozyrsky, A, Mayer TN. Sex differences in the use of health care services. *N Engl J Med* 1998; 338(23):1678–1683.

Myers CD, Wise EA, Riley JL, Robinson ME. Relative contributions of sex and gender to cardiovascular reactivity and experimental pain response. Poster presented at the 17th annual meeting of the American Pain Society, San Diego, California, November 1998.

Nolen-Hoeksema S. *Sex Differences in Depression*. Stanford: Stanford University Press, 1990.

Nolen-Hoeksema S, Morrow J, Fredrickson BL. Response styles and the duration of episodes of depressed mood. *J Abnorm Psychol* 1993; 102(1):20–28.

Osman A, Barrios FX, Kopper BA, et al. Factor structure, reliability, and validity of the Pain Catastrophizing Scale. *J Behav Med* 1997; 20(6):589–605.

Otto MW, Dougher MJ. Sex differences and personality factors in responsivity to pain. *Percept Motor Skills* 1985; 61:383–390.

Potter LB, Sacks JJ, Kresnow MJ, Mercy J. Nonfatal physical violence, United States, 1994. *Public Health Rep* 1999; 114:343–352.

Riley JL III, Robinson ME, Kvaal SA, Gremillion HA. Effects of physical and sexual abuse in facial pain: direct or mediated? *J Cranio Pract* 1998a; 16:1–8.

Riley JL III, Robinson ME, Wise E, Myers CD, Fillingim RB. Sex differences in the perception of noxious experimental stimuli: a meta-analysis. *Pain* 1998b; 74:181–187.

Robin O, Vinard H, Vernet-Maury E, Saumet JL. Influence of sex and anxiety on pain threshold and tolerance. *Funct Neurol* 1987; 2(2):173–179.

Robinson ME, Riley JL III. Role of negative emotions in pain. In: Gatchel RJ, Turk DC (Eds). *Psychosocial Factors in Pain*. New York: Guilford Press, 1998.

Robinson ME, Wise EA, Riley JL. Sex differences in clinical pain: a multi-sample study. *J Clin Psychol Med Set* 1998; 5:413–423.

Robinson ME, Riley JL III, Myers CD, et al. Gender role expectations: do they explain sex differences in pain? Poster presented at the 18th annual meeting of the American Pain Society, Ft. Lauderdale, Florida, October 1999.

Rollman GB. Culture and pain. In: Kazarian SS, Evans DR (Eds). *Cultural Clinical Psychology*. New York: Oxford University Press, 1998, pp 267–286.

Safran DG, Rogers WH, Tarlov AR, McHorney CA, Ware JE Jr. Gender differences in medical treatment: the case of physician-prescribed activity restrictions. *Soc Sci Med* 1997; 45(5):711–722.

Savedra M, Gibbons P, Tesler M, Ward J, Wegner C. How do children describe pain? A tentative assessment. *Pain* 1982; 14:95–104.

Spinhoven P, Ter Kuile MM, Linssen AC, Gazendam B. Pain coping strategies in a Dutch population of chronic low back pain patients. *Pain* 1989; 37(1):77–83.

Strong J, Ashton R, Stewart A. Chronic low back pain: toward an integrated psychosocial assessment model. *J Consult Clin Psychol* 1994; 62(5):1058–1063.

Sullivan MJL, D'Eon JL. Relation between catastrophizing and depression in chronic pain patients. *J Abnorm Psychol* 1990; 99(3):260–263.

Tota-Faucette ME, Gil KM, Williams DA, Keefe FJ, Goli V. Predictors of response to pain management treatment. The role of family environment and changes in cognitive processes. *Clin J Pain* 1993; 9(2):115–123.

Turk DC, Okifuji A. Does sex make a difference in the prescription of treatments and the adaptation to chronic pain by cancer and non-cancer patients? *Pain* 1999; 82(2):139–148.

Turk DC, Rudy TE. Assessment of cognitive factors in chronic pain: a worthwhile enterprise? *J Consult Clin Psychol* 1986; 54(6):760–768.

Turkat ID, Guise BJ. Test of reliability of perception of parental and childhood illness behavior. *Percept Mot Skills* 1983; 57(1):101–102.

Turkat ID, Guise BJ, Carter KM. The effects of vicarious experience on pain termination and work avoidance: a replication. *Behav Res Ther* 1983; 21(5):491–493.

Turner JA, Clancy S. Strategies for coping with chronic low back pain: relationship to pain and disability. *Pain* 1986; 24(3):355–364.

Unger RK. Toward a redefinition of sex and gender. *Am Psychol* 1979; 34:1085–1094.

Unruh AM. Gender variations in clinical pain experience. *Pain* 1996; 65(2-3):123–167.

Unruh AM, Ritchie J, Merskey H. Does gender affect appraisal of pain and pain coping strategies? *Clin J Pain* 1999; 15(1):31–40.

van den Akker OB, Eves FF, Service S, Lennon B. Menstrual cycle symptom reporting in three British ethnic groups. *Soc Sci Med* 1995; 40(10):1417–1423.

Verbrugge LM. Female illness rates and illness behavior: testing hypothesis about sex differences in health. *Womens Health* 1979; 4:61–79.

Verbrugge LM, Patrick DL. Seven chronic conditions: their impact on US adults' activity levels and use of medical services. *Am J Public Health* 1995; 85(2):173–182.

Vingerhoets AJ, Van Heck GI. Gender, coping and psychosomatic symptoms. *Psychol Med* 1990; 20(1):125–135.

Vlaeyen JW, Kole-Snijders AM, Boeren RG, van Eek H. Fear of movement/(re)injury in chronic low back pain and its relation to behavioral performance. *Pain* 1995; Sept, 62(3):363–72

Wade JB, Price DD, Hamer RM, Schwartz SM. An emotional component analysis of chronic pain. *Pain* 1990; 40:303–310.

Wall PD, Jones M. *Defeating Pain: The War Against a Silent Epidemic*. New York: Plenum Press, 1991.

Watson D, Pennebaker JW. Health complaints, stress, and distress: exploring the central role of negative affectivity. *Psychol Rev* 1989; 96:234–254.

Wallbott HG, Scherer KR. Stress specificities: differential effects of coping style, gender, and type of stressor on autonomic arousal, facial expression, and subjective feeling. *J Pers Soc Psychol* 1991; 61(1):147–156.

Weir R, Browne G, Tunks E, Gafni A, Roberts J. Gender differences in psychosocial adjustment to chronic pain and expenditures for health care services used. *Clin J Pain* 1996; 12(4):277–290.

Weisenberg M, Tepper I, Schwarzwald J. Humor as a cognitive technique for increasing pain tolerance. *Pain* 1995; 63(2):207–212.

Williams DA, Keefe F. Pain beliefs and the use of cognitive-behavioral coping strategies. *Pain* 1991; 46(2):185–190.

Wise EA, Papas RK, Campbell LC, Riley JL III, Robinson ME. A quantitative review of cultural differences in experimental pain. Poster presented at the 18th annual meeting of the American Pain Society, Ft. Lauderdale, Florida, October 1999.

Zatzick DF, Dimsdale JE. Cultural variations in response to painful stimuli. *Psychosom Med* 1990; 52:544–557.

Zborowski M. Cultural components in response to pain. *J Soc Issues* 1952; 8:16–30.

Zola I. Culture and symptoms—an analysis of patients' presenting complaints. *Am Sociol Rev* 1966; 31:615–630.

Correspondence to: Michael E. Robinson, PhD, Department of Clinical and Health Psychology, University of Florida, Box J-165 HSC, Gainesville, FL 32610, USA. Tel: 904-392-4551; Fax: 904-395-0468; email: merobin@nersp.nerdc.ufl.edu.

Part II

Sex-Related Differences in Experimental Pain Responses

Sex, Gender, and Pain, Progress in Pain Research and Management, Vol. 17, edited by R.B. Fillingim, IASP Press, Seattle, © 2000.

5

Experimental Studies of Sex-Related Factors Influencing Nociceptive Responses: Nonhuman Animal Research

Wendy F. Sternberg and Melissa W. Wachterman

Department of Psychology, Haverford College, Haverford, Pennsylvania, USA

Gender as a source of variability in human pain responses has gained a great deal of attention among pain clinicians and researchers. The explanatory power of the social, cultural, and biological issues associated with gender in humans can account for the rather consistent observations of gender-related variability in the clinic, and the rather inconsistent observations of gender-related variability in the laboratory (see Berkley 1997, Riley et al. 1998, and Unruh 1996 for reviews). However, the focus on sex-related factors in addressing nociceptive variability in the laboratory animal has only recently come to the forefront of research. This chapter serves as a review and synthesis of studies investigating sex-related differences in nociceptive responses, involving both ascending and descending pain-processing pathways.

Although addressing the question of the existence of sex-differences in pain behavior in laboratory animals would appear relatively straightforward, the highly variable nature of pain behavior makes conclusions somewhat difficult. In most cases, individual variability far outweighs the contributions of sex-related variables, although hormonal factors play an important role in determining some aspects of nociceptive and antinociceptive responses. Further complications are the multiple methodologies that have been applied to the study of nociception. Sex differences are apparent on only a subset of algesiometric assays. Thus, before tackling the literature on sex differences in nociceptive processing and the hormonal determinants of sex differences, it is necessary to understand the methods used to study these variables in the laboratory setting.

When discussing responses to noxious stimuli in nonhuman animals, researchers commonly avoid the term "pain" and describe these responses as "nociceptive," reflecting an apparent inability to directly assess a perceptual construct such as pain in all but human subjects. Nociception describes activity in peripheral sensory pathways that respond to tissue-damaging (actual or impending) stimuli. However, it is my contention that as with any subjective perceptual process in any organism (human or nonhuman), observation of behavior (including verbal report, in humans) is the only noninvasive way to determine whether contact with a noxious stimulus has resulted in a pain response in a conscious subject. Clearly, if the dependent variable is the recording of activity in peripheral afferents in isolated preparations, or in anesthetized or spinalized subjects (or reflexive responses in these subjects), nociception is the appropriate term. But operationally defined pain behaviors in any subject (such as paw-licking, paw-shaking, jumping, guarding, favoring, abdominal constriction, vocalization, or verbal report) represent functionally equivalent markers of "pain." Therefore, where appropriate I use the terms nociception and pain interchangeably (and I consider antinociception equivalent to analgesia when the observation is a reduction in pain behaviors), even when discussing nonhuman subject populations.

COMMONLY USED NOCICEPTIVE ASSAYS FOR STUDYING SEX DIFFERENCES IN PAIN

The noxious stimuli that are most often used in tests of pain processing in nonhuman animals are thermal, electrical, mechanical, and chemical. Behavioral responses to thermal noxious stimuli are assessed on the hot-plate test, in which the animal is placed on a surface maintained at a constant noxious temperature (50°–58°C), and latency to a pain behavior (hindpaw lick, flick, shake) is recorded. Differences in response latency between or within subjects is interpreted to represent differences in nociceptive processing. The tail-flick test also measures latency to withdrawal behavior from noxious heat, but this test commonly employs a radiant heat stimulus that rapidly rises to nociceptive threshold. The dependent measure is a reflexive withdrawal response that is believed to be wholly mediated at the spinal level, since the response occurs in spinalized or anesthetized subjects (Morgan et al. 1989). Another variant of the tail-flick test involves withdrawal from a water bath (tail-immersion test) at a constant noxious temperature, also a reflexive response. In contrast, hot-plate responding is an organized, supraspinally mediated pain behavior that is not believed to be reflexive (Morgan et al. 1989). One feature of the hot-plate and tail-flick tests (and variants of the latter) is that the animal is often restrained, immobilized, or has its movement partially restricted to prevent excessive exploration of the thermal surface or to keep the tail in contact with the noxious stimulus. The dependent measure in both of these tests is the time required to elicit a pain behavior; latency measurements are taken as an indication of pain threshold, and the animal is removed from the noxious stimulus upon making a response.

Nociceptive threshold assays may also employ electrical noxious stimuli. The jump test assays pain behavior to a cutaneous electrical stimulus applied to the feet, typically in the rat. The stimulus intensity at which the subject first displays a pain response (generally jumping from a charged grid through which the noxious stimulus is passed) is considered to represent nociceptive threshold.

The algesiometric assays described above share certain sensory characteristics; they all assess thresholds for responsivity to brief, phasic noxious stimuli. Such models of acute, cutaneous pain differ from models of tonic, continuous pain (e.g., the formalin and abdominal constriction tests) in sensory characteristics and in their neurochemical and neuroanatomical substrates.

Phasic pain models typically use noxious stimuli such as radiant heat or electricity that are brief, escapable (the stimulus ceases as soon as pain behavior is observed), and high in intensity, and usually employ some sort of "cutoff," an arbitrarily set time point or maximum stimulus intensity, after which the noxious stimulus is removed from a nonresponding animal to avoid possible tissue damage. The noxious stimuli presented in models of tonic pain, however, are typically longer in duration, inescapable, moderate in intensity, and are often associated with inflammation and/or tissue damage. For these reasons, models of tonic pain may be more relevant to clinical pain conditions than phasic pain tests. The formalin test and abdominal constriction test are two examples of assays that measure behavioral responses to ongoing painful stimuli.

In the formalin test, a small amount of a dilute formalin solution (5–10%) is injected into one of the hindpaws (which are not usually licked during normal grooming); the time that the animal spends licking the affected paw is the quantified pain behavior. Visceral pain is assessed in the abdominal constriction (also called writhing) test, in which one of several noxious chemical substances (such as dilute acetic acid or hypertonic saline) is injected into the peritoneal cavity; the number of abdominal constrictions exhibited by the subject is assessed over a fixed period of time following injection.

Tonic pain tests are thought to differ from phasic pain assays not only in their sensory characteristics, but also in their neurochemical and neuroanatomical substrates. However, given their ease of use, phasic pain tests are far more frequently used to address the question of sex differences in pain behavior.

SUMMARY OF LITERATURE ON SEX DIFFERENCES IN PAIN BEHAVIOR

As part of an investigation into sex and strain differences in pain behavior and morphine sensitivity, our group recently conducted a thorough survey of the literature on sex differences, pain, and analgesia (Mogil et al., in press). Part of the difficulty in synthesizing the literature stems from the inclusion of various species and strains of rodents and the multiple methodologies used to assess pain, all of which are considered to represent a singular phenomenon. In our synopsis, we attempted to account for overall patterns of sex differences by identifying subtle variations in experimental parameters, subject populations, hormonal manipulations, and experimental power. We reviewed the results of all investigations that had tested for (and reported the results of) basal nociceptive responses of male and female rodents in several different experimental contexts. Some of these investigations measured sex differences in response to noxious stimuli as the primary dependent variable, while others simply reported these data as part of a larger study on responses to analgesic manipulation.

One clear conclusion that we were able to draw was that sex differences are more frequently noted in some nociceptive assays than in others. For example, sensitivity to electric shock is consistently higher in female rats than in males, as evidenced by shorter latencies and lower thresholds to flinching or jumping in response to shock, independent of sex differences in body size (Pare 1969; Beatty and Beatty 1970; Marks and Hobbs 1972; Beatty and Fessler 1976, 1977; Romero and Bodnar 1986; Romero et al. 1987, 1988a,b; Arjune 1989; Kepler et al. 1991; Kiefel and Bodnar 1991). Females also display more pain behavior than males in the formalin test, especially at high concentrations of formalin (Aloisi et al. 1994, 1995). Thus, if behavioral responses to noxious electrical and chemical stimuli are taken as the dependent measures, the overwhelming conclusion would be that females are indeed more sensitive to noxious stimuli than males, supporting the conventional wisdom on this topic. However, the exact opposite conclusion may be drawn from studies using reflexive withdrawal responses to noxious heat as the dependent variable. In the tail-flick test and tail-immersion test, when sex differences are observed, the more frequent observation is that male rats display faster responses than females, indicating greater pain sensitivity in males (Romero et al. 1987, 1988a,b; Arjune 1989; Forman et al. 1989; Islam et al. 1993; Molina 1994; Bartok and Craft 1997; Craft and Mulholland 1998; Craft et al. 1999).

Just as commonly reported as findings of sex differences (in either direction) in the response to noxious thermal stimuli are studies that detect no apparent sex differences (Kepler et al. 1989, 1991; Kavaliers and Colwell 1991; Kiefel and Bodnar 1991; Aloisi et al. 1994; Cicero et al. 1996). Failure to demonstrate an effect is difficult to interpret in the scientific literature, because it is not always clear whether between-group differences do not exist or are simply undetected due to insufficient experimental power; this could result from small sample size or failure to control for extraneous sources of variability. For example, on the hot-plate test, only a few studies report sex differences (mostly in the direction of shorter latencies in females than in males; Kavaliers and Innes 1987a, 1990), whereas most studies report no differences in latency (Kavaliers and Innes 1987b, 1988; Lipa and Kavaliers 1990; Kavaliers and Galea 1995; Kavaliers et al. 1998a). All of these studies reporting differences in hot-plate responding were conducted on mice (inbred strains of *Mus musculus* or *Peromyscus maniculatus*). Experiments conducted on rats have shown no sex differences in hot-plate latency, although the studies are often characterized by relatively small samples.

Aside from the obvious methodological variability associated with using distinctly different pain assays, we were unable to account for the presence or absence of sex differences simply by considering differences in methodology between laboratories. For example, the presence or absence of sex differences apparently does not depend on phase of the light cycle during which animals are tested—sex differences are inconsistently reported, despite the fact that most investigators test subjects during the light phase. Likewise, subtle variations in the parameters of the assays (such as exact temperature settings of the hot-plate device) cannot account for discrepancies in the literature, as inconsistencies are prevalent even in studies conducted in the same laboratory.

Our motivation for undertaking the extensive review was the observation, in a survey of sex differences in nociception in various inbred mouse populations, of male-female differences in some strains, but not in others (Kest et al. 1999). Furthermore, molecular genetic analyses suggest that some variability in pain responses can be accounted for genetically (see Chapter 3 for a review of genetic factors underlying sex differences in nociception). Although we did not find the existing literature to be confounded by strain differences (due to almost exclusive reliance on a few outbred strains of rodents), our review included an experimental component in which we conducted a sex comparison among commonly used outbred strains of rats and mice in the tail-withdrawal assay. The existence and direction of sex differences were directly related to strain. Among Sprague Dawley rats, consistent with the existing literature, males were more sensitive than females; however, among Long Evans rats, females were more sensitive than males. No differences were observed in tail-withdrawal latencies among Wistar rats (Mogil et al., in press). Although these conclusions are limited by their reliance on one nociceptive assay, they highlight the importance of considering both sex and strain in future studies on sex differences in nociceptive processing.

SEX DIFFERENCES IN ANALGESIA

Pain behavior does not simply reflect activity in peripheral nociceptive pathways, but also is heavily influenced by descending modulation from the brain. Descending influences from the brain modulate activity in the pain pathways arising in the periphery so as to diminish or enhance pain perception, depending on situational factors. Thus, at any given time, the experience of pain is subserved by activity in both ascending and descending pathways. The activity of descending pain-modulatory pathways may be assessed by stimulating them electrically, pharmacologically, or by environmental stress (which is believed to be the natural trigger for endogenous pain inhibition). Although no cross-sex comparisons have been published for electrical stimulation-produced analgesia, a substantial literature indicates sex differences in the response to analgesic drugs and the analgesic response to stress.

Experimental observations of sex differences in opioid analgesia are far more consistent than those of basal pain sensitivity. When differences are observed, the overwhelming majority of studies report that effects of analgesic pharmaceuticals are greater in males than in females. These sex differences are most consistently observed for morphine analgesia (an endogenous opioid agonist; Cicero et al. 1996, 1997), although other drugs that influence different neurotransmitter systems (e.g., pilocarpine, a muscarinic cholinergic agonist; clonidine, an α_2-adrenergic agonist; and SCH 34826, an enkephalinase inhibitor) also produce similar sex differences (Kiefel and Bodnar 1991; Kavaliers and Innes 1993). Interestingly, one of the few studies reporting greater analgesia in females than in males was an experiment assessing κ-opioid analgesic effects (Bartok and Craft 1997), which were also shown to be greater in women than men in a clinical setting (Gear et al. 1996).

Descending pain-modulatory pathways also can be activated by environmental stressors, and several studies have addressed sex differences in the degree of activation of endogenous pain-modulatory systems by assessing stress-induced analgesia (SIA) as a dependent variable. Given the reliable sex differences in opioid analgesic responsiveness noted in pharmacological studies, it would be reasonable to expect that males would exhibit greater levels of opioid (i.e., naloxone-reversible) SIA, since both pharmacological and environmental stress methods of analgesia induction are believed to activate the same underlying neuroanatomical substrate. Indeed, male rodents exhibit greater levels of analgesia than females following various stressful manipulations, such as immobilization, swim stress, and exposure to novel situations as assessed in deer mice (Kavaliers and Innes 1987b, 1988; Kavaliers and Galea 1995), opioid analgesia in deer mice resulting from exposure to a predator (although non-opioid, predator-induced analgesia is greater in females than males; Kavaliers and Colwell 1991), and cold-water swim stress in Sprague Dawley rats (Romero and Bodnar 1986).

Thus, the literature clearly suggests that male rodents (rats and deer mice) exhibit greater analgesia than females following morphine administration and opioid-mediated SIA. The finding that males experience greater analgesia than females from opioid agonists (independent of pharmacokinetic factors) implies that the endogenous pain-modulatory pathways are more sensitive or active in males.

HORMONAL FACTORS IN PAIN AND PAIN INHIBITION

Despite the conflicting evidence, it is clear that at least in some strains, and in some pain modalities, differences do exist between males and females in sensitivity to noxious stimuli. More convincingly, sex differences are clearly apparent in the degree of analgesia exhibited following administration of analgesic drugs or exposure to environmental stress. Since a major source of gender-related variability is that associated with gonadal hormonal influences (both developmentally and in adulthood), it is useful to consider the effects of sex hormones as a determinant of these differences. Binding sites for gonadal steroid hormones are ubiquitously distributed throughout central nervous system regions involved in pain perception and pain inhibition, such as the periaqueductal gray, rostroventral medulla, and spinal cord dorsal horn (Papka et al. 1996, Scott et al. 1998, VanderHorst et al. 1998). Thus, it is not unreasonable to suspect that sex hormones lie at the root of sex differences in pain.

One obvious hormone-related sex difference is the fluctuation associated with the ovulatory cycle in females. The estrous cycle in rats, the animal used by the overwhelming majority of researchers in this field, consists of four stages: proestrus, estrus, metestrus, and diestrus (Martínez-Gómez et al. 1994). Estrogen and progesterone fluctuate through the estrous cycle, and both reach peak levels 24 hours prior to estrus and are comparatively low for 1 or 2 days in diestrous rats. Estrus is the period of peak sexual receptivity, whereas rats in diestrus are generally nonreceptive (Ryan and Maier 1988). The size of peripheral receptive fields varies within females across the estrous cycle (e.g., Bereiter and Barker 1980), which suggests that nociceptive thresholds would also be affected. However, a review of the literature on the estrous cycle and pain reveals inconsistent findings, despite similar methodologies (nearly all studies employ phasic noxious stimuli such as tail-flick and electric shock). Other possible sources of variability include strain of rodent used and subtle differences in separation of experimental groups by estrous phase, as described below.

Some studies do not report differences in pain sensitivity on the tail-flick test across the estrous cycle. For example, no differences in basal nociceptive thresholds were noted between estrous and diestrous female albino rats (derived from the Holtzman Sprague Dawley strain) on the tail-flick test (Ryan and Maier 1988), although this study did not report pain thresholds during proestrus and metestrus. However, Martínez-Gómez et al. (1994), found significantly shorter tail-flick latencies (lower pain threshold) in Wistar rats during the estrous and metestrous phases compared to the proestrous and diestrous periods, indicating that data collection during all four phases is essential in such studies. Kepler et al. (1989) measured pain thresholds on the tail-flick test during the proestrous, estrous, and combined metestrous/diestrous phases in female Sprague Dawley rats. They found that females in proestrus had shorter latencies (lower pain thresholds) than did females in the estrous or the combined metestrous/diestrous phase. The merging of the metestrous and diestrous phases into one phase may be problematic if in fact, as Martínez-Gómez et al. showed, pain thresholds differ significantly between these phases. Adding to the inconsistency is a study by Frye et al. (1992) in which tail-flick latencies were measured in Long Evans rats at each of the four estrous stages. Females in diestrus had significantly longer tail-flick latencies (higher pain thresholds) than those in proestrus. No other phases were significantly different. Strain differences may account for the disparate findings, as outbred rats of various genetic origins were used in these experiments, although this explanation is unlikely because differences exist even in studies using the same strain of rats.

Ovarian hormones are at their peak during proestrus, and it would seem advantageous for animals to have a mechanism that would diminish pain sensitivity when copulation (a potentially painful event) is most likely. However, the results of the tail-flick studies described above are far too inconsistent to confirm such a mechanism; sensitivity to noxious electric shock was lower during proestrus compared to metestrus (during the trough in ovarian hormone levels) in some studies (e.g., Leer et al. 1988), but others have reported no estrous phase differences in jump thresholds (e.g., Kepler et al. 1989).

This lack of consensus regarding estrous cycle effects leads to the conclusion that the differences in hormone levels exhibited by female rodents during the 4–5-day cycle are not responsible for overall sex differences. If it were the case that the inconsistent findings in sex difference studies are due to a failure to control for estrous cycle phase (with some investigators testing females during the troughs in ovarian hormones, and others during the peaks), then we would expect to observe consistent differences in basal pain threshold within females across the cycle. Clearly, this is not the case. Overall, estrous cyclicity can explain little of the variability in sex differences in basal pain threshold. For example, Kepler et al. (1989) found that while tail-flick and jump thresholds varied across the estrous cycle in females, males and females did not differ overall in pain thresholds.

Estrous cycle comparisons have also been conducted to investigate the possibility that hormonal fluctuations are responsible for sex differences in analgesia. Here, the studies are more conclusive, with more reliable estrous cycle effects observed for opioid than non-opioid analgesia. However, as with the basal pain threshold literature, inconsistent findings are characteristic. In these studies, opioid analgesia refers to the pain-inhibitory effects of opioid pharmaceuticals (such as morphine or other opioid-receptor agonists) or SIA that can be blocked or attenuated by the opioid antagonist naloxone. Non-opioid analgesia, conversely, is defined as analgesia (pharmacological or stress-induced) that is naloxone-insensitive.

Studies of non-opioid analgesia have consistently shown no significant differences across the estrous cycle. For example, Romero and Bodnar (1986) found that different phases of the estrous cycle did not affect the magnitude of continuous cold-water swim analgesia on tail-flick and jump tests, a form of non-opioid SIA in Sprague Dawley rats. Likewise, Ryan and Maier (1988) failed to show any effect of estrous cycle stage (comparison of estrous and diestrous females) on non-opioid analgesia induced by tail-shock stress. However, in this same study, naloxone-sensitive (i.e., opioid) tail-shock SIA was of far greater magnitude in diestrous females compared to those in estrus.

Studies of estrous cycle effects on opioid pharmacological analgesia reveal divergent findings. Frye et al. (1992) showed no estrous cycle effects on analgesia from morphine (7.5 mg/kg) in Long Evans rats using the tail-flick method. Conversely, other studies have detected variations in morphine analgesia across the estrous cycle. Direct intracerebroventricular administration of morphine to female rats in proestrus or estrus resulted in significantly higher levels of analgesia than those exhibited by rats in a combined metestrous/diestrous phase (Kepler et al. 1989). In a more powerful within-subjects design, Banerjee et al. (1983) found that sensitivity to morphine varied at different stages of the estrous cycle. There was no statistically significant difference in sensitivity to morphine between day 1 (ovulation) and day 2 of the estrous cycle. On the afternoon of day 3 (presumably, diestrus) morphine sensitivity increased significantly compared to days 1 and 2. Maximum sensitivity was reached at 14:00 hours of day 4, and at 19:00 of day 4, the sensitivity to morphine notably decreased.

Therefore, although analgesia levels vary somewhat across the estrous cycle in females, these fluctuations are unlikely to explain cross-sex variability in analgesic responses to morphine and environmental stress. Far more impressive are the effects of gonadectomy and hormone replacement on the presence or absence of sex differences (particularly in studies of analgesic magnitude or quality), suggesting that the effects of gonadal hormones are not subtle ones. Rather, gross alterations in sex hormones can influence the activity of the ascending and descending pain pathways.

NEONATAL AND ADULT HORMONE MANIPULATIONS INFLUENCE BASAL PAIN THRESHOLDS AND ANALGESIA

In most sexually dimorphic systems studied, the organizing effects of hormonal exposure in early life can render the system sensitive to the activating effects of gonadal steroid hormones. The ascending and descending components of the pain perception pathway can be influenced by early life hormone manipulations (such as neonatal gonadectomy or hormone exposure, or indirect hormone manipulations resulting from prenatal stress) and by adult gonadectomy. The results of such manipulations suggest that the organizational and activational effects of sex hormones play a role in sex differences in pain behavior and analgesia.

One commonly used procedure for affecting changes in the hormonal milieu in utero is creating prenatal stress. Exposing pregnant rats to stress disrupts the testosterone surge of late pregnancy (Ward 1972) and has demasculinizing effects on male offspring. Abnormal copulatory behavior, increased maternal behavior, and decreased aggression have all been observed in prenatally stressed male rodents (Ward and Ward 1972; Kinsley and Svare 1986, 1988). Other investigators have reported masculinizing effects of prenatal stress on female fetuses (Herrenkohl and Scott 1984; Sachser and Kaiser 1996). Our laboratory has demonstrated a decrease in hot-plate latencies (suggesting an increase in pain sensitivity) induced by prenatal stress in mice of both sexes, particularly in young adult subjects (Sternberg 1999). Other studies have demonstrated no effect of prenatal stress on basal pain sensitivity on the tail-flick test in rats (Szuran et al. 1991), which suggests that if prenatal stress does affect pain sensitivity, then it does so at supraspinal loci. More studies are needed to confirm this hypothesis.

The effects of prenatal stress on the descending components of the pain pathway have been studied in both stress-induced and morphine-induced analgesia paradigms. Szuran and colleagues (1991) demonstrated a significant reduction in cold-water swim SIA in prenatally stressed rats of both sexes compared to nonstressed controls. Other investigators have shown that exposure to prenatal stress reduces cold-water swim SIA in females but not males (Kinsley et al. 1988). Morphine analgesic responses are also sensitive to prenatal stress in a sex-dependent manner; prenatal stress increases morphine (5 mg/kg) analgesia in females, but decreases analgesic magnitude in males (Kinsley et al. 1988). These effects of prenatal stress on opioid analgesia are attributed to disruptions in the fetal development of endogenous opioid systems, alterations that persist into adulthood. The same pattern of an increased analgesic effect limited to prenatally stressed females was also noted in a study of naloxone-insensitive SIA conducted in our laboratory (Sternberg 1999).

Adult gonadectomy manipulations may also influence some aspects of pain and analgesia expression and might reveal the activational effects of sex hormones on these behaviors. However, the effects of gonadectomy have not been reliably observed in tests of basal pain threshold. In studies that show no sex differences in pain threshold, a consistent observation is that gonadectomy has no effect (Romero et al. 1988a; Kepler et al. 1991; Kiefel and Bodnar 1991; Candido et al. 1992; Mogil et al. 1993). Females typically display lower nociceptive thresholds to noxious electrical stimuli, and this sex difference persists in gonadectomized subjects (Beatty and Beatty 1970; Marks and Hobbs 1972; Beatty and Fessler 1977). Ovariectomy has similarly small effects on morphine analgesia magnitude, even in studies that show an overall sex difference, with males showing greater analgesia (Krzanowska 1999). Both opioid and non-opioid SIA magnitudes (which are larger in males than females) are reduced by gonadectomy in both sexes and are restored by testosterone (Romero et al. 1988a). Given that adult gonadectomy effects are noted in SIA but not typically in morphine analgesia paradigms, it is possible that the activating effects of sex hormones are related to the overall stress response regardless of the pain/analgesia pathway.

QUALITATIVE SEX DIFFERENCES IN STRESS-INDUCED ANALGESIA

Thus far, this chapter has been primarily concerned with sex differences and hormonal effects on quantitative aspects of pain—the magnitude of pain behavior displayed, or the degree of reduction of pain behavior from analgesic manipulation. Of potentially greater clinical importance are sex differences in qualitative aspects of pain processing. Promising new analgesic manipulations may capitalize on the knowledge gained from the study of endogenous analgesia pathways in animal subjects. However, if important differences exist in the mechanisms of pain inhibition (above and beyond any magnitudinal differences that are seen in the degree of activation of these pathways), then treatments that are developed may not be equally effective in both sexes. Already, human research has indicated a different degree of analgesia achieved by equivalent doses of analgesic drugs between the sexes in a clinical setting (Gear et al. 1996). This discrepancy may reflect an underlying difference in the predominant pathways mediating pain inhibition (Mogil and Kest 1994).

Over the past decade, a trend in identifying qualitative differences in pain-inhibitory mechanisms has emerged in animal studies. Bodnar's group demonstrated in the late 1980s that cold-water swim, which produced opioid-mediated, naloxone-reversible SIA in male rats, produced an analgesia that was insensitive to naloxone antagonism in females (Romero et al. 1988). Wong (1987) observed the opposite phenomenon—an opioid analgesia in female mice, but non-opioid analgesia in males. In 1993, while working in the laboratory of the late John Liebeskind at the University of California at Los Angeles, Mogil, Sternberg, and others noted similar qualitative sex differences in the neurochemical mediation of SIA. Focusing on a form of naloxone-insensitive (non-opioid) SIA induced in mice by forcing them to swim in cold water, we implicated excitatory amino acids binding at the *N*-methyl-D-aspartate (NMDA) receptor as putative neurochemical mediators of SIA. The noncompetitive NMDA antagonist MK-801 (MK) selectively blocks non-opioid components of SIA, leaving opioid SIA and morphine analgesia unaffected (Marek et al. 1992). However, this characterization is only true for male mice. As described below, this basic sex difference in

NMDA mediation of analgesia has been confirmed by research conducted by Kavaliers and colleagues using different SIA paradigms.

Female mice display equivalent amounts of naloxone-insensitive SIA (induced by swimming or by exposure to biting flies) when compared to males, but the analgesia exhibited by females is also insensitive to the NMDA antagonist, suggesting an alternative neurochemical mechanism (Mogil et al. 1993; Kavaliers and Galea 1995; Kavaliers et al. 1998b). Females are not deficient in NMDA-mediated analgesia circuitry, however. When hormonal influences are removed through gonadectomy (or during times of low reproductive capacity in mice that are seasonal breeders), females *do* show MK-reversible analgesia (Mogil et al. 1993; Kavaliers and Galea, 1995). Estrogen replacement over a period of 7 days reinstates the female pattern of MK insensitivity of SIA, indicating hormonal dependence of the sex difference and suggesting that under normal hormonal conditions, females have a neurochemically distinct mechanism for inhibiting pain during times of stress. In male mice, gonadectomy (which reduces the level of analgesia overall) and subsequent estrogen replacement do not change the antagonistic property of MK-801 on swim SIA. Thus, the hormonally dependent analgesia mechanism appears to be female-specific in an organizational sense—that is, it cannot be induced in males by adult gonadectomy manipulations.

The presence of a "female-specific" SIA mechanism is believed to depend on the neonatal hormonal milieu. When exposed to testosterone on the day of their birth, females exhibit MK-reversible analgesia in adulthood (Sternberg et al. 1995). Furthermore, no sex difference in MK reversibility is apparent in 30-day-old prepubescent mice; MK blocks analgesia in mice of both sexes at that stage of development (Sternberg 1994).

Investigations of the sex difference in neurochemical mediation of non-opioid analgesia have been based on a psychopharmacological approach to studying the neurochemical basis of behavior. Since MK (an NMDA antagonist) blocks analgesia in males, but not in females, researchers have concluded that analgesia is mediated by NMDA in males, but must rely on alternative neurochemical mechanisms in females. The gonadectomy and hormone-replacement studies suggest that the alternative mechanism in females is dependent on hormonal status. When hormonally intact, females display non-opioid, non-NMDA-mediated analgesia; when gonadectomized, they express the NMDA-mediated mechanism. Our original formulation of these systems proposes that in females, the hormonally dependent system and the NMDA-mediated analgesia mechanism are mutually inhibitory, or else intact females would display *greater* levels of analgesia than males. Since females and males display essentially equivalent levels of analgesia, the difference appears to be solely one of quality, not of quantity.

A recent parametric study of SIA in females in our laboratory (W.F. Sternberg et al., unpublished manuscript) confirms the inability of MK to block analgesia at several doses of the drug, following swim stressors of various durations and temperatures, and tested at several time intervals following stress. Our group previously conducted a similar parametric study in male mice (Mogil et al. 1996) in which we demonstrated that as swim temperature decreased or swim duration increased, the resultant analgesia became naloxone-insensitive. We thus provided support for the stressor-severity hypothesis in which more severe parameters of a stressor produce non-opioid (i.e., naloxone-insensitive) analgesia. As displayed in Fig. 1, female mice consistently displayed naloxone-insensitive, MK-insensitive analgesia, even following swim stressors that produced opioid analgesia in male subjects (Mogil et al. 1996). The results of these parametric investigations suggest that the default analgesia mechanism in females is a non-opioid one (defined by naloxone insensitivity), and its inability to be antagonized by MK lends support to the notion that females exhibit a qualitatively (i.e., neurochemically) distinct analgesia mechanism following swim stress. In addition, it seems that our inability to block analgesia in

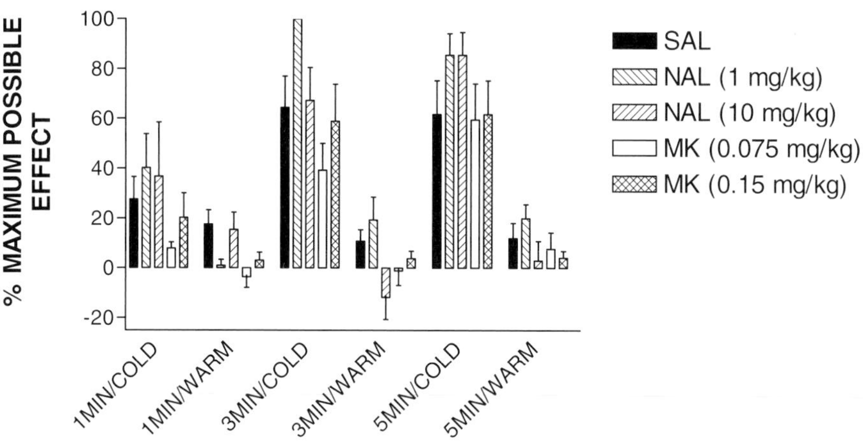

Fig. 1. Neither naloxone (NAL; 1 and 10 mg/kg) nor MK-801 (MK; 0.15 and 0.075 mg/kg) antagonized analgesia in female mice (only 2-minute post-swim data are presented) following swims of any duration and at either temperature. None of the drug-treated subjects were significantly different from saline-treated subjects (with the exception of a potentiation of analgesia in subjects given either dose of NAL in the cold-water swim condition). SAL = saline; n = 4–13 subjects per group. Data are from W.F. Sternberg (unpublished manuscript).

females with MK-801 is a more general phenomenon, and is not limited to the experimental situation in which we first observed it. That is, at differing doses and swim stressor parameters, sex differences in MK sensitivity of SIA are still observed.

That males and females may have evolved different mechanisms for the inhibition of pain is not surprising, given the different pain-related pressures facing males and females throughout evolution. The quality and magnitude of painful events clearly differs for males and females, and the frequency of painful events is certainly associated with hormonal events in females. Studies currently underway in our laboratory are aimed at understanding the hormonal regulation of female-specific analgesia mechanisms and elucidating the neurotransmitters that are responsible for producing analgesia following swim stress in female rodents.

CONCLUSIONS

The laboratory animal has served as a useful model for the study of mechanisms of pain sensation and pain inhibition and for research into the potential efficacy of analgesic manipulation. As is typical of biomedical research, the usual subject is the adult male. Although sex differences in the magnitude of pain behavior are modest and inconsistently observed, the important qualitative differences that are observed in mechanisms of pain inhibition must be considered when planning future studies in the laboratory or clinic. Research into sex differences such as those described in this chapter highlight why the single-sex approach is inappropriate and may contribute misleading information regarding the best way to manage pain.

REFERENCES

Aloisi AM, Albonetti ME, Carli G. Sex differences in the behavioural response to persistent pain in rats. *Neurosci Lett* 1994; 179:79–82.

Aloisi AMS, Albonetti P, Emanuela M, Giancarlo C. Sex-related effects on behavior and Beta-endorphin of different intensities of formalin pain in rats. *Brain Res* 1995; 699:242–249.

Arjune DB, Richard J. Post-natal morphine differentially affects opiate and stress analgesia in adult rats. *Psychopharmacology* 1989; 98:512–517.

Banerjee P, Chatterjee TK, Ghosh JJ. Ovarian steroids and modulation of morphine-induced analgesia and catalepsy in female rats. *Eur J Pharmacol* 1983; 96:291–294.

Bartok RE, Craft RM. Sex differences in opioid antinociception. *J Pharmacol Exp Ther* 1997; 282:769–778.

Beatty WW, Beatty PA. Hormonal determinants of sex differences in avoidance behavior and reactivity to electric shock in the rat. *J Comp Physiol Psychol* 1970; 16:413–417.

Beatty WW, Fessler RG. Ontogeny of sex differences in open field behavior and sensitivity to electric shock in the rat. *Physiol Behav* 1976; 16:413–417.

Beatty WW, Fessler RG. Gonadectomy and sensitivity to electric shock in the rat. *Physiol Behav* 1977; 19:1–6.
Bereiter DA, Barker DJ. Hormone induced enlargements of receptive fields in trigeminal mechanoreceptive neurons: 1. Time course, hormone, sex, and modality specialty. *Brain Res* 1980; 184:395–410.
Berkley K. Sex differences in pain. *Behav Brain Sci* 1997; 20:371–380.
Candido J, Lufty K, Billings B, et al. Effect of adrenal and sex hormones on opioid analgesia and opioid receptor regulation. *Pharmacol Biochem Behav* 1992; 42:685–692.
Cicero TJ, Nock B, Meyer ER. Gender-related differences in the antinociceptive properties of morphine. *J Pharmacol Exp Ther* 1996; 279:767–773.
Cicero TJ, Nock B, Meyer ER. Sex-related differences in morphine's antinociceptive activity: relationship to serum and brain morphine concentrations. *J Pharmacol Exp Ther* 1997; 282:939–944.
Craft RM, Mulholland RB. Sex differences in cocaine- and nicotine-induced antinociception in the rat. *Brain Res* 1998; 809:137–140.
Craft RM, Stratmann JA, Bartok RE, Walpole TI, King SJ. Sex differences in development of morphine tolerance and dependence in the rat. *Psychopharmacology (Berl)* 1999; 143(1):1–7
Forman LJ, Tingle V, Estilow S, Cater J. The response to analgesia testing is affected by gonadal steroids in the rat. *Life Sci* 1989; 45:447–454.
Frye CA, Bock BC, Kanarek RB. Hormonal milieu affects tailflick latency in female rats. *Physiol Behav* 1992; 52:699–706.
Gear RW, Gordon NC, Heller PH, et al. Gender difference in analgesic response to the kappa-opioid pentazocine. *Neurosci Lett* 1996; 205:207–209.
Herrenkohl LR, Scott S. Prenatal stress and postnatal androgen: effects on reproduction in female rats. *Experientia* 1984; 40:101–103.
Islam AK, Cooper ML, Bodnar RJ. Interactions among aging, gender and gonadectomy effects upon morphine antinociception in rats. *Physiol Behav* 1993; 54:45–53.
Kavaliers M, Colwell DD. Sex differences in opioid and non-opioid mediated predator-induced analgesia in mice. *Brain Res* 1991; 568:173–177.
Kavaliers M, Galea LAM. Sex differences in the expression and antagonism of swim stress-induced analgesia in deer mice vary with the breeding season. *Pain* 1995; 63:327–334.
Kavaliers M, Innes DGL. Sex and day-night differences in opiate induced responses of insular wild deer mice. *Pharmacol Biochem Behav* 1987a; 27:477–482.
Kavaliers M, Innes D. Stress-induced opioid analgesia and activity in deer mice: sex and population differences. *Brain Res* 1987b; 425:49–56.
Kavaliers M, Innes DGL. Novelty-induced opioid analgesia in deer mice (*Peromyscus maniculatus*): sex and population differences. *Behav Neural Biol* 1988; 49:54–60.
Kavaliers M, Innes DGL. Developmental changes in opiate-induced analgesia in deer mice: sex and population differences. *Brain Res* 1990; 516:326–331.
Kavaliers M, Innes DGL. Sex differences in the antinociceptive effects of the enkephalinase inhibitor, SCH 34826. *Pharmacol Biochem Behav* 1993; 46:777–780.
Kavaliers M, Colwell DD, Choleris E. Sex differences in opioid and N-methyl-D-aspartate mediated non-opioid biting fly exposure induced analgesia in deer mice. *Pain* 1998b; 77:163–171.
Kepler KL, Kest B, Kiefel JM, Cooper ML, Bodnar RJ. Roles of gender, gonadectomy and estrous phase in the analgesic effects of intracerebroventricular morphine in rats. *Pharmacol Biochem Behav* 1989; 34:119–127.
Kepler KL, Standifer KM, Paul D, et al. Gender effects and central opioid analgesia. *Pain* 1991; 45:87–94.
Kest B, Wilson SG, Mogil JS. Sex differences in supraspinal morphine analgesia are dependent on genotype. *J Pharmacol Exp Ther* 1999; 289(3):1370–1375.
Kiefel JM, Bodnar RJ. Roles of gender and gonadectomy in pilocarpine and clonidine analgesia in rats. *Pharmacol Biochem Behav* 1991; 41:153–158.

Kinsley CH, Svare BB. Prenatal stress reduces inter-male aggression in mice. *Physiol Behav* 1986; 36:783–786.

Kinsley C, Svare B. Prenatal stress alters maternal aggression in mice. *Physiol Behav* 1988; 42:7–13.

Kinsley CH, Mann PE, Bridges RS. Prenatal stress alters morphine-and stress-induced analgesia in male and female rats. *Pharmacol Biochem Behav* 1988; 30:123–128.

Krzanowska EK, Bodnar RJ. Morphine antinociception elicited from the ventrolateral periaqueductal gray is sensitive to sex and gonadectomy differences in rats. *Brain Res* 1999; 821(1):224–230.

Leer MN, Bradbury A, Maloney JC, Stewart CN. Elevated shock threshold in sexually receptive female rats. *Physiol Behav* 1988; 42:617–620.

Lipa SM, Kavaliers M. Sex differences in the inhibitory effects of the NMDA antagonist MK-801 on morphine and stress-induced analgesia. *Brain Res Bull* 1990; 24:627–630.

Marek P, Mogil JS, Sternberg WF, Panocka I, Liebeskind JC. N-methyl-D-aspartic acid (NMDA) receptor antagonist MK 801 blocks non-opioid stress-induced analgesia. II. Comparison across three swim-stress paradigms in selectively bred mice. *Brain Res* 1992; 578:197–203.

Marks HE, Hobbs SH. Changes in stimulus reactivity following gonadectomy in male and female rats of different ages. *Physiol Behav* 1972; 8:1113–1119.

Martinez-Gomez M, Cruz Y, Salas M, Hudson R, Pacheco P. Assessing pain threshold in the rat: changes with estrus and time of day. *Physiol Behav* 1994; 55:651–657.

Mogil JS, Kest B. Sex differences in opioid analgesia: of mice and women. *Pain Forum* 1994; 8:48–50.

Mogil JS, Sternberg WF, Kest B, Marek P, Liebeskind JC. Sex differences in the antagonism of swim stress-induced analgesia: effects of gonadectomy and estrogen replacement. *Pain* 1993; 53:17–25.

Mogil JS, Sternberg WF, Balian H, et al. Opioid and nonopioid swim stress-induced analgesia: a parametric analysis in mice. *Physiol Behav* 1996; 59:123–132.

Mogil JS, Chesler EJ, Wilson SG, Juraska JM, Sternberg WF. Sex differences in thermal nociception and morphine antinociception in rodents depend on genotype. *Neurosci Biobehav Rev* 2000; 24:375–389.

Molina N. Sex-related differences in the analgesic response to the rat tail immersion test. *Braz J Med Biol Res* 1994; 27:1669–1672.

Morgan MM, Sohn JH, Liebeskind JC. Stimulation of the periaqueductal gray matter inhibits nociception at the supraspinal as well as spinal level. *Brain Res* 1989; 502:61–66.

Papka RE, Williams S, Miller KE, Copelin T, Puri P. CNS location of uterine-related neurons revealed by trans-synaptic tracing with pseudorabies virus and their relation to estrogen receptor-immunoreactive neurons. *Neuroscience* 1998; 84:935–952.

Pare WP. Age, sex, and strain differences in the aversive threshold to grid shock in the rat. *J Comp Physiol Psychol* 1969; (2):214–218

Riley JL, Robinson ME, Wise EA, Myers CD, Fillingim RB. Sex differences in the perception of noxious experimental stimuli: a meta-analysis. *Pain* 1998; 74:181–187.

Romero MT, Bodnar RJ. Gender differences in two forms of cold water swim analgesia. *Physiol Behav* 1986; 37:893–897.

Romero MT, Kepler KL, Cooper ML, Komisaruk BR, Bodnar RJ. Modulation of gender specific effects upon swim analgesia in gonadectomized rats. *Physiol Behav* 1987; 40:39–45.

Romero MT, Cooper ML, Komisaruk BR, Bodnar RJ. Gender-specific and gonadectomy-specific effects upon swim analgesia: role of steroid replacement therapy. *Physiol Behav* 1988a; 44:257–265.

Romero MT, Kepler KL, Bodnar RJ. Gender determinants of opioid mediation of swim analgesia in rats. *Pharmacol Biochem Behav* 1988b; 29:705–709.

Ryan SM, Maier SF. The estrous cycle and estrogen modulate stress-induced analgesia. *Behav Neurosci* 1988; 102:371–380.

Sachser N, Kaiser S. Prenatal social stress masculinizes the females' behavior in guinea pigs. *Physiol Behav* 1996; 60:589–594.

Scott CJ, Rawson JA, Pereira AM, Clarke IJ. The distribution of estrogen receptors in the brainstem of female sheep. *Neurosci Lett* 1998; 241:29–32.

Sternberg WF. Sex differences in pain perception and pain inhibition. PhD Dissertation. Los Angeles: University of California, 1994.

Sternberg WF. Sex differences in the effects of prenatal stress on stress-induced analgesia. *Physiol Behav* 1999; 68:63–72.

Sternberg WF, Mogil JS, Kest B, et al. Neonatal testosterone exposure influences neurochemistry of non-opioid swim stress induced analgesia in adult mice. *Pain* 1995; 63:321–326.

Szuran TZE, Pliska V, Pfister HP, Welzl H. Prenatal stress effects on exploratory activity and stress-induced analgesia in rats. *Dev Psychobiol* 1991; 24:361–372.

Unruh AM. Gender Variations in clinical pain experience. *Pain* 1996; 65:123–167.

VanderHorst VG, Schasfoort FC, Meijer E; Le euwen FW, Holstege G. Estrogen receptor-alpha-immunoreactive neurons in the periaqueductal gray of the adult ovariectomized female cat. *Neurosci Lett* 1998; 240:13–16.

Ward IL. Prenatal stress feminizes and demasculinizes the behavior of males. *Science* 1972; 172:82–84.

Ward IL, Ward OB. Reproductive behavior and physiology in prenatally stressed males. In: Weiner H, Florin I, Murison R (Eds). *Frontiers of Stress Research: Neural Control of Bodily Function: Basic and Clinical Aspects.* Stuttgart: Hans Huber, 1972, pp 9–20.

Wong CL. Sex difference in naloxone antagonism of swim stress-induced antinociception in mice. *Methods Find Exp Clin Pharmacol* 1987; 9:275–278.

Correspondence to: Wendy F. Sternberg, PhD, Department of Psychology, Haverford College, 370 Lancaster Avenue, Haverford, PA 19041, USA. Tel: 610-896-1237; Fax: 610-896-4963; email: wsternbe@haverford.edu.

Sex, Gender, and Pain, Progress in Pain Research and Management, Vol. 17, edited by R.B. Fillingim, IASP Press, Seattle, © 2000.

6

Ovarian Sex Steroids Activate Antinociceptive Systems and Reveal Gender-Specific Mechanisms

Alan R. Gintzler and Nai-Jiang Liu

Department of Biochemistry, State University of New York, Downstate Medical Center, Brooklyn, New York, USA

In all cultures and societies, pain is a primary component of late pregnancy and labor. If not modulated, such pain would impose an additional increment of stress on an already highly stressful and energy-consuming physiological process. Consequently, modulation of pregnancy- and labor-related pain produces physiological effects that are salutary for mother and infant. Not surprisingly, endogenous pain-attenuating pathways have evolved by which the pain and discomfort of pregnancy and labor can be significantly mitigated, although not abolished. The neural substrates and mechanisms that mediate gestational antinociception provide a unique window into gender-specific determinants of antinociception.

Pregnancy-related antinociception was first demonstrated in rats in which nociceptive response thresholds to an electric foot shock progressively increased as gestation progressed, peaking just prior to parturition (Gintzler 1980) (Fig. 1A). Subsequently, pregnancy-induced analgesia was observed in rats and sows in response to somatic stimuli (Gintzler 1980; Toniolo et al. 1987; Kristal et al. 1990; Jarvis et al. 1997) and to visceral noxious stimuli (Iwasaki et al. 1991). Pregnant women also manifest gestational antinociception (Cogan and Spinnato 1986; Whipple et al. 1990). During the last 10 days of pregnancy, quantification of verbally reported discomfort thresholds revealed significantly greater tolerance of the progressive inflation of a blood pressure cuff than was observed in control, nonpregnant women (Cogan and Spinnato 1986).

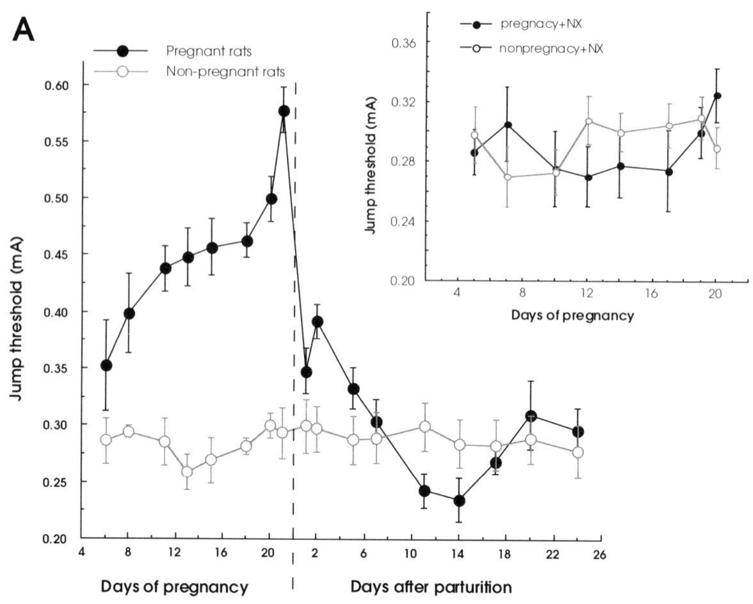
A
Pregnant rats
Non-pregnant rats
Jump threshold (mA)
Days of pregnancy
Days after parturition
pregnacy+NX
nonpregnacy+NX
Jump threshold (mA)
Days of pregnancy

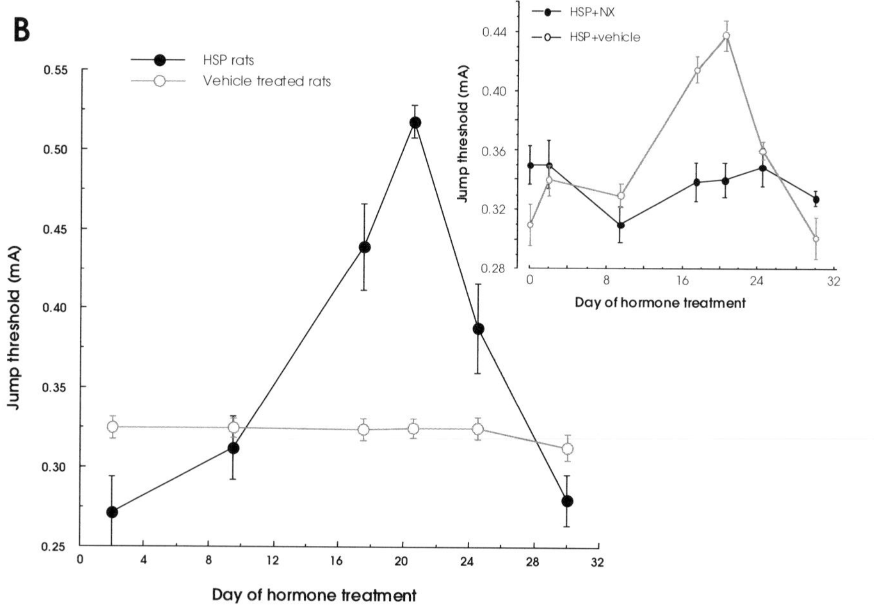
B
HSP rats
Vehicle treated rats
Jump threshold (mA)
Day of hormone treatment
HSP+NX
HSP+vehicle
Jump threshold (mA)
Day of hormone treatment

SPINAL VERSUS SUPRASPINAL OPIOID CONTRIBUTIONS

In rats, the antinociception associated with pregnancy is multifactorial and involves both central (spinal and supraspinal) and peripheral components. Multiple opioid antinociceptive systems comprise the predominant spinal component and are the final mediators of gestational antinociception.

Assessment of the effects of peripheral application of the opioid antagonist naltrexone in rats first revealed that the elevated nociceptive response thresholds of gestation are mediated by endogenous opioids (inset to Fig. 1A). The ability of naltrexone to virtually abolish the entire pregnancy-associated increase in pain thresholds, coupled with the absence of any effect of naltrexone on pain thresholds of nonpregnant animals, indicated that pregnancy-induced antinociception results from the activation of one or more opioid analgesic systems that are quiescent under basal physiological conditions (Gintzler 1980).

Anatomically discrete administration of naltrexone indicates that activation of spinal, but not supraspinal, opioid antinociceptive systems is essential for pregnancy-related antinociception. This conclusion is based on two observations. First, intracerebroventricular application of naltrexone did not attenuate gestational nociceptive response thresholds. On the contrary, at the earliest time point examined, this treatment paradoxically resulted in a further elevation in pain thresholds (J.L. Steinman and A.R. Gintzler, unpublished observations). In contrast, blockade of spinal opioid receptors not only attenuated the analgesia of pregnancy but abolished it (Sander and Gintzler 1987; Dawson-Basoa and Gintzler 1997, 1998). Moreover, this consequence of spinal opioid receptor blockade is selective of opioid receptor type.

← **Fig. 1.** Influence of (A) physiological gestation and (B) hormone-simulated pregnancy (HSP) on nociceptive response thresholds. (A) Nociceptive response thresholds were determined on the indicated days of physiological pregnancy and the postpartum period (ordinate). (B) Nociceptive response thresholds were determined throughout the course of treatment with estrogen (E_2) and progesterone (P). Each point represents the mean ± SEM jump threshold that was observed during each hormone treatment period and is plotted as the midpoint of that period ($n = 7$ for each group). Inset to Fig. 1A illustrates jump thresholds obtained in pregnant and nonpregnant rats each receiving systemic naltrexone (NX). Inset to Panel B illustrates jump thresholds obtained in HSP animals with or without systemic naltrexone. During physiological gestation and HSP, there is increased activity of an opioid system(s) that is quiescent under normal physiological conditions but is activated by the pregnancy blood concentration profile of E_2 and P. As a consequence, thresholds for responsiveness to aversive stimuli are increased.

PREGNANCY-RELATED ANALGESIA IS SELECTIVE OF SPINAL OPIOID RECEPTOR TYPE

Pharmacological experiments using a variety of opioid agonists have shown that three distinct types of opioid receptor, termed μ, δ, and κ, are present in the central nervous system (CNS) (Lord et al. 1977; Leslie et al. 1981; Tung and Yaksh 1982). All three types have been cloned (Evans et al. 1992; Li et al. 1993; Wang et al. 1993; Yasuda et al. 1993). The use of opioid receptor antagonists that can differentiate between μ-, δ-, and κ-opioid receptors can reveal the relative contribution of each receptor type to antinociceptive phenomena (see Table I) and to other physiological functions.

Intrathecal (i.t.) administration of the δ-opioid receptor antagonists 7-benzylidenenaltrexone (BNTX; Sofuoglu et al. 1993) or naltriben (NTB; Sofuoglu et al. 1991; Stewart and Hammond 1993) to rats essentially abolished pregnancy-related elevations in pain thresholds, which were on the order of 75–100% (Dawson-Basoa and Gintzler 1997). A comparable reduction in nociceptive response thresholds was observed (Dawson-Basoa and Gintzler 1998) following i.t. application of the κ-opioid-receptor-selective antagonist nor-binaltorphimine (nor-BNI; Takemori et al. 1988). In contrast, and much to our surprise, the robust and predominant spinal μ-opioid receptor analgesic system does not appear to contribute to gestational antinociception. This was indicated by the inability of the μ-selective antagonist D-Phe-Cys-Tyr-D-Trp-Arg-Thr-Pen-Thr-NH_2 (CTAP; Kramer et al. 1993) to diminish the pain thresholds of pregnancy (Dawson-Basoa and Gintzler 1996). It should be noted that blockade of spinal κ- or δ-opioid receptors has no effect on nociceptive response thresholds of nonpregnant animals.

Table I
Effect of spinal opioid receptor blockade on gestational antinociception

		Consequence	
Receptor	Antagonist	Pregnant	Control
μ	CTAP	None	None
δ	BNTX or NTB	Abolish	None
κ	nor-BNI	Abolish	None

Note: On gestational day 20, jump thresholds were determined after which CTAP (34 nmol), BNTX (10 pmol), NTB (250 pmol), or nor-BNI (87 nmol) was intrathecally administered. Jump thresholds were redetermined and compared with those obtained prior to mating (Dawson-Basoa and Gintzler 1997, 1998).

These results demonstrate that gestational antinociception depends on the recruitment of two relatively minor spinal opioid analgesic systems (δ and κ) that are quiescent under basal (nonpregnant) conditions.

OVARIAN STEROID MILIEU OF PREGNANCY IS CRITICAL FOR ACTIVATION OF κ/δ ANALGESIA

One critical peripheral component of the mechanisms underlying gestational antinociception is the pregnancy blood concentration profile of 17-β-estradiol (estrogen, E_2) and progesterone (P). The relevance of these hormones to gestational analgesia was confirmed by experiments that determined the effect on pain thresholds of nonpregnant rats of simulating pregnancy blood levels of E_2 and P. Pregnancy blood levels of E_2 and P were achieved either by inducing a condition known as pseudopregnancy or by systemically administering E_2 and P following ovariectomy.

Intermittent 5-minute mechanostimulation of the vaginal cervix of rats during the estrous phase induces a pseudopregnant state lasting for ~9–14 days (deFeo 1966). During this period, changes in circulating E_2 and P levels parallel those that occur during physiological gestation (deFeo 1966; Pepe and Rothchild 1974). The mean jump thresholds to electric shock of rats rendered pseudopregnant are significantly elevated (mean increase of ~60%) relative to the period immediately preceding the onset of pseudopregnancy or subsequent to its offset (Gintzler and Bohan 1990). Moreover, the entire pseudopregnancy-induced increase in pain thresholds can be abolished by the systemic administration of naltrexone (Gintzler and Bohan 1990). These results indicate that endogenous opioid antinociceptive systems can be activated by peripheral ovarian sex steroids, whose circulating concentration profile is altered during pseudopregnancy (and during actual pregnancy).

This inference was confirmed by direct simulation of the pregnancy blood concentration profile of circulating E_2 and P in nonpregnant, ovariectomized rats. Hormone blood concentration profiles were manipulated via the subcutaneous implantation of Silastic tubing filled with either a solution of E_2 (in sesame oil) or crystalline P (Bridges 1984). The resulting hormone-simulated pregnancy (HSP) produced a statistically significant elevation in pain thresholds (Dawson-Basoa and Gintzler 1993) that was strikingly similar in both temporal pattern and magnitude to that observed during actual gestation (compare Figs. 1A and 1B). Administration of pregnancy levels either of E_2 or P alone or of E_2 with the delayed addition of P (starting on day 15 of hormone treatment, when analgesia is first apparent) produced no increase in pain threshold. Therefore, the entire pregnancy profile of steroid hormones is required for the manifestation of analgesia. Chronic administration of naltrexone blocks the increase in pain threshold associated with HSP, indicating that this type of analgesia is mediated by an endogenous opioid system or systems, as is the analgesia of actual pregnancy.

The types of opioid receptor that mediate HSP analgesia and their CNS localization parallel those observed for the analgesia of pregnancy. Blockade of spinal κ-opioid (Dawson-Basoa and Gintzler 1996, 1998) or δ-opioid receptors (Dawson-Basoa and Gintzler 1997) abolished the analgesia produced by ovarian hormones (Table II), as was observed for pregnancy. Also, as in pregnancy, the antinociception of HSP is independent of spinal μ-opioid receptor activity (Dawson-Basoa and Gintzler 1996).

The striking similarities between the analgesia of HSP and actual gestation reaffirm that the profile of change in plasma E_2 and P is an essential parameter for the manifestation of elevated pain thresholds during pregnancy. Additionally, these data underscore the existence of a spinal opioid analgesic system that is subject to gender-specific hormonal modulation.

One striking feature of the antinociception of gestation and its hormonal simulation is that although both result from the recruitment of κ- and δ-opioid analgesic systems, blockade of each, individually, is sufficient to completely abolish the increase in nociceptive response thresholds. This finding indicates a special relationship between the spinal κ- and δ-opioid receptors, and suggests that it is their combined activity that mediates gestational and HSP antinociception.

Table II
Effect of spinal opioid receptor blockade on E_2/P-induced antinociception in female rats

		Consequence	
Receptor	Antagonist	E_2/P-Treated	Control
μ	CTAP	None	None
δ	BNTX or NTB	Abolish	None
κ	nor-BNI	Abolish	None

Note: On day 19 of steroid treatment, the effect of pharmacological blockade of spinal cord μ- , δ-, and κ-types of opioid receptor were determined as described for Table I except that post-injection jump thresholds were compared with those obtained prior to the onset of ovarian steroid hormone treatment (Dawson-Basoa and Gintzler 1996, 1997, 1998).

MULTIPLICATIVE SPINAL κ/δ INTERACTIONS DURING GESTATION AND HORMONE-STIMULATED PREGNANCY

Gestational and HSP antinociception could theoretically result from three types of interaction between spinal κ- and δ-opioid antinociceptive systems: (1) Antinociception could result from the parallel activation of κ and δ types of opioid receptor, each of which, alone, would be sufficient to mediate the full extent of the analgesia. (2) Antinociception could result from the parallel activation of spinal κ- and δ-opioid systems, each of which would independently contribute a portion of the total analgesia. (3) Activation of spinal κ- and δ-opioid receptors alone may not be sufficient to elevate maternal pain thresholds; in this scenario, the manifestation of pregnancy- or HSP-induced analgesia would require their coincident activation.

The first putative mechanism requires that the analgesia of pregnancy not be antagonized unless more than one type (or subtype) of opiate receptor is blocked (Watkins et al. 1992) because the untargeted receptor type should remain fully functional and continue to mediate antinociception. This, however, is not consistent with the ability of i.t. nor-BNI, BNTX, or NTB, individually at doses in which they interact with a single population of receptor, to not only attenuate but abolish the gestational- or HSP-induced increase in pain thresholds. Consequently, mediation of gestational or HSP antinociception via the first putative mechanism is not a viable possibility. Similarly, the second putative mechanism is not viable because it requires that individual blockade of a single opioid receptor type produce only a partial reduction in pregnancy- or HSP-induced antinociception, i.e., the untargeted receptor should continue to mediate the portion of the total antinociception that results from its activity. Only the third mechanism is consonant with the ability of individual spinal opioid receptor type-selective blockade to eliminate the increase in nociceptive response thresholds.

Direct evidence that the antinociception of gestation and HSP derives from κ/δ antinociceptive synergy comes from comparing the effect on jump thresholds of gestational or HSP rats of interrupting spinal κ- and δ-opioid transmission individually versus concomitantly. The rationale for this approach is that if an additive interaction underlies the analgesia of pregnancy and HSP, the magnitude of reduction in pain thresholds produced by concomitant elimination of spinal κ- and δ-receptor activity should be greater than that produced by eliminating each individually. Alternatively, equivalent effects on pain thresholds resulting from either measure would indicate that coincident activation of more than one type is a prerequisite for the analgesia of pregnancy or HSP.

During both physiological pregnancy (day 20) and HSP (day 19), the magnitude of reduction in jump thresholds produced by the i.t. application of combinations of κ and δ antagonists, each at submaximal doses, was indistinguishable from that observed following their individual i.t. application (Dawson-Basoa and Gintzler 1998). This finding strongly suggests that gestational and ovarian-steroid-induced antinociception is not simply the sum of the independent analgesic effects of spinal κ- and δ-opioid systems, but requires their coincident activation and resultant antinociceptive synergy. Thus the effect of various medicinal therapies on the interactive spinal κ/δ opioid analgesia of gestation should be considered in the clinical management of pregnant women.

Mediation of endogenous antinociception by a mechanism that utilizes analgesic synergy between its component parts would be consistent with the considerable evidence that "cross-talk" among different types of opioid receptor can modulate analgesic responsiveness to the exogenous administration of opioid agonists. For example, simultaneous i.t. administration of opioid agonists that act selectively at κ- and δ-opioid receptor sites produces analgesic synergy (Miaskowski et al. 1990). Evidence also suggests analgesic synergy between δ and μ opioids (Lee et al. 1980; Jiang et al. 1990; Sutters et al. 1990; Horan et al. 1992) and between κ and μ opioids (Sutters et al. 1990). More recent evidence indicates that activation of multiple subtypes of spinal cord δ receptor (δ_1 and δ_2) may be required to suppress responses in the hotplate test (activation of δ_2 receptors alone is not sufficient) (Stewart et al. 1994).

The multiplicative nature of gestational and ovarian-steroid-induced antinociception indicates that predominant mechanisms that underlie pharmacologically induced analgesia are not necessarily those utilized by endogenous opioid antinociceptive pathways. Although activation of a single opioid receptor type by an exogenous opioid results in substantial antinociception, concomitant activation of multiple opioid receptor types is a prerequisite for the naturally occurring analgesia of pregnancy (and HSP).

CONTRIBUTION OF SPINAL α_2-NORADRENERGIC PATHWAYS TO GESTATIONAL AND HSP ANTINOCICEPTION

Analgesic responsiveness to exogenous opioids is influenced by monoaminergic tone. The same applies to the antinociception of gestation and HSP, i.e., the spinal antinociception that results from spinal κ/δ opioid synergy is further magnified by ongoing spinal monoaminergic activity (Liu and Gintzler 1999).

Nociceptive response thresholds of pregnant or HSP animals can be significantly reduced (by ~60%) following blockade of spinal α_2 (but not α_1) noradrenergic receptors (Liu and Gintzler 1999). No effect of spinal α_2-noradrenergic blockade was observed in nonpregnant rats or ovariectomized rats treated with placebo Silastic implants. This finding indicates that spinal α_2-noradrenergic antinociceptive mechanisms do not contribute to basal nociceptive response thresholds but are activated by the E_2/P profile of pregnancy.

Spinal opioid receptor blockade has no effect on the antinociception produced by activation of spinal α_2-noradrenergic receptors (Ossipov et al. 1989), but it abolishes the analgesia associated with both pregnancy and HSP (Dawson-Basoa and Gintzler 1997, 1998; Liu and Gintzler 1999). Thus, it is unlikely that spinal noradrenergic systems would directly contribute to the antinociception associated with pregnancy or HSP. Instead, attenuation of the analgesia of these conditions following spinal noradrenergic α_2-receptor blockade most likely derives from the interruption of the multiplicative antinociceptive consequences of concomitant activation of spinal α_2 and opioid receptors.

Antinociceptive synergy following the concomitant activation of spinal α_2 and opioid receptors was originally demonstrated following the exogenous (i.t.) application of clonidine (an α_2 agonist) and κ- or δ-opioid agonists (Wang et al. 1980; Yaksh and Reddy 1981; Hylden and Wilcox 1983; Ossipov et al. 1989, 1990). The antinociception of pregnancy and HSP suggests that an analogous analgesic synergy also occurs between their endogenous counterparts and subserves a significant component of the antinociception of each condition. Such a mechanism would be consistent with previous reports that spinal α_2-receptor activation is required for the full manifestation of the antinociception produced by the systemic, supraspinal (Yaksh 1979; Camarata and Yaksh 1985), or i.t. (Ossipov et al. 1989) administration of morphine. It would also be consonant with the absence of analgesic synergy following the i.t. application of α_2 and opioid agonists in α_2-receptor knockout mice (Stone et al. 1997).

Although spinal α_2-noradrenergic tone is a prerequisite for the full manifestation of gestational and HSP antinociception, it is not required for the spinal κ/δ antinociceptive synergy that partially subserves this analgesia. Following blockade of spinal α_2 receptors, the remaining increase in pain thresholds (~40%) can be abolished by blockade of either spinal κ- or δ-opioid receptors, individually. Thus, the component of ovarian-steroid-induced antinociception that persists despite the absence of α_2-noradrenergic receptor activity results from κ/δ antinociceptive synergy and not from the additive, independent analgesic contributions of these opioid pathways.

The absence of any dependence of the HSP-induced spinal κ/δ analgesic synergy on spinal α_2 noradrenergic tone has significant mechanistic implications. This finding indicates that the attenuation of HSP- and pregnancy-induced increases in nociceptive response thresholds following i.t. yohimbine (an α_2-receptor antagonist) results from the removal of an additional level of antinociceptive synergy. Thus, multiple levels of analgesic synergy appear to underlie the antinociception associated with HSP and gestation: the analgesic synergy between spinal κ/δ-opioid antinociceptive pathways is amplified by an additional synergy between endogenous opioid systems and descending noradrenergic pathways (Fig. 2).

Decreased pain sensitivity that results from endogenous opioid analgesic synergy has decided benefits. This mechanism allows for significant physiological effects to be achieved with concentrations of endogenous dynorphin and enkephalin that for either peptide alone would produce minimal opioid receptor activation (and analgesia). Lowering the concentrations of endogenous opioids that are required to produce significant levels of antinociception would decrease the propensity for developing opioid tolerance and dependence. In other words, when multiple independent receptor systems (κ, δ, and α_2) are activated concomitantly to achieve analgesia, each receptor type is less likely to develop tolerance. For example, in primates, the analgesic potency of i.t. morphine is substantially diminished over a period of 3–5 days. In contrast, antinociceptive responses to i.t. combinations of morphine and the α_2 agonist ST-91 do not seem to decrease over a 21-day period (Wang et al. 1980; Yaksh and Reddy 1981).

THE HYPOGASTRIC NERVE IS INVOLVED IN SPINAL α_2-NORADRENERGIC ANTINOCICEPTIVE MECHANISMS

An intact hypogastric nerve (a major uterine afferent) is essential for the full manifestation of gestational (Gintzler et al. 1983) and HSP (Liu and Gintzler 1999) antinociception. In HSP animals subjected to bilateral hypogastric neurectomy, the magnitude of the increase in nociceptive response thresholds was reduced by ~60%. Interestingly, this reduction is comparable to that observed following blockade of spinal α_2-noradrenergic receptors. Moreover, in HSP rats following bilateral hypogastric neurectomy, spinal α_2-receptor blockade had no effect on HSP pain thresholds (Liu and Gintzler 1999). These results suggest that during pregnancy and its hormonal simulation, activation of spinal α_2 receptors is secondary to increased hypogastric neuronal function. The ability of hypogastric neurectomy to lower pain thresholds of pregnancy and HSP presumably results from the loss of augmented spinal α_2-noradrenergic tone.

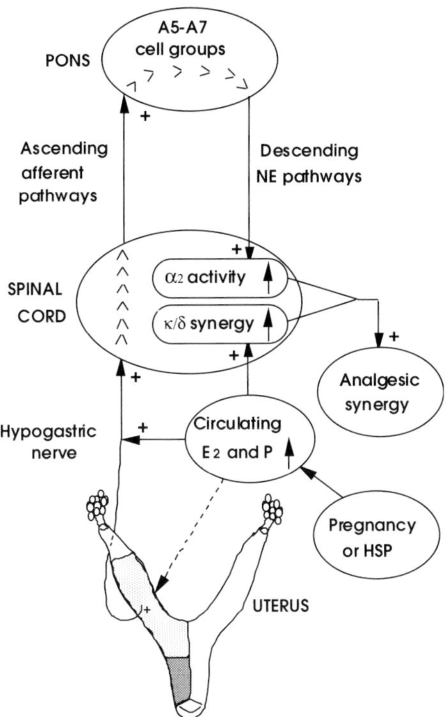

Fig. 2. Summary of known peripheral and central components of gestational antinociception. The former include changes in the blood concentration profile of ovarian sex steroids and activity of the hypogastric nerve. The latter include augmented activity of spinal κ- and δ-opioid receptors as well as α_2-noradrenergic receptors. A predominant characteristic of gestational and HSP antinociception is that it results from analgesic synergy between spinal δ- and κ-opioid receptor activity and an additional α_2-noradrenergic/opioid synergy. The former synergy is resistant to hypogastric nerve transection and thus could result from a direct spinal action of estrogen (E_2) or progesterone (P). In contrast, since cutting the hypogastric nerve eliminates the α_2-noradrenergic component of hormone-simulated pregnancy (HSP), it is suggested that HSP activates hypogastric neurotransmission, which in turn results in the increased activity of one or more spinal ascending pathways. This, directly or indirectly, results in increased activity of one or more descending noradrenergic pathways. The consequent augmentation of spinal α_2 activity would result in analgesic synergy with ongoing spinal κ/δ neurotransmission. Dark and light gray areas show differential uterine innervation by pelvic and hypogastric nerves, respectively.

The involvement of the hypogastric nerve in HSP-related antinociception processes underscores the dichotomous relationship of afferent input to nociceptive processing. In a recent study (Temple et al. 1999), bilateral hypogastric neurectomy eliminated escape responses to uterine distension, which suggests that this nerve transmits aversive uterine afferent input. This finding contradicts demonstrations that the hypogastric nerve is critical to the antinociception of gestation as well as its hormonal simulation (Gintzler et al. 1983; Liu and Gintzler 1999) and that uterine afferent stimuli augment the analgesic consequences of endogenous spinal opioid (κ/δ) activity. Also, although neuropathic pain is relatively insensitive to opioids (Arnér and Meyerson 1988; Portenoy et al. 1990; Dubner 1991; Chemy et al. 1994), the antinociceptive ability of opioids can be significantly enhanced by concomitant i.t. administration with low doses of substance P (Kream et al. 1993). Moreover, spinal (κ) opioids have an increased ability to attenuate hyperalgesia in rats subjected to chronic inflammation (Neil et al. 1986; Hylden et al. 1991). Collectively, these observations indicate that afferent input can play a dual role in the processing of nociceptive stimuli, the nature of which is determined by the type of afferent information transmitted. Moreover, uterine distension elicits escape responses during diestrus or metestrus but is not aversive during proestrus and estrus (Bradshaw et al. 1999). Together with the observation that antinociception mediated by ovarian steroids is dependent, in part, on the hypogastric nerve, this finding underscores the importance of the female-specific endocrine milieu to the influence of visceral (pelvic) afferent activity on nociceptive processing.

SUPRASPINAL COMPONENTS OF GESTATIONAL AND HSP ANTINOCICEPTION

The involvement of spinal α_2-noradrenergic receptor activity in the antinociception of gestation and HSP is the first indication of a supraspinal contribution to these phenomena. All noradrenergic terminals in the spinal cord originate from descending pathways. The cell bodies of these neurons are located in the A5–A7 cell groups of the pons in the locus ceruleus, subceruleus, the medial and lateral parabrachial and the Kolliker-Fuse nuclei, and adjacent to the superior olivary nucleus (Westlund et al. 1983). Furthermore, noradrenergic terminals in lamina I and the outer layer of lamina II of the dorsal horn, the spinal region in which α_2-noradrenergic receptors would be expected to modulate nociception, do not make synaptic contact with primary afferent terminals (Hagihira et al. 1990). Consequently, exclusive involvement of increased activity at the terminal of noradrenergic spinal projection neurons would not be consonant with the ability of hypogastric neurectomy to abolish the spinal noradrenergic component of gestational and HSP antinociception. Thus, it is likely that increased activity in descending noradrenergic pathways occurs during pregnancy and its hormonal simulation, resulting in an augmentation of spinal α_2-receptor activity (see Fig. 2). This underscores the relevance of pontine nuclei to the processing of pelvic afferent stimuli and the endogenous regulation of spinal κ/δ antinociceptive systems.

PUTATIVE MECHANISMS OF OVARIAN STEROID-PRODUCED ANALGESIA IN PREGNANCY

The mechanisms by which pregnancy levels of E_2 and P activate spinal α_2/opioid and κ/δ antinociception are unknown. The dependence of the former, but not the latter mechanism of analgesia, on pelvic afferent stimuli suggests a peripheral (hypogastric nerve) as well as a central locus of E_2/P action. Regarding α_2/opioid activity, there is precedent for ovarian steroid regulation of hypogastric function. Functionality of the hypogastric nerve varies across the estrous cycle (Robbins et al. 1992). For example, the minimum uterine pressure required to evoke multi-unit activity of the hypogastric nerve is highest in diestrus and significantly lower during both proestrus and estrus (Robbins et al. 1992). This finding suggests that the increasing concentrations of E_2 and P that characterize HSP (and pregnancy) could similarly lower the threshold for hypogastric nerve impulse propagation, i.e., increase hypogastric nerve responsiveness. In the full-term pregnant rat, a profound uterine neuronal degeneration has been reported (Haase et al. 1997), which would imply that the involvement of the hypogastric nerve in the antinociception of HSP and pregnancy derives from the ability of E_2 and P to directly augment hypogastric nerve activity.

Since the yohimbine-resistant spinal κ/δ antinociception of HSP persists after hypogastric neurectomy, its steroid activation would appear to be independent of hypogastric afferent activity and could be a consequence of a direct E_2/P action on spinal neurons. This formulation would be consistent with the recent finding that the α isoform of the estrogen receptor colocalizes with enkephalin in many neurons of the superficial lamina of the spinal dorsal horn (Amandusson et al. 1996) and is also found in cells scattered among laminae I, II, VI, and VII (Shughrue et al. 1997). Additionally, cells expressing the β isoform of the estrogen receptor have been identified in lamina II of the dorsal horn (Shughrue et al. 1997). Thus, there is a biochemical basis for postulating that the antinociception associated with gestation and sustained ovarian steroid treatment results, in part, from a direct action on spinal tissue.

Peripherally administered sex steroid hormones influence several parameters of central opioid activity. For example, opioid receptor binding density and β-endorphin concentration increased by 52% in the preoptic area of ovariectomized rats given pregnancy levels of E_2 and P (Hammer and Bridges 1987; Mateo et al. 1992). Additionally, estrogen has been shown to positively regulate proenkephalin mRNA levels in the ventrolateral aspect of the ventromedial hypothalamic nucleus within 1 hour of its administration (Romano et al. 1989). Treatment with progesterone attenuates the rapid decline in hypothalamic levels of proenkephalin mRNA that occurs following the cessation of estrogen administration (Romano et al. 1988). It is tempting to speculate that an analogous ovarian steroid action occurs in the spinal cord of pregnant animals. It is relevant to note that the pregnancy blood concentration profile of 17-β-estradiol and progesterone was recently shown to be a predominant facet of the pregnant condition responsible for the increase in the spinal cord content of prohormone convertase 2, a proteolytic enzyme capable of generating mature dynorphin $A_{(1-17)}$ from its prohormone (Varshney et al. 1999).

SEQUENTIAL ACTIVATION AND SUMMATION OF MULTIPLE PAIN-ATTENUATING PATHWAYS

Pelvic afferent stimuli can also activate non-opioid antinociceptive processes. In nonpregnant rats and humans, vaginal and cervical mechanostimulation elevates pain thresholds (Komisaruk and Wallman 1977; Steinman et al. 1983; Cunningham et al. 1991; Komisaruk 1991), but this action is blocked in rats by transection of the hypogastric and pelvic nerves (Cunningham et al. 1991). Moreover, direct mechanostimulation of the uterine cervix also produces analgesia. Uterocervical mechanostimulation, applied via a Silastic disk implanted in the uterus and abutted against the cervix, produced an approximately twofold increase in tail-flick latency that was naloxone-insensitive (Gintzler and Komisaruk 1991). This antinociception, in contrast to that associated with pregnancy or HSP, was not altered by hypogastric neurectomy, but could be abolished by transection of the pelvic nerve. Uterine mechanostimulation activates the hypogastric nerve (Peters et al. 1987; Berkley et al. 1988; Robbins et al. 1990), but not the pelvic nerve (Peters et al. 1987), whereas vaginal mechanostimulation activates the pelvic nerve (Komisaruk et al. 1972), but not the hypogastric nerve (Peters et al. 1987). Both of these nerves are activated by cervical stimulation (Komisaruk et al. 1972; Peters et al. 1987; Berkley et al. 1988). During late pregnancy the growing fetus(es) might stimulate the uterine horns more than the cervix and thus activate predominantly the hypogastric nerve. However, during labor (parturition), stimulation of the cervix and thus the pelvic nerve would predominate. Thus, the antinociceptive mechanisms associated with parturition differ from those that underlie the analgesia characteristic of the gestational period.

The onset of activation of each of these mechanisms would be temporally distinct, but the analgesia that results would overlap and summate. Thus, during parturition, the analgesia that results from fetal stimulation of the uterine cervix and vagina would complement the augmentation of descending spinal noradrenergic pathways and activation of spinal κ/δ and α_2/opioid antinociceptive synergy that occur in response to changes in circulating E_2/P. Analgesia resulting from ingestion of amniotic fluid and placenta by parturient rats would potentiate the ongoing opioid antinociception (Kristal et al. 1985, 1990). Thus, as pregnancy progresses to parturition and birth there appears to be a crescendo of activated analgesic mechanisms.

The relevance of gender-specific physiology to pain-coping mechanisms is underscored by the phenomena of gestational and HSP antinociception. Gender-dependent differences in the modulation of and responsiveness to nociceptive stimuli have long been the subject of speculation and investigation (see Berkley 1997 for review). Women are more likely than men to experience recurrent pain, and to have severe and long-lasting pain (Unruh 1996). These differences in nociception have been reported for various modalities of aversive stimuli. For example, females (1) have lower response thresholds to thermal (Fillingim et al. 1998) and electrical (Walker and Carmody 1998) stimuli, (2) manifest greater temporal summation of thermal pain (Fillingim et al. 1998), and (3) experience greater pain at high levels of pressure stimulation (Ellermeier and Westphal 1995). The biological basis for gender-specific vulnerability to pain is not understood. However, the nature of the interactions among the various components of gestational and HSP analgesia could provide a useful starting point.

As a consequence of a multiplicative antinociceptive mechanism, such as that which is activated during gestation and HSP, a disproportionately large decrease in pain sensitivity would result from relatively small increase in the activity of one or more of its component processes. However, the converse would also be true, i.e., a relatively minor impairment of one or more contributing systems would result in a disproportionate increase in pain perception. Thus, the mechanisms of gestational and HSP antinociception could provide a rational framework with which to understand the male/female dichotomy of painful experience, documentation of which is rapidly expanding (see Berkley 1997 for review). Pharmacological targeting of some of the components of ovarian-steroid-regulated multiplicative antinociceptive systems, particularly during pregnancy, could provide a new starting point for medicinal treatment of pain syndromes in women.

GENDER-SPECIFIC MECHANISMS OF ANTINOCICEPTION

Spinal opioid antinociceptive responsiveness to E_2/P is not gender-specific. In a recent study (Liu and Gintzler 2000), treatment of orchidectomized, sexually mature male rats with the same regimen of E_2 and P used in females elicited a profound antinociception, comparable in robustness and temporal profile to that previously observed in females. However, the neurobiological substrates and interactive antinociceptive mechanisms that underlie ovarian sex steroid antinociception differ among males and females. In males, the analgesia resulting from ovarian steroid treatment derives from the independent contributions of spinal κ and μ (not δ) opioid receptor pathways. Moreover, their respective contributions are additive, not synergistic (see Table III). Spinal α_2-noradrenergic receptor activity and its attendant analgesic synergy with spinal opioid systems, essential components of ovarian-steroid-activated antinociception in females, do not contribute to analgesia in males. This is in contrast to the previous demonstrations that ovarian sex-steroid-induced antinociception in females results from antinociceptive synergy between activated spinal κ/δ opioid as well as α_2-noradrenergic receptor systems. Thus, ovarian-steroid-activated "high gain" multiplicative spinal antinociceptive pathways are prominent in females but do not appear to be present in males.

In summary, the antinociception of pregnancy and its hormonal simulation involves central (spinal opioid and noradrenergic pathways) as well as peripheral components, some of which are female-specific (e.g., circulating levels of estrogen and progesterone). Although many of the components are

Table III
Effect of spinal opioid receptor blockade on E_2/P-induced antinociception in male rats

		Consequence	
Receptor	Antagonist	E_2/P-Treated	Control
δ	BNTX or NTB	None	None
μ	CTAP	Partial reduction	None
κ	nor-BNI	Partial reduction	None
$\mu + \kappa$	CTAP + nor-BNI	Additivity resulting in abolishment	None

Note: The effect of pharmacological blockade of spinal cord μ-, δ-, and κ-types of opioid receptor on antinociceptive response thresholds of E_2/P-treated male rats was determined on day 19 as described for Table II. Ovarian-steroid-induced antinociception in males differs from that observed in females in both the identities of the spinal opioid receptors involved and in their interaction, i.e., additive versus synergistic (Liu and Gintzler 2000).

present in males as well as females (hypogastric nerve, spinal opioid and descending noradrenergic pathways), antinociceptive responsiveness to the simulation of a female-specific endocrine milieu in males as well as females reveals gender-specific interactions among them. These interactions have broad functional implications beyond those directly related to reproductive processes and heighten the utility of developing gender-specific strategies of pain management.

REFERENCES

Amandusson PJ, Hermanson O, Blomqvist A. Colocalization of estrogen receptor immunoreactivity and preproenkephalin mRNA expression to neurons in the superficial laminae of the spinal and medullary dorsal horn of rats. *Eur J Neurosci* 1996; 8:2440–2445.

Arnér S, Meyerson BA. Lack of analgesic effects of opioids on neuropathic and idiopathic forms of pain. *Pain* 1988; 33:11–23.

Berkley KJ. Sex differences in pain. *Behav Brain Sci* 1997; 20:371–380.

Berkley K, Robbins A, Sato Y. Afferent fibers supplying the uterus in the rat. *J Neurophysiol* 1988; 59:142–163.

Bradshaw HB, Temple JL, Wood E, Berkley KJ. Estrous variations in behavior responses to vaginal and uterine distension in the rat. *Pain* 1999; 82:187–197.

Bridges RS. A quantitative analysis of the roles of dosage, sequence, and duration of estradiol and progesterone exposure in the regulation of maternal behavior in the rat. *Endocrinology* 1984; 114:930–940.

Camarata PJ, Yaksh TL. Characterization of spinal adrenergic receptors mediating the spinal effects produced by microinjection of morphine into the periaqueductal gray. *Brain Res* 1985; 336:133–142.

Chemy NI, Thaler HT, Friedlander KH, et al. Opioid responsiveness of cancer pain syndrome caused by neuropathic or nociceptive mechanisms: a combined analysis of controlled, single dose studies. *Neurology* 1994; 44:857–861.

Cogan R, Spinnato JA. Pain and discomfort thresholds in late pregnancy. *Pain* 1986; 27:63–68.

Cunningham ST, Steinman JL, Whipple B, Mayer AD, Komisaruk BR. Differential roles of hypogastric and pelvic nerves in the analgesic and motoric effects of vaginocervical stimulation in rats. *Brain Res* 1991; 559:337–343.

Dawson-Basoa ME, Gintzler AR. 17-β-Estradiol and progesterone modulate an intrinsic opioid analgesic system. *Brain Res* 1993; 601:241–245.

Dawson-Basoa ME, Gintzler AR. Estrogen and Progesterone activate spinal kappa-opiate receptor analgesic mechanisms. *Pain* 1996; 64:607–615.

Dawson-Basoa ME, Gintzler AR. Involvement of spinal cord δ opiate receptors in the antinociception of gestation and its hormonal simulation. *Brain Res* 1997; 757:37–42.

Dawson-Basoa ME, Gintzler AR. Gestational and ovarian sex steroid antinociception: synergy between spinal κ and δ opioid systems. *Brain Res* 1998; 794:61–67.

deFeo VJ. Vaginal-cervical vibration: a simple and effective method for the induction of pseudopregnancy in the rat. *Endocrinology* 1966; 79:440–442.

Dubner R. A call for more science, not more rhetoric, regarding opioids and neuropathetic pain. *Pain* 1991; 47:1–2.

Ellermeier W, Westphal W. Gender differences in pain ratings and pupil reactions to painful pressure stimuli. *Pain* 1995; 61:435–439.

Evans CJ, Keith DE Jr, Morrison H, Magendzo K, Edwards RH. Cloning of a delta opioid receptor by functional expression. *Science* 1992; 258:1952–1955.

Fillingim RB, Maixner W, Kincaid S, Silva S. Sex differences in temporal summation but not sensory-discriminative processing of thermal pain. *Pain* 1998; 75:121–127.

Gintzler AR. Endorphin-mediated increases in pain threshold during pregnancy. *Science* 1980; 210:193–195.

Gintzler AR, Bohan MC. Pain thresholds are elevated during pseudopregnancy. *Brain Res* 1990; 507:312–316.

Gintzler AR, Komisaruk BR. Analgesia is produced by uterocervical mechanostimulation in rats: roles of afferent nerves and implications for analgesia of pregnancy and parturition. *Brain Res* 1991; 566:299–302.

Gintzler AR, Peters LC, Komisaruk BR. Attenuation of pregnancy-induced analgesia by hypogastric neurectomy in rats. *Brain Res* 1983; 227:186–188.

Haase EB, Buchman J, Tietz AE, Schramm LP. Pregnancy-induced uterine neuronal degeneration in the rat. *Cell Tissue Res* 1997; 288:293–306.

Hagihira S, Senba E, Yoshida S, Tohyama M, Yoshiya I. Fine structure of nor-adrenergic terminals and their synapses in the rat spinal dorsal horn: an immunohistochemical study. *Brain Res* 1990; 526:73–80.

Hammer RP, Bridges RS. Preoptic area opioids and opiate receptors increase during pregnancy and decrease during lactation. *Brain Res* 1987; 420:48–56.

Horan P, Tallarida RJ, Haaseth RC, et al. Antinociceptive interactions of opioid delta receptor agonists with morphine in mice: supra- and sub-additivity. *Life Sci* 1992; 50:1535–1541.

Hylden JLK, Wilcox GL. Pharmacological characterization of substance P-induced nociception in mice: modulation by opioid and noradrenergic agonists at the spinal level. *J Pharmacol Exp Ther* 1983; 226(2):398–404.

Hylden JLK, Thomas DA, Iadarola MJ, Dubner R. Spinal opioid analgesic effects are enhanced in a model of unilateral inflammation/hyperalgesia: possible involvement of noradrenergic mechanisms. *Eur J Pharm* 1991; 194:135–143.

Iwasaki H, Collins JG, Saito Y, Kerman-Hinds A. Naloxone-sensitive, pregnancy-induced changes in behavioral responses to colorectal distention: pregnancy-induced analgesia to visceral stimulation. *Anesthesiology* 1991; 74:927–933.

Jarvis S, McLean KA, Chirnside J, et al. Opioid-mediated changes in nociceptive threshold during pregnancy and parturition in the sow. *Pain* 1997; 72:153–159.

Jiang Q, Mosberg HI, Porreca F. Modulation of the potency and efficacy of mu-mediated antinociception by delta agonists in the mouse. *J Pharmacol Exp Ther* 1990; 254:683–689.

Komisaruk BR. Vaginocervical afference as a trigger for analgesic, behavioral, autonomic and neuroendocrine processes. In: Archer T, Ahlenius S, Hansen S, Sodersten P (Eds). *Biological Psychology: Neuroendocrine Axis.* Hillsdale, NJ: Lawrence Erlbaum Associates, 1991.

Komisaruk BR, Wallman J. Antinociceptive effects of vaginal stimulation in rats: neurophysiological and behavioral studies. *Brain Res* 1977; 137:85–107.

Komisaruk BR, Adler NT, Hutchison J. Genital sensory field: enlargement by estrogen treatment in female rats. *Science* 1972; 178:1295–1298.

Kramer TH, Shook JE, Kazmierski W, et al. Novel peptidic mu opioid antagonists: pharmacologic characterization in vitro and in vivo. *J Pharmacol Exp Ther* 1993; 249:544–550.

Kream RM, Kato T, Shimonaka H, Marchand JE, Wurm WH. Substance P markedly potentiates the antinociceptive effects of morphine sulfate administered at the spinal level. *Proc Natl Acad Sci USA* 1993; 90:3564–3568.

Kristal MB, Thompson AC, Grishkat HL. Placenta ingestion enhances opiate analgesia in rats. *Physiol Behav* 1985; 35:481–486.

Kristal MB, Thompson AC, Abbott P, et al. Amniotic-fluid ingestion by parturient rats enhances pregnancy-mediated analgesia. *Life Sci* 1990; 46:693–698.

Lee NM, Leybin L, Chang JK, Loh HH. Opiate and peptide interaction: effect of enkephalins on morphine analgesia. *Eur J Pharmacol* 1980; 68:181–185.

Leslie FM, Chavkin C, Cox BM. Opioid binding properties of brain and peripheral tissue: evidence for heterogeneity in opioid ligand binding sites. *J Pharmacol Exp Ther* 1981; 214:395–402.

Li S, Zhu J, Chen C, et al. Molecular cloning and expression of a rat κ opioid receptor. *Biochem J* 1993; 295:629–633.

Liu N-J, Gintzler AR. Gestational and ovarian sex steroid antinociception: relevance of uterine afferent and spinal α_2-noradrenergic activity. *Pain* 1999; 83:359–368.

Liu N-J, Gintzler AR. Prolonged ovarian sex steroid treatment of male rats produces antinociception: identification of sex-based divergent analgesic mechanisms. *Pain* 2000; 85:273–281.

Lord JA, Waterfield AA, Hughes J, Kosterlitz HW. Endogenous opioid peptides: multiple agonists and receptors. *Nature (Lond)* 1977; 267:495–499.

Mateo AR, Hijazi M, Hammer RP. Dynamic patterns of medial preoptic μ-opiate receptor regulation by gonadal steroid hormones. *Neuroendocrinology* 1992; 55:51–58.

Miaskowski C, Taiwo YO, Levine JD. κ- and δ opioid agonists synergize to produce potent analgesia. *Brain Res* 1990; 509:165–168.

Neil A, Kayser V, Gacel G, Besson J-M, Guilbaud G. Opioid receptor types and antinociceptive activity in chronic inflammation: both kappa and mu opiate agonistic effects are enhanced in arthritic rats. *Eur J Pharmacol* 1986; 130:203–208.

Ossipov MH, Suarez LJ, Spaulding TC. Antinociceptive interactions between alpha 2-adrenergic and opiate agonists at the spinal level in rodents. *Anesth Analg* 1989; 68:194–200.

Ossipov MH, Lozito R, Messineo E, et al. Spinal antinociception synergy between clonidine and morphine, U69593, and DPDPE: isobolographic analysis. *Life Sci* 1990; 47(16):PL71–PL76.

Pepe GJ, Rothchild FA. A comparative study of serum progesterone levels in pregnancy and in various types of pseudopregnancy in the rat. *Endocrinology* 1974; 95:275–279.

Peters LC, Kristal MB, Komisaruk BR. Sensory innervation of the external and internal genitalia of the female rat. *Brain Res* 1987; 408:199–204.

Portenoy RK, Foley KM, Inturrisi CE. The nature of opioid responsiveness and its implications for neuropathetic pain: new hypotheses derived from studies of opioid infusions (see comments). *Pain* 1990; 43:273–286.

Robbins A, Sato Y, Berkley K. Response of hypogastric nerve afferent fibers to uterine distention in estrous or metestrous rats. *Neurosci Lett* 1990; 110(No. 1–2):82–85.

Robbins A, Berkley K, Sato Y. Estrous cycle variation of afferent fibers supplying reproductive organs in the female rat. *Brain Res* 1992; 596:353.

Romano GJ, Harlan RE, Shiverst BD, Howels RD, Pfaff DW. Estrogen increases proenkephalin messenger ribonucleic acid levels in the ventromedial hypothalamus of the rat. *Mol Endocrinol* 1988; 2:1320–1328.

Romano GJ, Mobbs CV, Howels RD, Pfaff DDW. Estrogen regulation of proenkephalin gene expression in the ventromedial hypothalamus of the rat: temporal qualities and synergism with progesterone. *Mol Brain Res* 1989; 5:51–58.

Sander HW, Gintzler AR. Spinal cord mediation of the opioid analgesia of pregnancy. *Brain Res* 1987; 408:389–393.

Shughrue PJ, Lane MV, Merchenthaler I. Comparative distribution of estrogen receptor α and β mRNA in the rat central nervous system. *J Comp Neurol* 1997; 388:507–525.

Sofuoglu M, Portoghese PS, Takemori AE. Differential antagonism of delta opioid agonists by naltrindole and its benzofuran analog (NTB) in mice: evidence for delta receptor subtypes. *J Pharmacol Exp Ther* 1991; 257:676–680.

Sofuoglu M, Portoghese PS, Takemori AE. 7-Benzylidenenaltrexone (BNTX): a selective δ_1 opioid receptor antagonist in the mouse spinal cord. *Life Sci* 1993; 52:769–775.

Steinman JL, Komisaruk BR, Yaksh TL, Tyce GM. Spinal cord monoamines modulate the antinociceptive effects of vaginal stimulation in rats. *Pain* 1983; 16:155–166.

Stewart PE, Hammond DL. Evidence for delta opioid receptor subtypes in rat spinal cord: studies with intrathecal naltriben, cyclic [D-pen^2,D-pen^5] enkephalin and [D-ala^2,glu^4] deltorphin. *J Pharmacol Exp Ther* 1993; 266:820–828.

Stewart P, Holper EM, Hammond DL. δ Antagonist and κ agonist activity of naltriben: evidence for differential interaction with δ_1 and δ_2 opioid receptor subtypes. *Life Sci* 1994; 55(4):79–84.

Stone LS, MacMillan LB, Kitto KF, Limbird LE, Wilcox GL. The alpha2a adrenergic receptor subtype mediates spinal analgesia evoked by alpha2a agonists and is necessary for spinal adrenergic-opioid synergy. *J Neurosci* 1997; 17:7157–7165.

Sutters KA, Miaskowski C, Taiwo YO, Levine JD. Analgesic synergy and improved motor function by combinations of μ-δ and μ-κ opioids. *Brain Res* 1990; 530:290–294.

Takemori AE, Ho BY, Naeset JS, Portoghese PS. Nor-binaltorphimine, a highly selective kappa-opioid antagonist in analgesic and receptor binding assays. *J Pharmacol Exp Ther* 1988; 246:255–258.

Temple JL, Bradshaw HB, Wood E, Berkley KJ. Effects of hypogastric neurectomy on escape responses to uterine distention in the rat. *Pain* 1999; (Suppl) 6:S13–S20.

Toniolo MV, Whipple BH, Komisaruk BR. Spontaneous maternal analgesia during birth in rats. *Proc NIH Centennial MBRS-MARC Symp* 1987; 15.

Tung AS, Yaksh TL. In vivo evidence for multiple opiate receptors mediating analgesia in the rat spinal cord. *Brain Res* 1982; 247:75–83.

Unruh AM. Gender variations in clinical pain experience. *Pain* 1996; 65:123–167.

Varshney C, Rivera MR, Gintzler AR. Modulation of prohormone convertase 2 in spinal cord during gestation and hormone-simulated pregnancy. *Neuroendocrinology* 1999; 70:268–279.

Walker JS, Carmody JJ. Experimental pain in healthy human subjects: gender differences in nociception and in response to ibuprofen. *Anesth Analg* 1998; 86:1257–1262.

Wang JB, Imai Y, Eppler CM, et al. Opiate receptor: cDNA cloning and expression. *Proc Natl Acad Sci USA* 1993; 90:10230–10234.

Wang JY, Yasuoka S, Yaksh TL. Studies on the analgetic effect of intrathecal ST-91 (2-[2,6-diethylphenylamino]-imidazooine): antagonism, tolerance and interaction with morphine. *Pharmacologist* 1980; 22:302.

Watkins LR, Wiertelak EP, Grisel JE, Silbert LH, Maier SF. Parallel activation of multiple spinal opiate systems appears to mediate 'non-opiate' stress-induced analgesias. *Brain Res* 1992; 594:99–108.

Westlund KN, Bowker RM, Ziegler MG, Coutler JD. Noradrenergic projections to the spinal cord of the rat. *Brain Res* 1983; 263:15–31.

Whipple B, Josimovich JB, Komisaruk BR. Sensory thresholds during the antepartum, intrapartum, and postpartum periods. *Int J Nurs Stud* 1990; 27(3):213–221.

Yaksh TL. Direct evidence that spinal serotonin and noradrenaline terminals mediate the spinal antinociceptive effects of morphine in the periaqueductal gray. *Brain Res* 1979; 160:180–185.

Yaksh TL, Reddy SVR. Studies in the primate on the analgetic effects associated with intrathecal actions of opiates, α-adrenergic agonists and baclofen. *Anesthesiology* 1981; 54:451–467.

Yasuda K, Raynor K, Kong H, et al. Cloning and functional comparison of κ and δ opioid receptors from mouse brain. *Proc Natl Acad Sci USA* 1993; 90:6736–6740.

Correspondence to: Alan R. Gintzler, PhD, Box 8, Department of Biochemistry, SUNY HSCB, 450 Clarkson Avenue, Brooklyn, NY 11203, USA. Tel: 718-270-2129; Fax: 718-270-3316; email: agintzler@netmail.hscbklyn.edu.

Sex, Gender, and Pain, Progress in Pain Research and Management, Vol. 17, edited by R.B. Fillingim, IASP Press, Seattle, © 2000.

7

How Does Vaginal Stimulation Produce Pleasure, Pain, and Analgesia?

Barry R. Komisaruk[a] and Beverly Whipple[b]

[a]*Department of Psychology, and* [b]*College of Nursing, Rutgers, The State University of New Jersey, Newark, New Jersey, USA*

Vaginal stimulation produces pleasure, pain, and analgesia. Is this assertion internally inconsistent? Data from extensive behavioral, neurophysiological, and pharmacological studies in rats and from perceptual studies in women (Komisaruk and Whipple 1995) provide clear evidence that vaginal and cervical mechanostimulation can produce analgesia. Furthermore, when women self-apply vaginal stimulation in a way that feels pleasurable, the magnitude of the analgesia increases (Whipple and Komisaruk 1988). However, vaginal stimulation can also be painful, as in the case of dyspareunia (Meana and Binik 1994; Meana et al. 1997) and cervical dilatation for curettage. In addition, recent studies have shown that rats will perform escape responses to vaginal or uterine distension (Berkley et al. 1995), indicating that such stimulation can be aversive. (For a diagram of the properties associated with vaginal stimulation, see Fig. 1.)

Given the extensive evidence that a wide variety of stressors, e.g., nociceptive stimuli, can produce analgesia, could the antinociception that is produced by vaginal or cervical stimulation be a form of nociceptive stress-induced analgesia? Not necessarily, for stressors need not be aversive, and indeed can be appetitive. An intense stress response that is characterized by a doubling of the heart rate and blood pressure, indicating activation of the sympathetic division of the autonomic system, can occur during orgasm (Whipple and Komisaruk 1988; Whipple et al. 1992)—an example of a pleasurable stress response.

This chapter addresses the multiple characteristics of vaginal, cervical, and uterine afferent activity, and the extent to which the effects of afferent activity from each of these sites and their underlying mechanisms are distinct from each other.

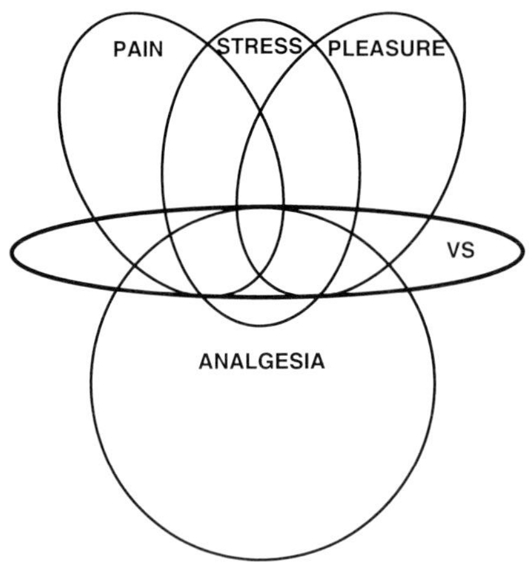

Fig. 1. Venn diagram to represent conceptually both the independence and overlap among the processes discussed in the present chapter. Vaginocervical stimulation (VS) can produce pleasure, stress, pain, and analgesia. Each of the other processes can also produce analgesia. Stress can be pleasurable as well as painful, and can produce analgesia.

VAGINAL AFFERENCE IN HUMANS CAN BE PLEASURABLE, BUT ALSO PAINFUL

In women, mechanical stimulation of the vagina (Ladas et al. 1982; Alzate and Londono 1984; Whipple et al. 1992) and/or the uterine cervix (Komisaruk et al. 1997) can be sufficient to generate pleasurable feelings and orgasm. Excision of the uterine cervix significantly reduces the incidence of orgasm (Kilkku et al. 1983).

However, vaginal stimulation can produce pain under certain pathological conditions, including dyspareunia ("difficult coitus"), which has been distinguished from vaginismus (Meana and Binik 1994), in addition to vulvar vestibulitis, vaginal atrophy as a result of hormonal changes, chronic infections of the genital tract, and malignant and nonmalignant growths (Meana and Binik 1994; Meana et al. 1997). Vaginal stimulation can also produce pain of nonpathological origin—the pain of parturition has been described as among the most severe forms of pain experienced by humans (Melzack 1984).

AVERSIVE RESPONSE TO VAGINAL STIMULATION IN RATS: A MODEL OF PATHOLOGY?

Aversive responses to vaginal stimulation have been demonstrated in rats trained to perform an operant response (moving the head to break a photocell circuit) to escape from stimulation produced by inflating a balloon in the vagina or uterus (Berkley et al. 1995). The rats were less sensitive to the balloon (i.e., they showed escape responses at a higher magnitude of balloon distension) during proestrus and estrus than during metestrus and diestrus (Bradshaw et al. 1999). The authors interpret these findings to indicate that vaginal and uterine stimulation are aversive, but less so during proestrus and estrus, when estrogen levels are relatively high. Transection of the hypogastric nerves, which provide sensory innervation of the uterus (Peters et al. 1987; Berkley et al. 1988), attenuated the escape responses of rats to uterine distension (Temple et al. 1999).

If we conclude from the above studies that vaginal stimulation is aversive or painful and thereby elicits escape behavior, then we must ask whether that phenomenon generalizes to the natural life of the rat. The obvious question that arises is: If the vaginal stimulation that occurs during natural mating is also aversive, why do not female rats learn to avoid mating? It would seem maladaptive for mating to be aversive, for it would inhibit the behavior pattern—mating—that is essential to procreation of the species. On the contrary, it would seem more likely that the vaginal stimulation that is generated by mating would be positively reinforcing rather than aversive, thereby tending to ensure reproduction. Consequently, this paradigm of *aversive* vaginal stimulation would seem to be a model of reproductive tract *pathology,* rather than of normal reproductive behavior.

VAGINAL AFFERENCE IN HUMANS AND RATS: A POTENT PAIN SUPPRESSANT

The mechanostimulation that occurs during natural mating behavior in rats produces a potent analgesia, equivalent to more than 15 mg/kg morphine sulfate (Gomora et al. 1994). The analgesic effect is abolished by transection of the pelvic and hypogastric nerves, but sexual receptivity persists in neurectomized individuals. This finding demonstrates that the analgesia results from the vaginal stimulation per se, rather than from other components of the mating interaction, e.g., arousal and lordosis in response to the male's mounts. This analgesic effect of natural mating can be mimicked by artificial vaginocervical mechanostimulation (VS) (e.g., Komisaruk and Larsson 1971; Komisaruk et al. 1976; Komisaruk and Wallman 1977).

In women, vaginal self-stimulation produces profound analgesia (Whipple and Komisaruk 1985, 1988). Pain threshold, measured by asking subjects to rate pressure applied to the fingers, increased by over 50% during self-applied vaginal pressure. When the women applied the vaginal pressure in a way that they stated felt pleasurable, their pain threshold increased by over 75%. In women who experienced orgasm during this self-stimulation, the pain threshold increased by over 100%. Tactile thresholds, measured concurrently at the hand, did not change significantly. The more pleasurable the vaginal self-stimulation, the greater was the degree of analgesia (Whipple and Komisaruk 1985), which indicates that vaginal self-stimulation-induced analgesia is distinctly different from the class of nociception-induced forms of analgesia (Mayer and Watkins 1984).

As reviewed below, an increase in pain threshold has also been demonstrated in rats during pregnancy (Gintzler 1980; see Chapter 6 of this volume for a detailed review) and parturition (Toniolo et al. 1987), and during parturition in women (Whipple et al. 1990). In rats, the analgesia of pregnancy was significantly reduced by hypogastric nerve transection (Gintzler and Komisaruk 1991), and analgesia produced by mechanostimulation of the uterine cervix was significantly reduced by pelvic nerve transection (Gintzler et al. 1983). These findings suggest that the *natural, gradual* distension of the uterus produced by the developing fetuses during pregnancy produces analgesia, because uterine denervation markedly attenuated analgesia (Gintzler and Komisaruk 1991).

If there is one clear conclusion about the nature of vaginal, cervical, and uterine sensory activity, it is that this activity can produce all three qualities: pleasure, pain, and analgesia. Appreciation of this fact leads to the question, not which is the "real" effect of this afferent activity, but instead: Under which conditions and by which mechanisms does this sensory activity produce each of its effects?

EVIDENCE THAT VAGINOCERVICAL MECHANOSTIMULATION PRODUCES ANALGESIA

EVIDENCE FROM ANIMAL STUDIES

Our laboratory was the first to demonstrate that VS blocks responses to noxious stimulation *but not innocuous stimulation,* on the basis of the following behavioral, neurophysiological, and functional neuroanatomical evidence in the rat: (1) Vaginal and cervical stimulation, applied separately, each blocked the leg-withdrawal reflex to foot pinch, even after total transection of the spinal cord at the mid-thoracic level (Komisaruk and Larsson 1971). (2) Vocalization responses (squeaks) were generated in response to noxious and innocuous sensory stimulation; VS blocked the vocalization to the noxious but not the innocuous stimulation, indicating that VS inhibited the pain, rather than the ability to vocalize (Komisaruk and Wallman 1977). (3) The threshold for electrical current applied to the tail to elicit a vocalization response was increased by VS (Crowley et al. 1976), and VS also increased the latency to flick the tail away from a radiant heat source (Steinman et al. 1983). The magnitude of the pain-inhibitory effect was proportional to the force of VS, and was significantly and strongly augmented by estrogen treatment (Crowley et al. 1976). (4) When confronted with inescapable noxious skin shock, rats performed an appetitive, operant response selectively for VS (Ross et al. 1979). (5) In single neurons of the somatosensory thalamus that responded to innocuous, as well as noxious, sensory stimulation, VS blocked the response of the neurons to the noxious but not the innocuous stimulation (Komisaruk and Wallman 1977). (6) Responses in the (sensory) dorsal horn of the spinal cord to noxious stimulation of the foot were attenuated by VS, as measured by 2-DG, a marker for neuronal activity (Johnson et al. 1988; Johnson and Komisaruk 1996). These findings of a differential suppressive effect on noxious, but not innocuous, sensory stimulation provide evidence that VS produces *analgesia*, rather than anesthesia.

The ability of VS to suppress motor and sensory responses to noxious sensory stimulation is supported by evidence in cats, where VS inhibited responses of leg flexor muscles to foot pinch (Cueva-Rolon et al. 1993). Furthermore, in cats with spinal cord transection above L1, VS depressed the firing rate of spinal cord sensory neurons at L1 in response to noxious cutaneous stimulation (Henry 1983), providing further evidence of the antinociceptive property of VS.

EVIDENCE FROM HUMAN STUDIES

The most critical test of whether vaginal afferent activity produces analgesia requires a verbal report. Consequently, we ascertained the effect of vaginal self-stimulation on pain thresholds and tactile thresholds in women (Komisaruk and Whipple 1984; Whipple and Komisaruk 1985). Pain thresholds were measured using a Ugo Basile algometer, which applies a calibrated compressive force via a lucite pin (1 mm diameter) of gradually increasing intensity to the tips of the fingers, until the subject first reports that the force on the fingers feels painful (pain detection threshold), and then when it feels too uncomfortable to continue (pain tolerance threshold), at which time the force is discontinued. Tactile thresholds were measured by applying von Frey fibers (a set of nylon monofilaments of graded stiffness, calibrated according to the force required to just bend each one) to the dorsum of the hand. All vaginal pressure and pleasurable stimulation was self-applied with a specially developed pressure transducer assembly consisting of a hollow plastic cylinder (a facial-type massager with motor and batteries removed).

In our first study, pressure was self-exerted against the anterior vaginal wall using the stimulator rod. This stimulation significantly elevated pain detection thresholds by 53% over the no-stimulation control condition, but did not significantly affect tactile thresholds. Posterior vaginal wall pressure did not significantly affect pain thresholds. Controls for various forms of distraction did not significantly affect pain thresholds. This selective attenuation of pain, but not touch, and the lack of effect of distraction, confirmed in women that vaginal sensory activity produces analgesia rather than nonspecific anesthesia (Komisaruk and Whipple 1984; Whipple and Komisaruk 1985).

In a second study to determine whether vaginal self-stimulation might be a type of "counter-irritation" that would produce analgesia, we asked the women to apply the vaginal self-stimulation in a manner that felt pleasurable. Under that condition, the pain detection threshold increased significantly by 84%. Four of the 10 women in the study experienced orgasm during the pleasurable self-stimulation; their pain detection threshold increased significantly by 106.7% over the baseline level. The comparable elevation in pain detection threshold during vaginal self-stimulation applied as pressure in the same women (47.4%, confirming the first study) was also significant, but was significantly less than that during pleasurable vaginal self-stimulation or orgasm (Whipple and Komisaruk 1985). Distraction control conditions of watching an exciting movie segment or rubbing a fur mitt against the body surface in a manner that was perceived by the subject as pleasurable did not significantly affect pain thresholds. Two women described vaginal self-stimulation as uncomfortable; they showed the lowest magnitude of analgesia (Whipple and Komisaruk 1985, 1988).

IS VAGINAL STIMULATION-PRODUCED ANALGESIA A FORM OF STRESS-INDUCED ANALGESIA?

Intense sensory stimulation of many different types can produce analgesia, indicating that analgesia can act as a compensatory process that ameliorates the aversive properties of the stimulation (for reviews see Hayes et al. 1978; Terman et al. 1983; Mayer and Watkins 1984; Bodnar 1986; Amit and Galina 1988; Price 1988). This effect, termed stress-induced analgesia (SIA), can be produced by a variety of aversive stimuli, e.g., electric skin shock (Terman et al. 1983), pinching the skin (Ornstein and Amir 1981), or cold-water swim (Bodnar 1986). The question then arises as to whether VS *also* produces analgesia by acting as an aversive stimulus. The short answer is: no. Perhaps the best evidence in support of this contention is that cited just above—that the more pleasurable vaginal self-stimulation produced greater analgesia, and that orgasm produced the greatest magnitude of analgesia. The following section reviews some forms of SIA, and how they differ from VS-produced analgesia.

MECHANISMS OF STRESS-INDUCED ANALGESIA THAT DO NOT APPLY TO VAGINAL STIMULATION-PRODUCED ANALGESIA

OPIOID, DIFFUSE NOXIOUS INHIBITORY CONTROL

Diffuse noxious inhibitory control (DNIC) is a term that describes a form of analgesia produced by noxious somatic stimulation applied to widespread areas of the body in rats (LeBars et al. 1979a,b). VS-produced analgesia is different from DNIC with regard to the nature of the inducing stimulus, the nerves that mediate the response, the time course of the response, and the underlying pharmacology. A more detailed contrast between DNIC and VS-produced analgesia is as follows:

1) DNIC does not inhibit responses to noxious stimuli if they are applied below the level of a spinal cord transection in rats (LeBars et al. 1979b). By stark contrast, VS *does* block leg-withdrawal responses to foot pinch as well as tail-flick responses to radiant heat in rats given a total spinal cord transection at the mid-thoracic level (Komisaruk and Larsson 1971). A likely mechanism for this effect is that VS blocks footshock-induced substance P release into the spinal cord (Steinman et al. 1994). Substance P is released into the spinal cord from primary afferent terminals in response to noxious stimulation (Piercey et al. 1986; Go and Yaksh 1987). Thus, the ability of VS to block substance P release suggests that VS produces presynaptic inhibition of substance P, i.e., at primary afferents, at the level of the first synapse in the spinal cord (Steinman et al. 1994). This could provide a mechanism by which, in spinal-cord-transected rats, VS blocks withdrawal reflexes to noxious intensities of stimulation applied below the level of the transection.

2) DNIC occurs with a latency of "several seconds" (LeBars et al. 1981) in response to noxious pinch or shock applied to the foot or tail. By contrast, VS *immediately* blocks the leg-withdrawal responses to foot pinch; however, tail pinch, used as a control for VS, has no such inhibitory effect on the leg-withdrawal response to foot pinch (Komisaruk and Larsson 1971; Komisaruk and Wallman 1977).

3) DNIC has long-lasting analgesic effects (LeBars et al. 1981). By contrast, the analgesic effect of VS declines sharply within 10 seconds of termination of stimulation (Gomora et al. 1994), then continues to decline gradually over the next few minutes (Komisaruk and Wallman 1977).

4) DNIC can be elicited by noxious stimulation applied to the skin in a wide variety of body regions, including the muzzle, ears, legs, and tail. By contrast, while pressure against the cervix (innervated by the pelvic, hypogastric, and probably vagus nerves; Komisaruk et al. 1972, 1996; Peters et al. 1987) blocks leg withdrawal to foot pinch, the same pressure applied to the immediately surrounding perigenital skin (innervated by the pudendal nerves) does not inhibit the leg-withdrawal response (Komisaruk and Larsson 1971; Komisaruk and Wallman 1977). The profound analgesia that occurs in female rats when they receive intromittive stimulation or ejaculation (i.e., vaginal stimulation) is abolished by transection of the pelvic and hypogastric nerves (Gomora et al. 1994; Fig. 2). While these neurectomized females continue to show sexual responsiveness and to receive intromissions, the absence of analgesia demonstrates that the attendant somatic skin stimulation and arousal are not sufficient to produce analgesia. These findings demonstrate that the analgesia is specific to vaginal (and probably also cervical) stimulation (Gomora et al. 1994).

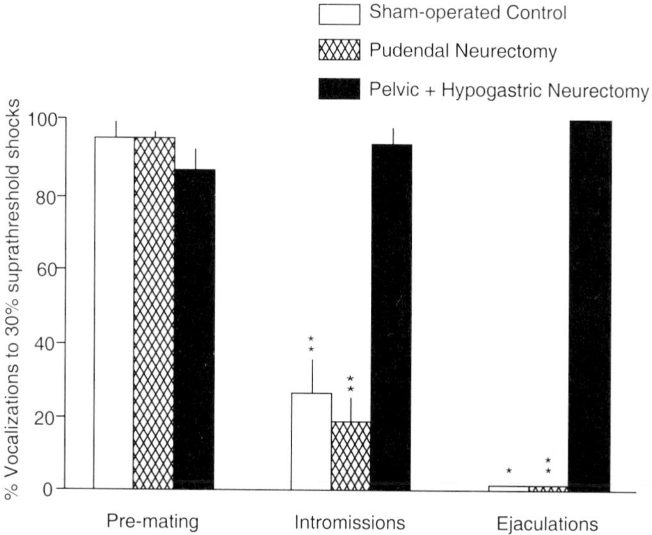

Fig. 2. Analgesia in normal female rats produced by the vaginal stimulation that occurs during natural mating. Vocalization was elicited in the females by 0.1-second tail shocks at a constant voltage, 30% over initial baseline threshold, and the ratio of vocalizations to shocks was recorded. Note that in the intact group, the females' vocalizations were strongly inhibited during intromissions and ejaculations by the males, but in the group in which vaginocervical denervation was produced by transection of the pelvic and hypogastric nerves, there was little or no inhibition. Note also that the females continued to mate after the denervation (Gomora et al. 1994). Asterisks denote * $P < 0.05$, ** $P < 0.002$ compared with corresponding pre-mating level.

5) Naloxone reduces the ability of DNIC to inhibit nociceptive responses of dorsal horn neurons, indicating that DNIC uses an endogenous opioid system (LeBars et al. 1981). By contrast, naloxone only minimally reduces the ability of VS to increase tail-flick latency (Hill and Ayliffe 1981; Steinman et al. 1982); even more noteworthy is the finding that neither naloxone nor induction of morphine tolerance affect the ability of VS to increase vocalization thresholds (Crowley et al. 1977). Specifically, naloxone administered intraperitoneally (10 mg/kg) attenuated VS-produced analgesia measured by tail-flick latency only by about a third, and had no significant effect on VS-produced analgesia when measured by the vocalization threshold (Crowley et al. 1977). Furthermore, rats rendered tolerant to morphine, to the extent that 25 mg/kg morphine sulfate no longer produced an increase in vocalization threshold, showed a completely normal elevation in vocalization threshold in response to VS (Crowley et al. 1977). This evidence clearly shows that VS produces a non-opioid-mediated form of analgesia.

NON-OPIOID, COLD-WATER-SWIM-PRODUCED ANALGESIA

Cold-water swim (CWS) produces a non-opioid form of analgesia (Bodnar 1986), and there is a significant degree of cross-tolerance between CWS- and VS-produced analgesia, in that rats made tolerant to CWS by repeated exposure became significantly less sensitive to VS-produced analgesia (Bodnar and Komisaruk 1984). However, naloxone *increased* CWS analgesia. To account for the findings, Bodnar (1986) proposed the existence of a reciprocal inhibition between opioid- and non-opioid- forms of SIA, such that if the opioid form is blocked, the non-opioid form is potentiated. Thus, the major component of analgesia produced by VS is non-opioid, and furthermore, VS-produced analgesia differs from CWS-produced analgesia in that the former does not show a reciprocal augmentation in response to naloxone.

NON-OPIOID, NMDA-MEDIATED ANALGESIA

The NMDA-receptor antagonist MK-801, when tested in male rats (females were not reported), blocked non-opioid SIA (Ben-Eliyahu et al. 1993). Testing the effect of the NMDA-receptor antagonist AP-5 on VS-produced analgesia, we found the opposite effect: AP-5 significantly and markedly *augmented* the analgesia-producing effect of VS (Caba et al. 1998) and of glycine injected directly to the spinal cord (Beyer et al. 1992). Because VS releases glycine in the spinal cord (Masters et al. 1993), and since glycine stimulates both the glycine (inhibitory) receptor and the NMDA (excitatory) receptor (see Beyer et al. 1992), we concluded that by blocking the excitatory component of glycine, we augmented its inhibitory action, thereby inhibiting responses to noxious sensory stimulation (Beyer et al. 1992; Caba et al. 1998). Consequently, VS evidently produces its non-opioid-mediated analgesia component by a mechanism other than by blocking the NMDA receptor.

Other forms of non-opioid analgesia are also evidently different from VS-produced analgesia. Thus, adrenalectomy, hypophysectomy, or dexamethasone treatment (which inhibits the release of ACTH and β-endorphin from the anterior pituitary) significantly attenuate non-opioid-mediated SIA (Mousa et al. 1983). However, since VS-produced analgesia occurs immediately upon application of VS (Komisaruk and Wallman 1977), the time constraint alone of activating the brain-pituitary-adrenal axis would render it unlikely that this axis is necessary for VS-produced analgesia.

Having ruled out the above mechanisms, how, then, does VS produce analgesia?

EVIDENCE THAT VAGINOCERVICAL STIMULATION ACTIVATES COMPONENTS OF THE STRESS-INDUCED ANALGESIA SYSTEM

PARALLELS BETWEEN SIA AND VS-PRODUCED ANALGESIA

Some of the brain regions that mediate sexual responses also mediate some forms of SIA, which suggests a convergence between the two mechanisms. In the medulla and forebrain, neural responses in rats to vaginal stimulation have been observed in the same regions in which electrical or pharmacological stimulation can attenuate responses to noxious stimulation. Thus, electrical stimulation of the nucleus reticularis paragigantocellularis (NRPG) of the medulla inhibits behavioral responses to noxious stimulation (Hammond and Yaksh 1984; Hammond 1986), and neuronal firing activity in the NRPG increases in response to VS (Hornby and Rose 1976). Furthermore, in rats, electrical stimulation of the medial preoptic area of the forebrain attenuates responses of trigeminal nucleus neurons to noxious stimulation (Mokha et al. 1987), and artificial VS increases levels of ^{14}C-2-deoxyglucose in the medial preoptic area (Allen et al. 1981). In response to mating, FOS protein increases in the medial preoptic area (Erskine 1993), and during parturition, the levels of both ^{14}C-2-deoxyglucose (Del Cerro et al. 1995) and *c-fos* (Komisaruk et al. 2000) increase in the medial preoptic area, both probably resulting from the natural vaginal stimulation.

Electrical stimulation of the midbrain periaqueductal gray matter (PAG) attenuates responses of spinal cord neurons to noxious heat, but not innocuous stimulation (Bennett and Mayer 1979). Local administration to the PAG of pharmacological agents that mimic or antagonize the action of the inhibitory neurotransmitter GABA respectively facilitate or attenuate sexual receptivity in rats (McCarthy et al. 1991).

A neural pathway has been identified that descends from the lower brainstem to the spinal cord and "gates" (i.e., attenuates) pain at the level of the spinal cord (Basbaum and Fields 1978). Transection of this pathway, the dorsolateral funiculus, blocks the ability of NRPG stimulation to attenuate responses of neurons in the spinal cord to noxious stimulation (Basbaum et al. 1978). Transection of the same descending pathway also attenuates the ability of VS to block behavioral responses to noxious stimulation (Watkins et al. 1984). Extensive evidence shows that this neural pathway utilizes norepinephrine and serotonin. These neurotransmitters are released into the spinal cord in response to VS; pharmacological antagonists of norepinephrine and serotonin attenuate the analgesia produced by electrical stimulation of this system at the level of the lower brainstem (for review see Hammond 1986). VS also releases norepinephrine and serotonin into the spinal cord (Steinman et al. 1983), and administration to the spinal cord of receptor antagonists of these agents attenuates the analgesic effect of VS (Steinman et al. 1983). These findings suggest that VS accesses and utilizes, at least in part, this major pain-gating endogenous neural system (see Fig. 3 for a schematic representation of these mechanisms).

Two types of neurons have been characterized in the raphe nuclei in the rat, termed "on" cells and "off" cells, on the basis that the cells either become active or inactive, respectively, when the tail flicks away from a radiant heat source (Heinricher et al. 1989). Without exception, "on" cells, while firing in response to noxious heat directed at the tail, were inhibited by VS, and "off" cells, while *not* firing when noxious heat was applied to the tail, were stimulated to fire by VS (Rojas-Piloni et al. 1998). Thus, the effects of VS on these raphe neurons were diametrically opposite to the effects of noxious heat applied to the tail. The "on" cells are interpreted to be pain-responsive cells (Heinricher et al. 1989). The interpretation by Cueva's group was that VS, while inhibiting these pain-responsive cells, activated pain-inhibitory cells (Rojas-Piloni et al. 1998). They speculated that the "off" cells are the serotonin-synthesizing cells of the median raphe that project to the spinal cord where they release serotonin, thereby producing antinociception. This interpretation is consistent with our previous findings (Steinman et al. 1983) that VS releases serotonin (and norepinephrine) into superfusates of the spinal cord, and that the serotonin receptor antagonist, methysergide, attenuates the analgesic effect of VS.

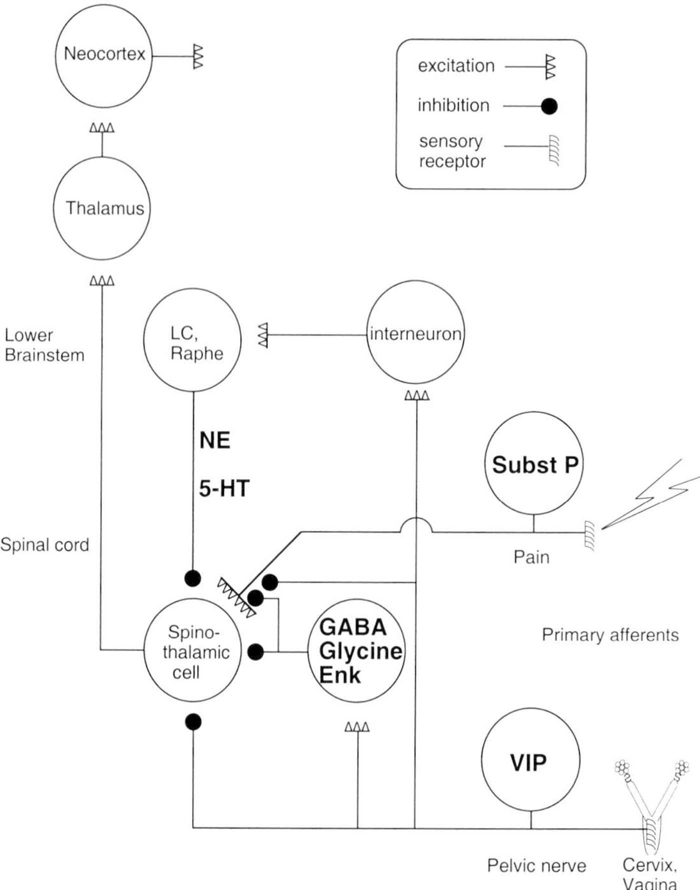

Fig. 3. Schematic representation of pathways and neurotransmitter neuromodulators that mediate vaginocervical stimulation (VS)-produced analgesia. Note that the descending serotoninergic and noradrenergic pathways are activated by VS, as in the Basbaum and Fields (1978) model of the endogenous analgesia system. Evidence indicates that the interneuronal transmitters GABA and glycine play a significant role, and that there is a minor endogenous opioid component. Since the release of substance P by noxious stimulation is inhibited by VS, we have postulated a presynaptic inhibitory effect of VS (Steinman et al. 1994). We suggest that vasoactive intestinal peptide (VIP) is a primary afferent trigger for the analgesic response to VS, on the basis that it is released into superfusates of the spinal cord by VS and produces analgesia when administered directly to the spinal cord (Komisaruk et al. 1988, 1989). Other abbreviations: Enk = enkephalin; NE = norepinephrine; 5-HT = serotonin; LC = locus ceruleus.

On the sensory side, there is some evidence, although scant, that the anterolateral columns, which convey nociceptive activity to the brain, also convey sensory input in the sexual system. In rats, transection of the anterolateral columns reduces the incidence of lordosis responding (Pfaff 1980).

In humans, a clinical report states that after anterolateral spinal cord transection was performed to control intractable pain in a male patient, he lost the ability to experience orgasm; however, several months later, the sensation of pain returned, and along with it, his ability to experience orgasm (Elliott 1969).

Thus, evidence suggests that the well-documented endogenous analgesia-producing system of the brain and spinal cord is accessed by sensory input evoked by both noxious stimulation and sexual stimulation. While it is commonly recognized that the endogenous analgesia-producing system is activated by noxious, stressful stimuli (for review see Hayes et al. 1978; Mayer and Watkins 1984; Price 1988), the studies reviewed above show that sensory stimulation of the reproductive tract, evoked naturally during mating and parturition, can also activate this system.

IS VAGINAL STIMULATION A "PLEASURABLE STRESSOR?"

The above evidence raises the question of whether VS-produced analgesia is a form of stress-induced analgesia. The answer is "yes" if it is acknowledged that stress is not necessarily aversive and can be pleasurable. Thus, the marked increases in heart rate and blood pressure that occur at orgasm in humans (Whipple et al. 1992) appear, from the physiological record, to be a significant stress, yet this experience can be intensely pleasurable. Similarly, sports, sky-diving, and roller coasters induce stress, but since they are voluntarily sought, they are, by definition, non-aversive; in fact, they are pleasurable in the excitement they produce (i.e., the activation of the sympathetic division of the autonomic system).

In female rats, VS produces an immediate and marked increase in heart rate, blood pressure, and pupil diameter (Catelli et al. 1987), the latter response occurring also during the intromissions and ejaculation that occur during natural mating (Szechtman et al. 1985). Since female rats "pace" the timing of their coming and going into the males' cage when provided the opportunity (Bermant 1961; Peirce and Nuttall 1961; Erskine 1992), this stress response related to mating behavior is evidently not aversive. Vaginal self-stimulation produces the same sympathetic-activating effects in women, i.e., markedly increasing heart rate and blood pressure, pupil dilatation, and higher pain thresholds (Whipple et al. 1992). Thus, pleasure can be a stressor, stress can be pleasurable, and vaginal stimulation can produce a pleasurable-stress-induced analgesia.

It should be noted that in female rats, the increase in blood pressure that occurs during VS-produced analgesia is neither necessary nor sufficient for the analgesia, because pharmacological blockade of the VS-produced blood pressure elevation by the ganglionic blocker chlorisondamine does not attenuate the analgesia. Furthermore, mimicking the magnitude of VS-produced blood pressure elevation with phenylephrine does not produce analgesia (Catelli et al. 1987). Thus, the sympathetic activation and the analgesia produced by VS are "in-parallel" rather than "in-series" responses to VS.

Evidently, VS can activate the same endogenous pain-suppression system as can noxious stimulation, without itself being aversive. To understand how a noxious and an innocuous stimulus could each activate the same endogenous analgesia-producing mechanism, an analogy may be instructive. The total heat *energy* contained in a bathtub full of warm water is greater than that in a cup of hot water, although the *temperature* of the water in the cup is higher. Thus, perhaps the vaginal afferent stimulation has a greater amount of energy input to the endogenous pain-suppression system, but at a lower intensity than painful stimulation, so that both types of input can provide an amount of energy that is adequate to activate the same analgesia-producing mechanism. In other words, the high *intensity* of the noxious stimulus is perceived as pain, while the lower intensity, but high total *energy* of the innocuous stimulus may be perceived as pleasure, and each can activate the same endogenous analgesia system.

TWO PARADOXES

CAN PLEASURE, PAIN, AND ANALGESIA BE ELICITED VIA THE SAME (PELVIC) NERVE?

Vaginal stimulation poses two paradoxes that if solved, could reveal an important process. The first is that vaginal stimulation can itself be painful (Meana and Binik 1994; Meana et al. 1997) or intensely pleasurable (Alzate and Londono 1984), and it can produce an immediate onset of analgesia without being aversive (Whipple and Komisaruk 1985). While the first of these effects would seem to be mutually exclusive with the other two, all three effects can evidently be conveyed to the central nervous system via the same, pelvic, nerve.

The pelvic nerve is the major vaginal afferent nerve, based on studies conducted to map the vaginal sensory field (Komisaruk et al. 1972; Peters et al. 1987; Berkley et al. 1990, 1993) and to ascertain the behavioral and physiological effects of transecting the pelvic nerve (Cunningham et al. 1991; Cueva-Rolon et al. 1996). The pelvic nerve predominantly contains small-diameter, unmyelinated C fibers (Patton 1961). In rats, neonatal injection of capsaicin, the pungent component of hot chili peppers, can irreversibly destroy this type of fiber in various peripheral nerves (as well as neurons in some regions of the spinal cord and brain) (Nagy 1982; Buck and Burks 1986).

We found that neonatal capsaicin attenuates or abolishes the effects of VS on analgesia and diminishes the extensor component of the sexual response in adult rats (Rodriguez-Sierra et al. 1988). This finding suggests that C fibers contain analgesia-triggering primary afferent neurotransmitters/neuromodulators. Furthermore, neonatal capsaicin treatment reduces the release of glycine, which contributes significantly to VS-produced analgesia (Beyer et al. 1992), into superfusates of the spinal cord (Masters et al. 1993). Consistent with its effect of disrupting vaginocervical sensory input, neonatal capsaicin treatment blocks neuroendocrine reflex responses to mating or artificial VS in female rats (Traurig et al. 1984, 1988; Nance et al. 1987).

In rats, capsaicin can exert neurotoxic effects via the gastric route (Pellicer et al. 1996). We speculated that early exposure to capsaicin via ingestion may exert disruptive effects on vaginocervical afference not only in rats, but in humans. We found that women who had consumed a diet high in hot chili peppers daily since childhood showed a significantly lower magnitude of VS-produced analgesia than did women whose diet was low in hot chili peppers (Whipple et al. 1989).

By destroying C fibers, neonatal capsaicin administration renders rats insensitive to various types of noxious stimuli, e.g., thermal and chemical (Nagy 1982; Buck and Burks 1986). However, capsaicin does not destroy Aδ fibers, which can also convey certain types of nociception, e.g., pinch. Our capsaicin-treated rats showed normal leg-withdrawal responses to foot pinch, but in diametric opposition to control rats, VS failed to block the withdrawal responses to foot pinch in the capsaicin-treated rats. In capsaicin-treated rats, VS also failed to facilitate the lordosis response, although all the control animals showed a strong facilitation of lordosis in response to VS. Consistent with our findings that neonatal capsaicin treatment blocks the effect of VS, Traurig et al. (1988) showed that rats treated neonatally with capsaicin mated, but failed to become pregnant. Their interpretation was that the capsaicin treatment blocked the requisite C-fiber afferent activity from the cervix that is necessary to release the hormones required for pregnancy (for review, see Komisaruk 1990).

Our interpretation of these findings is that leg withdrawal to foot pinch is mediated by Aδ fibers, whereas the critical vaginocervical afferent neurons, whose action was blocked, were C fibers. The paradox is that these findings suggest that pain and afferent signals that can block pain are *both* conveyed by C fibers. There is certainly VS-elicited pain (e.g., dyspareunia). There is certainly VS-produced pleasure (e.g., orgasm). There is certainly VS-produced analgesia.

An analogy to the possibility that the pelvic nerve conveys noxious as well as innocuous afferent activity is the case of allodynia (pain from innocuous stimulation). Extensive recent evidence suggests that nociceptive and non-nociceptive input can be conveyed along the same sensory nerves, as in the case of allodynia. We found that allodynia can result from a decrease in tonic GABAergic and/or glycinergic activity (Beyer et al. 1985; Roberts et al. 1986). Application directly to the spinal cord of receptor blockers of the inhibitory neurotransmitters GABA and glycine (e.g., bicuculline and strychnine, respectively) rendered rats exquisitely sensitive to the very mildest of stimuli (e.g., gently blowing on the fur) to the extent that they expressed intense distress vocalization in response to this gentle stimulus (Beyer et al. 1985; Roberts et al. 1986). Our interpretation has been supported in numerous recent reports by other laboratories (e.g., Yaksh 1989; Sivilotti and Woolf 1994). Thus, a change in the balance of neuromodulators in a neural system could drastically alter the subject's perception of afferent activity conveyed via a given nerve.

Three different nerves convey afferent activity from the region of the cervix: the pelvic, hypogastric, and vagus nerves (Komisaruk et al. 1972, 1996, 1997; Peters et al. 1987; Ortega-Villalobos et al. 1990; Robbins et al. 1990; Berkley et al. 1993; Bianca et al. 1994; Cueva-Rolon et al. 1994; Hubscher and Berkley 1995). Thus, it is quite possible that different perceptual qualities are elicited by different combinations of the input from these nerves. For example, direct electrical stimulation of just the vagus nerve elicited both nociceptive and analgesic responses that differed according to the stimulation parameters (Randich and Aicher 1988).

Our recent findings suggest that in women, afferent activity from the vagina and cervix can be conveyed via the vagus nerves, and this activity can induce a variety of perceptual responses. We studied women who were diagnosed with "complete" spinal cord injury (i.e., absence of cutaneous sensibility to pinprick or cotton wisp, and absence of voluntary movement below the level of the injury). Included in the study was a group of women whose injury was above the level of entry into the spinal cord of both the pelvic and hypogastric nerves (i.e., injury at or above T10). These women reported menstrual discomfort, and in response to vaginal or cervical self-stimulation they experienced analgesia (measured at the fingers), orgasm (Komisaruk et al. 1997), and cardiovascular responses (Whipple et al. 1996) (see Figs. 4, 5). In support of these findings, in rats after spinal cord transection at T5, we observed a persistence of responses to VS that are mediated above the level of the transection (i.e., algesic and pupillary). These responses were abolished by subsequent bilateral subdiaphragmatic vagotomy (Komisaruk et al. 1996).

Afferent activity generated in the genital system is strongly modulated by ovarian steroid hormones (e.g., Komisaruk et al. 1972; Robbins et al.

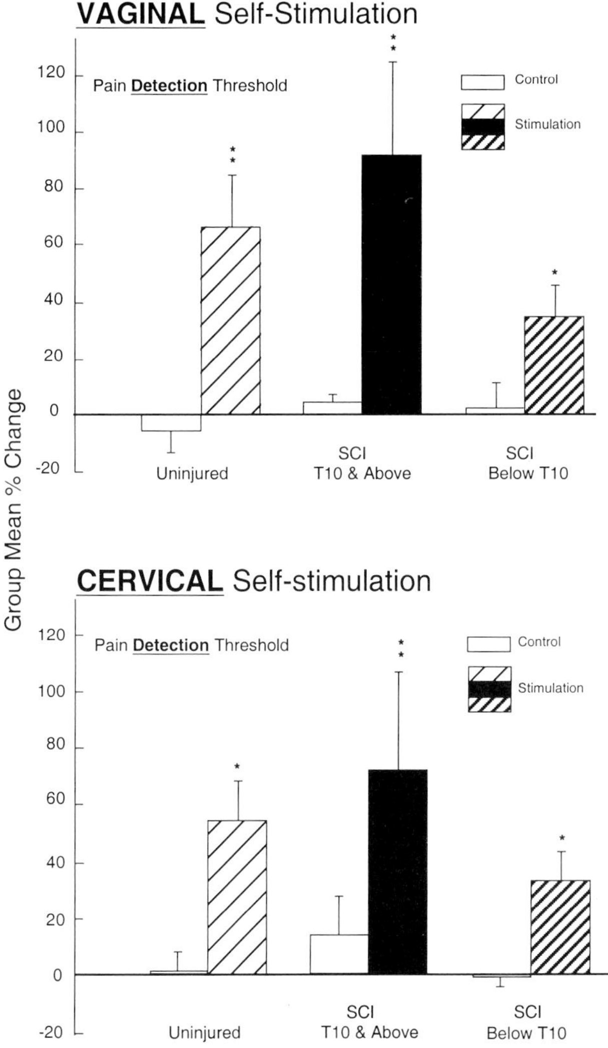

Fig. 4. Vaginal and cervical self-stimulation produced a significant elevation in pain detection threshold (measured at the finger tips), in women with "complete" spinal cord injury (SCI) at the two levels shown, and in non-injured women. The SCI at T10 and above would interrupt ascending activity conveyed via the hypogastric and pelvic nerves, whereas the SCI below T10 would allow at least some ascending activity conveyed via the hypogastric, but not the pelvic nerve. Since analgesia is produced in the women with complete SCI at and above T10, and since these women can experience menstrual discomfort (and in one in six cases, orgasm), we have postulated that vaginal and cervical afferent activity can also be conveyed via the vagus nerves (Whipple et al. 1996; Komisaruk et al. 1997).

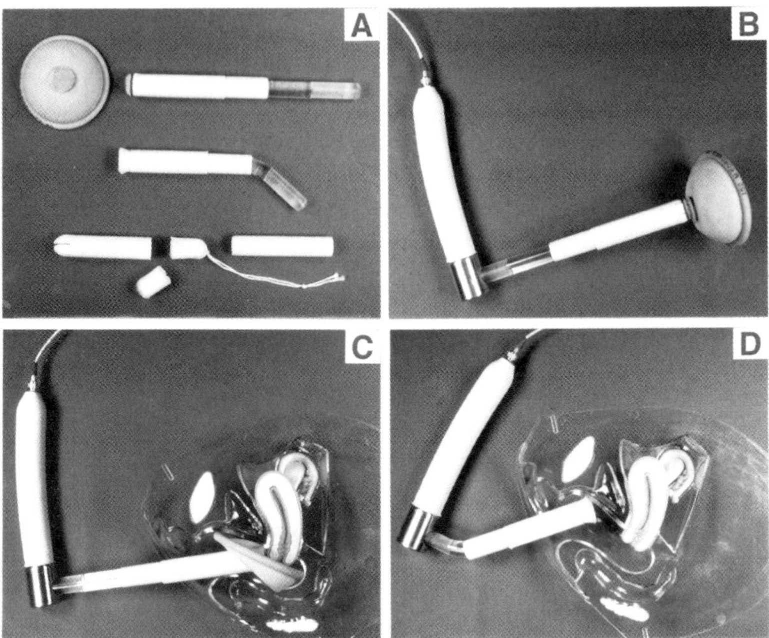

Fig. 5. Photograph of the vaginal and cervical self-stimulator, made from a modified tampon, and mounted on a passive (non-vibrating) handle, in the neck of which is mounted a force transducer. The cervical self-stimulator is attached to a gynecological diaphragm that protects the cervix and maintains the stimulator centered on the cervix (Komisaruk et al. 1997).

1992). Consequently, it should not be surprising that multiple perceptual qualities, including pleasure, pain, and analgesia, can each and all be produced by vaginal stimulation. And certainly, the central nervous system can provide additional "sculpting" of the hedonic quality of this afferent activity.

IS THE VAGINAL STIMULATION OF MATING BEHAVIOR IN RATS AVERSIVE? OR IS IT SATIATING?

A second interesting paradox concerns the nature of the effect of vaginal stimulation under natural mating conditions. A female rat, given the opportunity to enter the cage of a male rat and exit at will (the entrance being too small to allow the male to pass through), will vary the interval between freely entering and leaving as a function of whether she receives vaginal stimulation from the male (Erskine 1992; Coopersmith et al. 1996). That is, if the male mounts without intromission (penile insertion), the female either does not leave, or leaves and then returns with a shorter latency than if she received an intromission or ejaculation during the mount. These findings confirm and extend earlier findings (Bermant 1961; Peirce and Nuttall 1961). Consistent with these findings, if the pelvic nerves are transected, thereby producing a vaginal deafferentation, the females show a shorter latency to return to the male—a latency not significantly different from the latency to return after mounts without intromissions (Erskine 1992).

This finding is paradoxical, for it can be interpreted in two diametrically opposite ways—i.e., (1) the female rat waits until the aversiveness of the vaginal stimulation wanes before she returns for more, or (2) after a *non*-intromittive mount, the female rat does not leave, or else returns more quickly, because she did not receive the stimulation she was seeking, and is therefore trying to obtain it again sooner. In other words, the vaginal stimulation generated by an intromission could either be viewed as transiently aversive—more so than a non-intromittive mount—so the female waits until the stimulation subsides before returning to the male, or alternatively, an intromission could be viewed as transiently *satisfying*—more so than a non-intromittive mount—so the female is not motivated to return for another intromission as quickly. This apparent paradox has not been resolved.

Two findings that are probably based on a related process, but that present the same type of paradox, are that in female rats in which intromissions are blocked by a vaginal "mask" applied by the investigators, receptivity continues longer than in females that can receive intromissions (Hardy and Debold 1972). Similarly, if the pelvic nerves are transected, sexual receptivity continues longer than in intact females (Lodder and Zeilmaker 1976). Evidently, vaginal afferent activity is necessary to terminate the period of sexual receptivity in rats. This "refractory" effect of vaginal stimulation could be due to a nociceptive component, just as well as to an "appetitive satiation" process that is not necessarily aversive.

ADAPTIVE SIGNIFICANCE OF VAGINAL STIMULATION-PRODUCED ANALGESIA: PROCREATION

The above paradoxes raise the question: Is vaginal stimulation during mating aversive, but is the female so highly motivated to mate that she returns repeatedly for more stimulation despite the aversiveness? If it were so aversive, why would she not eventually learn to avoid the stimulation? Of course, if she learned to avoid vaginal stimulation, she would cease to procreate, a potentiality that evidently has not occurred. Indeed, Erskine (1992) has shown that the female's likelihood of becoming pregnant is greater if she paces her vaginal stimulation than if she receives uncontrolled mating stimulation from the male.

In the rat, VS elicits the female mating stance (the lordosis response), a dorsiflexion posture in which the pelvis is elevated and the lumbar region depressed, thereby exposing the vaginal orifice (Komisaruk and Diakow 1973). VS also induces sexual receptivity in previously unreceptive female rats tested with males (Rodriguez-Sierra et al. 1975). The lordosis-facilitating effect of 1-second application of VS persists for 2–3 hours (Rodriguez-Sierra et al. 1975). The receptivity-inducing and lordosis-facilitating effect of VS probably facilitates the impregnation process by increasing the likelihood that the female rat will accept the average number of eight intromissions prior to the male's ejaculation. These multiple intromissions are necessary to stimulate adequate levels of reflexive release of hormones (e.g., prolactin and progesterone) to prepare the uterus for implantation of the fertilized ovum. If the female rat receives too few intromissions prior to the male's ejaculation, inadequate levels of these hormones are released, and consequently, she fails to become pregnant (Adler 1969; Adler et al. 1970). In the context of mating, the analgesic effect of VS may increase the female rat's willingness to accept these multiple intromissions (Komisaruk and Whipple 1995), which are necessary for successful impregnation.

We speculate that one aspect of the adaptive significance of VS-produced analgesia is that it could reduce potentially aversive intensities of sensory stimulation that may occur naturally during coitus, and thereby increase the positive-reinforcing effects of the pleasurable component of the sensory stimulation. In this view, the pleasurable component of vaginal sensory activity would play a significant reinforcing role in coitus, and the pain-attenuating effect of vaginal sensory activity could facilitate that reinforcing effect by attenuating aversive components of the stimulation. These pain-attenuating and pleasure-inducing processes would, by acting in concert, facilitate the performance of coitus and thereby promote the process of reproduction.

In a different context, the VS-produced analgesia mechanism is evidently also activated during labor and delivery, when the contractions and the fetus-produced distension of the birth canal (uterus, cervix, and vagina) generate afferent activity via the sensory nerves of the reproductive tract.

CONCLUSIONS

The evidence presented in this chapter shows that the sensory input produced by vaginal stimulation produces a powerful analgesic effect. The function of this process may be to promote the behavioral patterns that result in fertilization, parturition, and maternal care of the young, thereby promoting procreation. Since sensory stimulation that occurs normally during mating and parturition could become sufficiently intense to reach aversive levels, it would seem adaptive for a mechanism to exist that could diminish the ability of aversive sensory activity from the genital system to interfere with mating behavior and perhaps with maternal behavior and nursing. In humans, the pleasurable component of vaginal stimulation could be an adaptive mechanism whose function is to promote and ensure procreation. In that sense, "sexual pleasure" could be a significant adaptive factor in the physiology of reproduction and the evolution of the species.

ACKNOWLEDGMENTS

Recent research reported herein was supported by grant 1 RO1 HD30156 from the Basic Rehabilitation Medicine Research Branch, National Center for Medical Rehabilitation Research, National Institute of Child Health and Human Development, The National Institutes of Health (B.R. Komisaruk and B. Whipple); by grant S06 GM08223, from the Minority Biomedical Research Support Program, National Institute of General Medical Sciences, the National Institutes of Health (Bethesda, MD) (B.R. Komisaruk and B. Whipple); and by the Charles and Johanna Busch Foundation (New Brunswick, NJ) (B.R. Komisaruk and B. Whipple).

REFERENCES

Adler NT. The effect of the male's copulatory behavior on successful pregnancy of the female rat. *J Comp Physiol Psychol* 1969; 69:613–622.

Adler NT, Resko JA, Goy RW. The effect of copulatory behavior on hormonal change in the female rat prior to implantation. *Physiol Behav* 1970; 5:1003–1007.

Allen TO, Adler NT, Greenberg JH, Reivich M. Vaginocervical stimulation selectively increases metabolic activity in the rat brain. *Science* 1981; 211:1070–1072.

Alzate H, Londono ML. Vaginal erotic sensitivity. *J Sex Marital Ther* 1984; 10:49–56.

Amit Z. Galina ZH. Stress induced analgesia plays an adaptive role in the organization of behavioral responding. *Brain Res Bull* 1988; 21:955–958.

Basbaum AI, Fields HL. Endogenous pain control mechanisms: review and hypothesis. *Ann Neurol* 1978; 4:451–462.

Basbaum AI, Clanton CH, Fields HL. Three bulbospinal pathways from the rostral medulla of the cat: an autoradiographic study of pain modulating systems. *J Comp Neurol* 1978; 178:209–224.

Ben-Eliyahu S, Page GG, Marek P, et al. The NMDA receptor antagonist MK-801 blocks nonopioid stress induced analgesia and decreases tumor metastasis in the rat. *Proc West Pharmacol Soc* 1993; 36:293–298.

Bennett CJ, Mayer DJ. Inhibition of spinal cord interneurons by narcotic microinjection and focal electrical stimulation in the periaqueductal central gray matter. *Brain Res* 1979; 172:243–257.

Berkley KJ, Hotta H, Robbins A, Sato Y. Functional properties of afferent fibers supplying reproductive and other pelvic organs in pelvic nerve of female rats. *J Neurophysiol* 1990; 63:256–272.

Berkley KJ, Robbins A, Sato Y. Afferent fibers supplying the uterus in the rat. *J Neurophysiol* 1988; 59:142–163.

Berkley KJ, Robbins A, Sato Y. Functional differences between afferent fibers in the hypogastric and pelvic nerves innervating female reproductive organs in the rat. *J Neurophysiol* 1993; 69:533–544.

Berkley KJ, Wood E, Scofield SL, Little M. Behavioral responses to uterine or vaginal distension in the rat. *Pain* 1995; 61:121–131.

Bermant G. Response latencies of female rats during sexual intercourse. *Science* 1961; 133:1771–1773.

Beyer C, Komisaruk BR, Lopez-Colome A-M, Caba M. Administration of AP5, a glutamate antagonist, unmasks glycine analgesic actions in the rat. *Pharmacol Biochem Behav* 1992; 41:229–232.

Beyer C, Roberts L, Komisaruk BR. Hyperalgesia induced by altered glycinergic activity at the spinal cord. *Life Sci* 1985; 37:295–301.

Bianca R, Sansone G, Cueva-Rolon R, et al. Evidence that the vagus nerve mediates a response to vaginocervical stimulation after spinal cord transection in the rat. *Soc Neurosci Abstracts* 1994; 20:961.

Bodnar R. Neuropharmacological and neuroendocrine substrates of stress-induced analgesia. *Ann NY Acad Sci* 1986; 467:345–360.

Bodnar R, Komisaruk BR. Reduction in cervical probing analgesia by repeated prior exposure to cold-water swims. *Physiol Behav* 1984; 32:653–655.

Bradshaw HB, Temple JL, Wood E, Berkley KJ. Estrous variations in behavioral responses to vaginal and uterine distention in the rat. *Pain* 1999; 82:187–197.

Buck SH, Burks TF. The neuropharmacology of capsaicin: review of some recent observations. *Pharmacol Rev* 1986; 38:179–226.

Caba M, Banas C, Komisaruk BR, Beyer C. Administration of AP-5, an NMDA antagonist, enhances analgesia produced by vaginocervical stimulation in rats. *Pharmacol Biochem Behav* 1998; 61:45–48.

Catelli JJ, Sved AF, Komisaruk BR. Vaginocervical stimulation elevates blood pressure and induces analgesia by separate mechanisms. *Physiol Behav* 1987; 41:609–612.

Coopersmith C, Candurra C, Erskine MS. Effects of paced mating and intromissive stimulation on feminine sexual behavior and estrus termination in the cycling rat. *J Comp Psychol* 1996; 110:176–186.

Crowley WR, Jacobs R, Volpe J, Rodriguez-Sierra JF, Komisaruk BR. Analgesic effect of vaginal stimulation in rats: Modulation by graded stimulus intensity and hormones. *Physiol Behav* 1976; 16:483–448.

Crowley WR, Rodriguez-Sierra JF, Komisaruk BR. Analgesia induced by vaginal stimulation in rats is apparently independent of a morphine-sensitive process. *Psychopharmacology* 1977; 54:223–225.

Cueva-Rolon R, Munoz-Martinez EJ, Delgado-Lezama R, Raya G. Prolonged inhibition of the flexor reflex by probing the cervix uteri in the cat. *Brain Res* 1993; 600:27–32.

Cueva-Rolon R, Sansone G, Bianca R, et al. Evidence that the vagus nerve mediates some effects of vaginocervical stimulation after genital deafferentation in the rat. *Soc Neurosci Abstracts* 1994; 20:961.

Cueva-Rolon R, Sansone G, Bianca R, et al. Vagotomy blocks responses to vaginocervical stimulation in genitospinal-neurectomized rats. *Physiol Behav* 1996; 60:19–24.

Cunningham ST, Steinman JL, Whipple B, Mayer AD, Komisaruk BR. Differential roles of hypogastric and pelvic nerves in the analgesic and motoric effects of vaginocervical stimulation in rats. *Brain Res* 1991; 559:337–343.

Del Cerro MCR, Perez Izquierdo MA, Rosenblatt JS, et al. Brain 2-deoxyglucose levels related to maternal behavior-inducing stimuli in the rat. *Brain Res* 1995; 696:213–220.

Elliott HC. *Textbook of Neuroanatomy*. Philadelphia: J.B. Lippincott, 1969.

Erskine MS. Pelvic and pudendal nerves influence the display of paced mating behavior in response to estrogen and progesterone in the female rat. *Behav Neurosci* 1992; 106:690–697.

Erskine MS. Mating-induced increases in FOS protein in preoptic area and medial amygdala of cycling female rats. *Brain Res Bull* 1993; 32:447–451.

Gintzler AR. Endorphin-mediated increases in pain threshold during pregnancy. *Science* 1980; 210:193–195.

Gintzler AR, Komisaruk BR. Analgesia produced by uterocervical mechanostimulation in the rat: role of afferent nerves and implications for analgesia of pregnancy and parturition. *Brain Res* 1991; 566:299–302.

Gintzler AR, Peters LC, Komisaruk BR. Attenuation of pregnancy-induced analgesia by hypogastric neurectomy in rats. *Brain Res* 1983; 277:186–188.

Go VL, Yaksh TL. Release of substance P from the cat spinal cord. *J Physiol (Lond)* 1987; 391:141–167.

Gomora P, Beyer C, Gonzalez-Mariscal G, Komisaruk BR. Momentary analgesia produced by copulation in female rats. *Brain Res* 1994; 656:52–58.

Hammond DL. Control systems for nociceptive afferent processing: the descending inhibitory pathways. In: Yaksh TL (Eds). *Spinal Afferent Processing*. New York: Plenum Press, 1986, pp 363–390.

Hammond DL, Yaksh TL. Antagonism of stimulation-produced antinociception by intrathecal administration of methysergide or phentolamine. *Brain Res* 1984; 298:329–337.

Hardy DFA, DeBold JF. Effects of coital stimulation upon behavior of the female rat. *J Comp Physiol Psychol* 1972; 78:400–408.

Hayes RL, Bennett GJ, Newlon PG, Mayer DJ. Behavioral and physiological studies of non-narcotic analgesia in the rat elicited by certain environmental stimuli. *Brain Res* 1978; 155:69–90.

Heinricher MM, Barbaro NM, Fields HL. Putative nociceptive modulatory neurons in the rostral ventromedial medulla of the rat: firing of on- and off-cells is related to nociceptive responsiveness. *Somatosens Mot Res* 1989; 6:427–439.

Henry JL. Low threshold mechanical stimulation of the vagina depresses dorsal horn unit activity in the spinal cat. *Neurosci Lett* 1983; 38:257–262.

Hill RG, Ayliffe SJ. The antinociceptive effect of vaginal stimulation in the rat is reduced by naloxone. *Pharmacol Biochem Behav* 1981; 14:631–632.

Hornby JB, Rose JD. Responses of caudal brain stem neurons to vaginal and somatosensory stimulation in the rat and evidence of genital-nociceptive interactions. *Exp Neurol* 1976; 51:363–376.

Hubscher CH, Berkley KJ. Spinal and vagal influences on the responses of rat solitary nucleus neurons to stimulation of uterus, cervix and vagina. *Brain Res* 1995; 702:251–254.

Johnson BM, Komisaruk BR. Antinociceptive action of vaginocervical stimulation in rat spinal cord: 2-DG analysis. *Physiol Behav* 1996; 60:979–983.

Johnson BM, Pott C, Siegel A, Adler NT, Komisaruk BR. Vaginocervical stimulation suppresses noxious sensory input at the spinal cord; 2-DG autoradiographic evidence. *Soc Neurosci Abstracts* 1988; (14):709.

Kilkku P, Gronroos M, Hirvonean T, Rauramo L. Supravaginal uterine amputation vs. hysterectomy. *Acta Obstet Gynecol Scand* 1983; 62:147–152.

Komisaruk BR. Vaginocervical afference as a trigger for analgesic, behavioral, autonomic and neuroendocrine processes. In: Archer T, Hansen S (Eds). *Behavioral Biology: Neuroendocrine Axis*. Hillsdale, NJ: Lawrence Erlbaum Associates, 1990, pp 123–137.

Komisaruk BR, Diakow C. Lordosis reflex intensity in rats in relation to the estrous cycle, ovariectomy, estrogen administration, and mating behavior. *Endocrinology* 1973; 93:548–557.

Komisaruk BR, Larsson K. Suppression of a spinal and a cranial nerve reflex by vaginal or rectal probing in rats. *Brain Res* 1971; 35:231–235.

Komisaruk BR, Wallman J. Antinociceptive effects of vaginal stimulation in rats: neurophysiological and behavioral studies. *Brain Res* 1977; 137:85–107.

Komisaruk BR, Whipple B. Evidence that vaginal self-stimulation in women suppresses experimentally-induced finger pain. *Soc Neurosci Abstracts* 1984; 10:675.

Komisaruk BR, Whipple B. The suppression of pain by genital stimulation in females. *Ann Rev Sex Res* 1995; 6:151–186.

Komisaruk BR, Adler NT, Hutchison J. Genital sensory field: enlargement by estrogen treatment in female rats. *Science* 1972; 178:1295–1298.

Komisaruk BR, Ciofalo V, Latranyi MB. Stimulation of the vaginal cervix is more effective than morphine in suppressing a nociceptive response in rats. In: Bonica JJ, Albe-Fessard D (Eds). *Advances in Pain Research and Therapy*. New York: Raven Press, 1976, pp 439–443.

Komisaruk BR, Banas C, Heller SB, et al. Analgesia produced by vasoactive intestinal peptide administered directly to the spinal cord in rats. *Ann NY Acad Sci* 1988; 527:650–654.

Komisaruk BR, Gintzler AR, Banas C, Blank MS. Vaginocervical stimulation releases vasoactive intestinal peptide-like immunoreactivity (VIP) into spinal cord superfusates in rats. *Soc Neurosci Abstracts* 1989; 15:216.

Komisaruk BR, Bianca R, Sansone G, et al. Brain-mediated responses to vaginocervical stimulation in spinal cord-transected rats: role of the vagus nerves. *Brain Res* 1996; 708:128–134.

Komisaruk BR, Gerdes C, Whipple B. "Complete" spinal cord injury does not block perceptual responses to genital self-stimulation in women. *Arch Neurol* 1997; 54:1513–1520.

Komisaruk BR, Rosenblatt JS, Barona ML, et al. Combined c-fos and ^{14}C-2-deoxyglucose analysis of maternal behavior in the rat: evidence of site-specific excitatory and inhibitory synaptic relationships. *Brain Res* 2000; 859:262–272.

Ladas AK, Whipple B, Perry JD. *The G Spot and Other Recent Discoveries about Human Sexuality*. New York: Holt, Rinehart and Winston, 1982.

LeBars D, Dickenson AH, Besson JM. Diffuse noxious inhibitory controls (DNIC). I. Effects on dorsal horn convergent neurones in the rat. *Pain* 1979a; 6:283–304.

LeBars D, Dickenson AH, Besson JM. Diffuse noxious inhibitory controls (DNIC). II. Lack of effect on non-convergent neurons, supraspinal involvement and theoretical implications. *Pain* 1979b; 6:305–327.

LeBars D, Chitour D, Kraus E, Dickenson AH, Besson JM. Effect of naloxone upon diffuse noxious inhibitory controls (DNIC) in the rat. *Brain Res* 1981; 204:387–402.

Lodder J, Zeilmaker GH. Role of pelvic nerves in the postcopulatory abbreviation of behavioral estrus in female rats. *J Comp Physiol Psychol* 1976; 90:925–929.

Masters DB, Jordan F, Beyer C, Komisaruk BR. Release of amino acids into regional superfusates of the spinal cord by mechano-stimulation of the reproductive tract. *Brain Res* 1993; 621:279–290.

Mayer DJ, Watkins LR. Multiple endogenous opiate and non-opiate analgesia systems. In: Kruger L, Liebeskind JC (Eds). *Advances in Pain Research and Therapy*. New York: Raven Press, 1984, pp 253–276.

McCarthy MM, Pfaff DW, Schwartz-Giblin S. Midbrain central gray GABA-A receptor activation enhances, and blockade reduces, sexual behavior in the female rat. *Exp Brain Res* 1991; 86, 108–116.

Meana M, Binik YM. Painful coitus: a review of female dyspareunia. *J Nerv Ment Dis* 1994; 182:264–272.

Meana M, Binik YM, Khalife S, et al. Dyspareunia: more than bad sex. *Pain* 1997; 71:211–212.

Melzack R. The myth of painless childbirth. *Pain* 1984; 19:321–337.

Mokha SS, Goldsmith GE, Hellon RF, Puri R. Hypothalamic control of nocireceptive and other neurones in the marginal layer of the dorsal horn of the medulla (trigeminal nucleus caudalis) in the rat. *Brain Res* 1987; 65:427–436.

Mousa S, Miller CHJ, Couri D. Dexamethasone and stress-induced analgesia. *Psychopharmacology (Berl)* 1983; 79:199–202.

Nagy JI. Capsaicin: a chemical probe for sensory neuron mechanisms. In: Iverson L, Iversen SD, Snyder SH (Eds). *Handbook of Psychopharmacology*. New York: Plenum Press, 1982, pp 185–235.

Nance DM, King TR, Nance PW. Neuroendocrine and behavioral effects of intrathecal capsaicin in adult female rats. *Brain Res Bull* 1987; 18:109–114.

Ornstein K, Amir S. Pinch-induced catalepsy in mice. *J Comp Physiol Psychol* 1981; 95:827–835.

Ortega-Villalobos M, Garcia-Bazan M, Solano-Flores LP, et al. Vagus nerve afferent and efferent innervation of the rat uterus: an electrophysiological and HRP study. *Brain Res Bull* 1990; 25:365–371.

Patton HD. Taste, olfaction and visceral sensation. In: Ruch TC, Patton HD, Woodbury JW, Towe AL (Eds). *Neurophysiology*. Philadelphia: W.B. Saunders, 1961.

Peirce JT, Nuttall RL. Self-paced sexual behavior in the female rat. *J Comp Physiol Psychol* 1961; 54:310–313.

Pellicer F, Picazo O, Gomez-Tagle B, de la Ol R. Capsaicin or feeding with red peppers during gestation changes the thermonociceptive response of rat offspring. *Physiol Behav* 1996; 60:435–438.

Peters LC, Kristal MB, Komisaruk BR. Sensory innervation of the external and internal genitalia of the female rat. *Brain Res* 1987; 408:199–204.

Pfaff DW. *Estrogen and Brain Function*. New York: Springer-Verlag, 1980.

Piercey MF, Moon MW, Blinn JR, Dobry-Schreur PJ. Analgesic activities of spinal cord substance P antagonists implicate substance P as a neurotransmitter of pain sensation. *Brain Res* 1986; 385:74–85.

Price DD. *Psychological and Neural Mechanisms of Pain*. New York: Raven Press, 1988.

Randich A, Aicher SA. Medullary substrates mediating antinociception produced by electrical stimulation of the vagus. *Brain Res* 1988; 445:68–76.

Robbins A, Sato Y, Hotta H, Berkley KJ. Responses of hypogastric nerve afferent fibers to uterine distension in estrous or metestrous rats. *Neurosci Lett* 1990; 110:82–85.

Robbins A, Berkley KJ, Sato Y. Estrous cycle variation of afferent fibers supplying reproductive organs in the female rat. *Brain Res* 1992; 20:353–356.

Roberts LA, Beyer C, Komisaruk BR. Nociceptive responses to altered GABAergic activity at the spinal cord. *Life Sci* 1986; 39:1667–1674.

Rodriguez-Sierra JF, Crowley WR, Komisaruk BR. Vaginal stimulation induces sexual receptivity to males, and prolonged lordosis responsiveness in rats. *J Comp Physiol Psychol* 1975; 89:79–85.

Rodriguez-Sierra JF, Skofitsch G, Komisaruk BR, Jacobowitz DM. Abolition of vagino-cervical stimulation-induced analgesia by capsaicin administered to neonatal, but not adult rats. *Physiol Behav* 1988; 44:267–272.

Rojas-Piloni G, Duran I, Cueva-Rolon R. The activity of ON and OFF cells at the rostroventromedial medulla is modulated by vagino-cervical stimulation. *Pain* 1998; 74:29–34.

Ross E, Komisaruk BR, O'Donnell D. Probing the vaginal cervix is analgesic in rats: evidence using an operant paradigm. *J Comp Physiol Psychol* 1979; 93:330–336.

Sivilotti L, Woolf CJ. The contribution of GABA-A and glycine receptors to central sensitization: disinhibition and touch-evoked allodynia in the spinal cord. *J Neurophysiol* 1994; 72:169–179.

Steinman JL, Roberts LA, Komisaruk BR. Evidence that endogenous opiates contribute to the mediation of vaginal stimulation-produced anti-nociception in rats. *Soc Neurosci Abstracts* 1982; 8:265.

Steinman JL, Komisaruk BR, Yaksh TL, Tyce GM. Spinal cord monoamines modulate the antinociceptive effects of vaginal stimulation. *Pain* 1983; 16:155–166.

Steinman JL, Hoffman SW, Banas C, Komisaruk BR. Vaginocervical stimulation attenuates hindpaw shock-induced substance P release into spinal cord superfusates in rats. *Brain Res* 1994; 647:204–208.

Szechtman H, Adler NT, Komisaruk BR. Mating induces pupillary dilatation in female rats: role of pelvic nerve. *Physiol Behav* 1985; 35:295–301.

Temple JL, Bradshaw HB, Wood E, Berkley KJ. Effects of hypogastric neurectomy on escape responses to uterine distention in the rat. *Pain* 1999; Suppl 6:S13–S20.

Terman GW, Lewis JW, Liebeskind JC. Opioid and non-opioid mechanisms of stress analgesia: lack of cross-tolerance between stressors. *Brain Res* 1983; 260:147–150.

Toniolo MV, Whipple B, Komisaruk BR. Spontaneous maternal analgesia during birth in rats. *Proceedings of the NIH Centennial MBRS-MARC Symposium*, 1987, p 100.

Traurig H, Saria A, Lembeck F. The effects of neonatal capsaicin treatment on growth and subsequent reproductive function in the rat. *Naunyn Schmiedebergs Arch Pharmacol* 1984; 327:254–259.

Traurig H, Papka RE, Rush ME. Effects of capsaicin on reproductive function in the female rat: role of peptide-containing primary afferent nerves innervating the uterine cervix in the neuroendocrine copulatory response. *Cell Tissue Res* 1988; 253:573–581.

Watkins LR, Faris PL, Komisaruk BR, Mayer DJ. Dorsolateral funiculus and intraspinal pathways mediate vaginal stimulation-induced suppression of nociceptive responding in rats. *Brain Res* 1984; 294:59–65.

Whipple B, Komisaruk BR. Elevation of pain threshold by vaginal stimulation in women. *Pain* 1985; 21:357–367.

Whipple B, Komisaruk BR. Analgesia produced in women by genital self-stimulation. *J Sex Res* 1988; 24:130–140.

Whipple B, Martinez-Gomez M, Oliva-Zarate L, Pacheco P, Komisaruk BR. Inverse relationship between intensity of vaginal self- stimulation-produced analgesia and level of chronic intake of a dietary source of capsaicin. *Physiol Behav* 1989; 46:247–252.

Whipple B, Josimovich JB, Komisaruk BR. Sensory thresholds during the antepartum, intrapartum, and postpartum periods. *Int J Nurs Stud* 1990; 27:213–221.

Whipple B, Ogden G, Komisaruk BR. Physiological correlates of imagery-induced orgasm in women. *Arch Sex Behav* 1992; 21:121–133.

Whipple B, Gerdes CA, Komisaruk BR. Sexual response to self-stimulation in women with complete spinal cord injury. *J Sex Res* 1996; 33:231–240.

Yaksh TL. Behavioral and autonomic correlates of the tactile evoked allodynia produced by spinal glycine inhibition: effects of modulatory receptor systems and excitatory amino acid antagonists. *Pain* 1989; 37:111–123.

Correspondence to: Barry R. Komisaruk, PhD, Department of Psychology, Rutgers, The State University of New Jersey, Newark, NJ, 07102 USA. Fax: 973-353-1102; email: brk@andromeda.rutgers.edu.

Sex, Gender, and Pain, Progress in Pain Research and Management, Vol. 17, edited by R.B. Fillingim, IASP Press, Seattle, © 2000.

8

Sex-Related and Hormonal Modulation of Visceral Pain

Maria Adele Giamberardino

Pathophysiology of Pain Laboratory, Department of Medicine and Science of Aging, "G. D'Annunzio" University of Chieti, Italy

The existence of sex differences in pain and the role played by sex hormones in the perception of painful symptoms have long been debated in the literature (Berkley 1997). In the past, reports of such differences, or their denial, were often anecdotal, with few studies using a systematic approach to address the issue. In recent years, however, this topic has gained increasing popularity in the scientific community, and the amount of research devoted to it has increased exponentially in both the experimental and clinical fields (Riley et al. 1998; Berkley and Holdcroft 1999).

Visceral pain represents a prominent medical problem. Clinical evidence has suggested for quite some time that its impact and modalities of presentation may differ between the sexes (Berkley 1997; Giamberardino 2000). Although much of the investigative effort has concentrated on somatic sensitivity (see references in Fillingim et al. 1998; Berkley and Holdcroft 1999), mostly due to the easier access to superficial structures than to internal organs (Arendt-Nielsen 1997), knowledge about sex and hormonal differences has also increased recently in the field of pain from internal organs (Berkley 1997).

After an indispensable introduction to the features of visceral pain and to the effects of sex hormones on pain perception, this chapter will focus on a number of painful conditions arising from the internal organs that show a different prevalence in the two sexes or are perceived differently depending on the patient's gender and on sex-hormonal fluctuations. The possible mechanisms underlying these differences will be discussed in light of the results of clinical and experimental studies. As underlined by LeResche (1999), much discussion has centered on the use of the terms "sex" and "gender," with some suggesting that "sex" be used to refer to biological aspects and "gender" to denote psychosocial identity. However, because this chapter will address ways in which both biological and psychosocial aspects of maleness and femaleness can affect the perception of visceral pain, the terms "sex" and "gender" will be used interchangeably.

VISCERAL PAIN

CLINICAL ASPECTS

Pain from internal organs is a highly prevalent condition in the clinical setting and is one of the most frequent reasons that patients seek medical care (Giamberardino 1999). The characteristics of visceral pain are typical, and differ from those of pain arising in superficial or deep somatic structures. They also tend to differ in the various phases of a visceral algogenic process. In the early stage of a painful episode, the symptom has a vague, poor localization, is perceived along the midline of the thorax or abdomen, whatever the viscus in question, and is accompanied by marked autonomic signs and strong alarm reactions (*true visceral pain*). In later phases of the first episode or in subsequent episodes, the symptom becomes better localized and sharper, i.e., qualitatively more similar to pain of somatic origin. It is perceived in different areas of the somatic body wall, depending on the specific viscus involved (areas usually segmentally related to the affected internal organ), and is no longer accompanied by emotional reactions or strong autonomic signs. At this stage the pain may or may not be accompanied by superficial or deep hyperalgesia of the somatic tissues of the area of referral (skin, subcutis, and muscle). Thus, two types of referred pain can be distinguished: a *referred pain without hyperalgesia* and a *referred pain with hyperalgesia,* the latter often being accompanied by sustained muscle contraction (Procacci et al. 1986). Several clinical studies on patients affected by different visceral pathologies (e.g., renal colics, biliary colics, and primary dysmenorrhea) have determined that this hyperalgesia mainly involves the muscle, as revealed by a significant decrease of pain thresholds to both mechanical and electrical stimuli (Vecchiet et al. 1989, 1990, 1992, 1996; Giamberardino et al. 1994, 1997b). In these studies, hyperalgesia appeared to be an early process; it tended to manifest as early as the first visceral episodes, was accentuated by reoccurrence of the visceral pain, and lasted for a long time (it not only lasted longer than the spontaneous pain from the internal organ, but sometimes even outlasted the primary focus in the viscus). In addition to the sensory changes (hyperalgesia), the somatic tissues in areas of referred pain from viscera are often the site of trophic changes, mostly in terms of increased thickness and consistency of the subcutaneous tissue and decreased thickness and section area of muscles (showing a tendency to muscle atrophy) (Procacci et al. 1986). Such trophic changes have been documented in patients using ultrasound evaluation (Vecchiet et al. 1996; Vecchiet and Giamberardino 1998; Giamberardino et al. 1999a).

PATHOPHYSIOLOGICAL ASPECTS

True visceral pain is usually felt around the midline because visceral organs are supplied with afferents bilaterally. Exceptions are the cecum, ascending colon, descending and sigmoid colon, kidneys, and ureters, whose innervation is strictly or predominantly unilateral (Bonica 1990). The poor localization and diffuse nature of the pain result from the low density of sensory innervation of the viscera, together with the extensive functional divergence of the visceral input within the central nervous system (CNS). A contribution to the relative nonspecificity of the visceral sensation in this phase (i.e., the difficulty in identifying its source) is also made by the viscero-visceral convergence at the central level. In fact, several experimental studies have documented the convergence of sensory inputs from different visceral domains onto the same second-order neurons (e.g., from the colon/rectum, bladder, vagina, and uterine cervix, or from the gallbladder and heart) (Berkley et al. 1993a,b; Foreman 1999; see also Giamberardino and Vecchiet 1996).

Referred pain without hyperalgesia is normally interpreted on the basis of the convergence-projection theory. Extensive experimental evidence indicates the convergence at central levels (spinal and supraspinal centers) of visceral and somatic afferent fibers onto the same neurons. The message from the viscera would thus be interpreted by higher brain centers as coming from the somatic structure because of memory traces of previous experiences of somatic pain (Cervero 1993, 1994, 1995a,b; Gebhart 1995a,b).

Referred pain with hyperalgesia, by far more common than the corresponding form without hyperalgesia, is more difficult to interpret, and the simple convergence-projection theory does not appear adequate to account for it. An increasing body of evidence from experimental studies demonstrates the contribution of central mechanisms to the generation of the hyperalgesia (Giamberardino et al. 1996, 1997c; Roza et al. 1998). The massive afferent barrage from the visceral domain triggers a number of neuroplastic changes in the CNS, involving hyperactivity and hyperexcitability of sensory neurons (receiving convergent viscerosomatic fibers), so that the normal input from the somatic periphery of pain referral would have an enhanced effect at the central level (convergence-facilitation). However, the intervention of further mechanisms cannot be ruled out, i.e., the activation of a number of reflex arcs of which the afferent branch is represented by the afferent fibers from the viscus and the efferent branch by sympathetic and/or somatic outputs toward the tissues of the peripheral area of referral. These outputs could be responsible for reflex sensitization of somatic nociceptors in this area, thus accounting for the hyperalgesia. Experimental evidence is so far scarce for this peripheral contribution to the generation of secondary hyperalgesia in the areas of referred pain from viscera. However, the hypothesis seems plausible, especially in light of clinical evidence that the areas of referred pain from viscera are the site of trophic alterations in addition to hyperalgesia; these objective changes cannot be the result of purely central processes (see Procacci et al. 1986; Giamberardino 1999, 2000).

SEX HORMONES AND PAIN

Although the three main sex hormones (estrogen, progesterone, and testosterone) are functionally active in both sexes (Goodman 1994), there are considerable differences between males and females in both absolute levels and temporal fluctuations of testosterone and of estrogen and progesterone (Berkley 1997). Females undergo periodic hormonal changes during the ovarian cycle in their reproductive years. Puberty, pregnancy, and menopause also bring tremendous hormonal changes. Males also undergo hormonal changes, but these are less extensive and more gradual than in women, especially after puberty (Berkley and Holdcroft 1999). On this basis, it seems logical to conceive that the hormonal differences between the sexes would entail a different way of perceiving a complex sensory experience such as pain throughout the lifespan.

Several painful conditions in women are indeed reported to vary in their incidence and prevalence as a function of puberty, pregnancy, menopause, and aging (reviewed in Berkley 1993; see Chapter 12, this volume). In men, likewise, some algogenic disorders show a different pattern in the various stages of life. Also, during the reproductive years, various forms of pain in women are reported to vary according to the phase of the menstrual cycle (Berkley 1997). The pathophysiology of these differences is still a matter of debate.

Progesterone has been associated with analgesia and anesthesia because some pain conditions (such as migraine) resolve or get better during pregnancy or during the mid-luteal phase of the menstrual cycle, and other types of pain are reduced in animals during lactation (when progesterone levels are high). Some anesthetics are progesterone-based (e.g., alphaxalone) (Berkley and Holdcroft 1999). Estrogen can accelerate wound healing and has also been associated with analgesia, because some pain conditions increase after menopause, when estrogen decreases (e.g., joint pain or vaginal pain) (Ashcroft et al. 1997). Similar considerations apply to testosterone, because some painful conditions, such as angina pain, become consistently more prevalent in men as testosterone concentrations decline with age (Berkley 1997).

As underlined by Berkley and Holdcroft (1999), however, for each of these examples either no effects or the opposite results can be found, such as the emergence in men at puberty (when testosterone increases) of cluster headaches, and the decrease in older men and postmenopausal women (when testosterone, estrogen, and progesterone levels decline) of abdominal pain (including irritable bowel disease), migraine, and tension headaches. These apparent contradictions can, at least in part, be explained by considering that the overall hormonal effects on the clinical manifestation of a painful syndrome probably depend not only on the absolute levels of a given hormone, but on its concentration relative to other hormones (Marcus 1995; Majewska 1996).

The exact mechanisms by which sex hormones influence pain perception are far from being fully elucidated, but among the many potentially important hormonal influences are those on metabolism (with implications for drug action), the immune system (with implications for painful autoimmune diseases, which are up to nine times more common in women; Fox 1995), trauma-induced inflammation (modulated by sex hormones; Ashcroft et al. 1997; Roof et al. 1997) and the hypothalamic-pituitary axis (with implications for the interactions among stress, pain, and cardiovascular variables; Fillingim and Maixner 1995; Aloisi 1997; Forslund et al. 1998).

Whatever their nature and mechanism, sex-hormonal effects on pain perception cannot be separated from the many other variables that have proven relevant to pain modulation. Social and cultural factors, in particular, are of undeniable importance as they can involve profound differences between men and women (both patients and physicians) in their attitude toward painful symptoms and their approach to treatment modalities (Bates 1987; Mendelson 1991; Strong et al. 1992).

SEX DIFFERENCES IN VISCERAL PAIN

In the specific field of visceral pain, the two sexes differ in several ways. One first, obvious, difference is that females and males have sex-specific viscera, i.e., the reproductive organs, and thus are subject to painful pathologies exclusive to their gender. Other differences concern prevalence and clinical expression of painful conditions from non-sex-specific viscera.

Lastly, another important difference is that during their fertile years, females, but not males, are subject to changes in pain perception from various visceral domains as a function of their ovarian cycle.

The following sections (visceral pain from sex-specific internal organs, visceral pain from non-sex-specific internal organs, and visceral pain fluctuations as a function of the female hormonal cycle) will describe some of the most common and paradigmatic visceral pain conditions belonging to each of the three categories of sex differences. Human studies will be reported in all cases and animal studies will be described where available, in an attempt to identify possible mechanisms underlying the observed differences.

VISCERAL PAIN FROM SEX-SPECIFIC INTERNAL ORGANS

Obvious absolute differences between females and males involve the characteristics of their reproductive structures, which are mainly visceral organs. Women have a vagina, clitoris, cervix, uterus, fallopian tubes, and ovaries; men have a penis, vas deferens, epididymis, prostate organ, seminal vesicles, and testes (Berkley 1997). Pain from sex-specific visceral organs (acute, recurrent, or chronic) appears to be more frequent in women than in men, given the more complex nature of the female pelvic region and the greater number of pathophysiological conditions directly or indirectly linked to female reproductive functions (Bonica 1990). Paradigmatic examples of such conditions are primary dysmenorrhea, labor pain, and post-partum pains, as well as pelvic inflammatory disease. Acute and chronic pain conditions also affect men's reproductive organs (e.g., prostatitis, prostate cancer, and epididymitis); one of the most demonstrative is chronic testicular pain. Although infrequent, this condition represents an important medical problem from both a diagnostic and a therapeutic point of view (Bonica 1990; Wesselmann et al. 1999).

PAIN FROM THE FEMALE REPRODUCTIVE ORGANS

Primary dysmenorrhea. Primary dysmenorrhea (cyclic pain associated with menses) is a highly prevalent clinical condition, estimated to occur in approximately 50% of all menstruating women (Ylikorkala and Dawood 1978). By definition not associated with pelvic or structural abnormalities, pain of primary dysmenorrhea is believed to be caused by relative uterine ischemia from hypercontractility of the myometrium, which in turn results from excess prostaglandins (which act by increasing uterine contractility and also by sensitizing nerve endings to the pain-producing effects of other compounds, such as bradykinins; see references in Bonica 1990).

The symptoms usually start a few hours or days before bleeding, worsen as the menstrual flow begins, and can last throughout the entire period of menses. Usually cramplike, the pain is typically perceived in the midportion of the lower abdomen, but can also involve the lower back and upper thighs. Autonomic signs and emotional reactions, typical of visceral pain perception, may precede or accompany the pain, i.e., nausea, vomiting, changes in heart rate, diarrhea, and anxiety. Some dysmenorrheic patients also have mittelschmerz (midcycle pain).

Pain of primary dysmenorrhea can be very intense and, like other forms of pain from internal organs, is usually accompanied by tissue hypersensitivity in the somatic area of referral. This phenomenon was quantified in a psychophysical study conducted by our group that compared dysmenorrheic versus nondysmenorrheic women (Giamberardino et al. 1997b).

In this study, pain thresholds to electrical stimulation were measured in the referred pain area (two symmetrical sites in the abdomen, 4 cm lateral to the navel) and also in two control sites on the limbs (at the deltoid and quadriceps level) in the skin, subcutis, and muscle. Thresholds were measured in four different phases of the menstrual cycle, i.e., in a 28-day cycle: menstrual, days 2–6; periovulatory, days 12–16; luteal, days 17–22; and premenstrual, days 25–28 (Giamberardino et al. 1997b). The most interesting results concerned the muscle. Thresholds varied throughout the cycle, with the lowest values always in the perimenstrual phase and the highest always in the luteal phase, whatever the body site. In dysmenorrheic women the monthly trend was accentuated, and the threshold decrease in the perimenstrual phase more pronounced. Thresholds in the abdomen in dysmenorrheic women were significantly lower than in nondysmenorrheic women, not only close to the painful period (perimenstrual phase) but also in the periovulatory and luteal phases. Muscle pain thresholds were significantly lower in the abdomen than in the limbs, particularly in dysmenorrheic women. There was also a direct linear correlation between the pain threshold decrease in the perimenstrual period and the intensity of the menstrual pain, both in nondysmenorrheic and dysmenorrheic women (normal women usually experience some degree of pain during menses, although of mild intensity). Further studies were conducted in different groups of women who had suffered from dysmenorrhea for a progressively higher number of years, which corresponds to a progressively higher number of painful episodes, given the recurrent nature of this condition (see Giamberardino et al. 1999a). The results showed that the decrease in pain threshold at the muscle level in the perimenstrual phase was greater in women who had suffered from dysmenorrhea for many years than in those who had experienced dysmenorrhea for only a few years. The characteristics of referred muscle hyperalgesia in primary dysmenorrhea were in line with those observed in patients affected with other painful pathologies from internal organs, i.e., the phenomenon mostly involves the muscle, its extent is a function of the pain previously experienced by the patient, and its duration is prolonged, i.e., goes beyond the phase of spontaneous pain.

Apart from hyperalgesia in the area of pain referral, dysmenorrheic women also showed a certain amount of muscle hypersensitivity in other body regions (diffuse muscle hyperalgesia), similar to the pattern observed in women with fibromyalgia (Vecchiet et al. 1994).

Labor pain. Pain during labor is a perfect model of acute pain. It is extremely intense and complex, with multiple components: somatic (both superficial and deep) and visceral (both direct and referred). The visceral (uterine) component is dominant; it appears first, in the early stages of labor, and results from dilatation of the cervix and from contraction and distension of the uterus and the peritoneal structures. In this phase, as for other intense forms of visceral pain, powerful autonomic signs and emotional reactions accompany the symptoms, and can include nausea, vomiting, shivering, sweating, brady- or tachycardia, anxiety, and often a feeling of impending death.

Visceral afferent fibers from the female reproductive area pass through the hypogastric plexus and the thoracic sympathetic chain to the 10th, 11th, and 12th thoracic and 1st lumbar nerves. Thus, as labor progresses, pain from the uterus is frequently referred to the somatic distribution of these segments in the lower abdomen, where it is accompanied by both superficial and deep hyperalgesia (referred pain with hyperalgesia) (Bonica 1990; Margaria et al. 1993).

The clinical picture of labor pain is complicated by somatic pain due to distension of the perineal tissues and birth canal; these regions often undergo trauma from spontaneous or surgical lesions. The somatic component becomes evident in the third and last period of delivery, when visceral symptoms are better tolerated, having reached the phase of referred pain (Margaria et al. 1993). The somatic component is transmitted by pudendal nerves that originate from the sacral plexus (S2–S4) and by other sensitive fibers from L1 (ileoinguinal nerve), L1–L2 (genitofemoral nerve), S1–S3 (posterior cutaneous nerve), and S4–S5 (sacrococcygeal nerve).

Analgesia that involves both neural and hormonal factors is induced during pregnancy. Hormones involved in parturition that have potential modulating effects on nociception include sex-steroid hormones, such as estrogen and progestogen, and peptides, such as β-endorphin and prolactin. As reported above, progesterone and its metabolites demonstrate both analgesic and sedative activity (Frye and Duncan 1994). Their increase during pregnancy may have a protective effect so as to attenuate pain experienced during labor. Labor also releases stress hormones such as cortisol and catecholamines from the adrenal gland, while antinociceptive mediators such as norepinephrine raise the pain threshold (Holdcroft 1999).

Despite all possible "protective" effects from the modulating action of hormones, labor remains an extremely painful event, in which for many hours the CNS is submitted to an intense barrage of afferent impulses from the uterus and other pelvic structures. Whether this exceptional experience has any permanent effect on sensory activity in the subsequent phases of a woman's life is still a matter of debate. Does it leave a residual and lasting hypersensitivity or a greater capacity for pain control? Do the involution of the uterus and its change to a more fibrous structure alter the structure and function of uterine sensory nerve fibers? (Holdcroft 1999).

Evidence indicates that, after the first labor, subsequent labors are not as painful (Melzack et al. 1981), but the explanation offered is that fear and anxiety are reduced because women know what to expect. In addition to these learned behaviors, however, and as has been hypothesized for other excruciatingly painful experiences (see Giamberardino et al. 1994), it cannot be excluded that the massive nociceptive input to the CNS during labor could also induce phenomena of altered pain processing, possibly responsible for a subsequent increase in women's susceptibility to algogenic conditions, especially of the pelvic domain.

Postpartum pain. Apart from labor, women also experience a number of visceral pains in the postpartum period. Holdcroft (1999) reports that in the first 10 days after delivery, the majority of women from a U.K. government-sponsored postnatal survey of 3570 mothers (with a 67% response rate) complained of pains in various parts of the body, mostly visceral in origin. For most of the women, these pains continued up to a month after delivery, and in a few, pain problems persisted for years. Holdcroft states:

> Pains after labor can be as severe as those experienced during labor, particularly the commonly occurring lower abdominal "after pains" that are associated with prolonged uterine contractions during breast feeding. Other causes of lower abdominal pain may not be physiologically based but are often direct complications of parturition, such as genital infection. The genital and urinary tract are, in fact, commonly traumatized during vaginal delivery; tissue trauma can lead to tissue ischemia, edema, and hematoma formation, followed by infection (Holdcroft 1999).

The lower abdominal "after pains" are normally perceived centrally on an intermittent basis and can be severe. Murray and Holdcroft (1989) studied such pains in 200 women, of whom half were primiparous. Half of the primiparous and 86% of multiparous women complained of pain (the difference in incidence was highly statistically significant). The pain reported as most intense ranged from menstrual pain to labor pain and was described most often as throbbing, cramping, and aching. Pain was relieved by simple measures of rest, changes in position, urination, and oral analgesics in half of the women. The pain was exacerbated by breast-feeding in more than 80% of the women, which provides evidence for a uterine origin (the stimulus of suckling triggers the production and release of oxytocin, which in turn promotes myometrial contractions; Holdcroft 1999).

Pelvic inflammatory disease. Pain associated with inflammation of the female reproductive organs is of great clinical significance. It is estimated that one in 10 American women has pelvic inflammatory disease during her reproductive years (Aral et al. 1991). As reported by Wesselmann and Lai (1997), each year at least a million American women are diagnosed with pelvic inflammatory disease and more than 200,000 are hospitalized, placing a high economic burden on society. An ascending genital infection is the primary cause of pelvic inflammatory disease in women. Serious sequelae of upper genital inflammations include chronic pelvic pain in about 23% of patients (for review see Lipscomb and Ling 1993). It is estimated that while overall a woman has about a 5% risk of having chronic pelvic pain in her lifetime, patients with a previous diagnosis of pelvic inflammatory disease have a fourfold increased risk of developing such pain (Ryder 1996). As with other forms of visceral pain, pelvic inflammatory disease often involves severe hyperalgesia in muscles of the lower abdominal quadrants and pelvic area. This hyperalgesia normally outlasts the spontaneous pain and persists for a long time, to the point that those affected may remain chronically hypersensitive in these somatic areas (Giamberardino 2000).

Animal models of persistent pain from the female reproductive organs have been particularly difficult to develop (see Giamberardino and Vecchiet 1994). One such model was recently set up by Wesselmann (Wesselmann and Lai 1997; Wesselmann et al. 1998), consisting of the injection of mustard oil into one uterine horn. Following this form of acute inflammation, the animals show repeated complex behavioral episodes indicative of visceral pain over 4 days post-intervention, along with evidence of muscle flank hypersensitivity, mostly ipsilateral to the inflamed uterine horn. This model mimics organic painful conditions of the reproductive organs in women—other than the situation occurring in primary dysmenorrhea—and it is extremely promising for study of pathophysiological mechanisms of persistent pain from the reproductive area.

A condition that could reproduce the characteristics of dysmenorrhea is endometriosis. The presence of endometrial tissue in ectopic locations in the pelvis is one of the most frequent causes of secondary dysmenorrhea in women (Bonica 1990). Experimental endometriosis has been developed in rats (Wood et al. 1995; Bradshaw and Berkley 1996), where, similar to the clinical condition, it promoted infertility and vaginal hypersensitivity. Apparently, it does not give rise to overt signs of visceral pain in rats, but is likely to provoke a latent algogenic condition in the pelvic area as it enhances the animals' pain behaviors in response to algogenic stimuli applied to the ureter, an organ with partially overlapping innervation (Giamberardino et al. 1998a; 1999b,c). This experimental pain is a phenomenon of viscero-visceral hyperalgesia (Giamberardino 1999, 2000), which will be discussed in detail below.

PAIN FROM THE MALE REPRODUCTIVE ORGANS

According to Wesselmann et al. (1997), one of the most vexing problems for men and most challenging for their treating physician can be *chronic orchialgia* (testicular pain). The incidence and prevalence of this chronic pain syndrome are not known. Most patients are in their mid- to late 30s (Davis et al. 1990; Costabile et al. 1991), but chronic testicular pain has been described from adolescence to old age (see references in Wesselmann et al. 1997). In many patients pain starts spontaneously, in the absence of a clear precipitating event (Wesselmann and Burnett 1999). Secondary causes of chronic orchialgia include infection, tumor, testicular torsion, varicocele, hydrocele, spermatocele, and trauma. Referred pain from the ureter or the hip has been reported as a cause of testicular pain, although other etiologies cannot be excluded (see Wesselmann et al. 1997 for a complete report).

Chronic orchialgia can be unilateral or bilateral. Some patients have constant pain; in others the pain is intermittent, either spontaneous or precipitated by certain movements or pressure on the testes. The pain can be confined to the scrotal contents or can radiate to the groin, penis, perineum, abdomen, legs, and back. Treatment requires identification of the underlying etiology. However, in nearly 25% of patients no obvious etiology can be found despite thorough evaluations; several treatments including sympathetic blocks have proven beneficial in these cases, but it is often difficult to resolve the symptoms completely.

Animal research would be helpful to clarify the pathophysiology of some forms of chronic orchialgia, in an attempt to find more effective (i.e., mechanism-based) treatments. Unfortunately, while acute noxious stimuli have often been applied to the testes (e.g., during electrophysiological studies; Kanui 1985; see also Cervero 1996), an animal model is still lacking that mimics the human condition of chronic testicular pain.

VISCERAL PAIN FROM NON-SEX-SPECIFIC INTERNAL ORGANS

Pain from visceral organs of the thoracic and abdominal cavity can manifest very differently in the two sexes. First, a different prevalence is reported for several potentially painful diseases of these organs. In particular, some conditions (1) have an age-dependent sex difference, a typical example being coronary heart disease, which prevails in men before the age of 55 (but then gradually reaches equal distribution in the two sexes); or (2) prevail either in women (i.e., esophagitis, reflux esophagitis with peptic ulcer, gallbladder disease, post-cholecystectomy syndrome, irritable bowel syndrome, interstitial cystitis, urethral syndrome, chronic constipation, and visceral pain of psychological origin) or in men (Pancoast's tumor, pancreatic disease, duodenal ulcer, and abdominal migraine) (Merskey and Bogduk 1994; see also Berkley 1997). Second, a different pattern of clinical expression (i.e., the way painful symptoms are perceived and reported) is often described in females and males for the same pathology affecting a specific organ (Berkley 1997).

Paradigmatic clinical examples of these differences are examined below.

Pain from the heart. Cardiac pain may result from several pathophysiological conditions. However, the most frequent cause is *coronary artery disease* (CAD) (Bonica 1990). CAD is estimated to constitute the single highest cause of death in the United States (Silverman 1999). CAD is prevalent in men until the age of 55, with mortality rates being four times those of women. After menopause, CAD increases progressively in women (Chiamvimonvat and Sternberg 1998), to reach equal distribution in the two sexes after age 65 (Roger et al. 1999). Risk factors also differ between men and women: diabetes is more prevalent in women with CAD, while overweight or external triggers such as exceptional stress are more prevalent in men (Behar et al. 1993; Seeman et al. 1993; Sullivan et al. 1994). Furthermore, among the elderly, hypertension is a stronger predictor of coronary heart disease in women than in men (Douglas and Ginsberg 1996). According to several authors, once established, CAD tends to evolve in a more aggressive fashion in women than in men, with a less favorable prognosis and less sensitivity to all kinds of treatments, both noninvasive and invasive (see references in Murabito et al. 1993; Orencia et al. 1993; Wenger 1998; Roger et al. 1999).

Several factors explain the various gender differences regarding CAD. The lower prevalence of CAD in women before menopause is commonly attributed to the protective effect of female sex hormones against atherosclerosis; atherosclerotic disease of coronary arteries accounts for 95% or more of patients with a CAD-related myocardial ischemia syndrome (Bonica 1990). However, further mechanisms, still unidentified, are probably involved in the "protection" against CAD during the fertile period, since in women the disease is strictly age-dependent and does not present any abrupt variation at the time of menopause, as would be expected if estrogens played an exclusive role (Roger et al. 1999).

The reportedly higher "aggressiveness" of CAD in women than in men, once the disease is established, is far from being clarified from a pathophysiological point of view. One possible reason for the apparently worse prognosis of CAD in women could lie in the different way painful symptoms are reported in the two sexes. The clinical picture of CAD appears more insidious and less promptly identifiable in women than in men, a circumstance that contributes to delays in correct diagnosis and appropriate treatment. As stated by Redberg in a recent article (1998): "coronary heart disease kills more women than all cancers combined, yet the clinical picture in women is different enough from men for the diagnosis to be missed or delayed." One first difference in symptomatology concerns chest pain. This is the most typical presenting symptom of CAD (Procacci et al. 1986; Bonica 1990). The relationship between heart disease and chest pain is nevertheless not straightforward; some patients with severe ischemia, to the point of myocardial infarction, do not experience any pain, while others complain of recurrent episodes of chest pain in the absence of significant cardiac disease. The poor correlation between CAD and chest pain is true for both sexes, but according to several researchers, is more pronounced for women, who not only are more likely than men to present with chest pain not motivated by heart disease, but are also more prone to "silent ischemia" (Hsia 1993; Sullivan et al. 1994). Foussas et al. (1998), for instance, examined patients with anginal pain who were subsequently found to have normal coronary arteries at diagnostic catheterization. Of patients referred with chest pain, women were more likely than men to have normal coronary arteries. Forslund et al. (1998) examined patients with stable angina pectoris versus healthy controls during an exercise test and with ambulatory ECG monitoring to evaluate signs of ischemia and ventricular arrhythmias in relation to gender. Although men and women showed similar frequencies of ST-depression and similar blood pressure and catecholamine responses on exercise testing, women had higher heart rates and were more prone to silent ischemia. While not all studies agree with these outcomes (see Adams et al. 1999), there is a general tendency in the literature to contend that chest pain is more predictive for coronary heart disease in men than it is in women (Garber et al. 1992; Sullivan et al. 1994; Scheuermann and Ladwig 1998).

When the samples studied consist of groups of patients with documented CAD, especially acute myocardial infarction, and the modalities of symptom presentation are retrospectively reconstructed (Goldberg et al. 1998; Meischke et al. 1998; Penque et al. 1998; Milner et al. 1999), it often appears that men and women have similar frequencies of chest pain or epigastric pain. However, women are significantly more likely than men to also complain of nausea as well as neck, back, and jaw pain. Thus, even in women with documented CAD, the overall clinical picture is often different to that of male patients. On the whole, as mentioned above, it appears that CAD symptoms in women tend to be underestimated by both patients and physicians, with the result that female patients are treated less promptly and less effectively than male patients. Foster and Mallik (1998) report that among patients who had experienced cardiac-related chest pain, men were admitted to the hospital more quickly than women. Men were more ready than women to believe that they might be having a heart attack, and thus sought treatment more promptly (Moser and Dracup 1993). Also, once hospitalized, women were less likely than men to undergo angiography and to receive i.v. nitroglycerin, heparin, and thrombolytic agents as part of the acute management of myocardial infarction (Penque et al. 1998).

The apparently more aggressive evolution and worse prognosis of CAD in women could also depend on organic factors, as suggested by the results of a recent study by Ossei-Gerning et al. (1998). These authors investigated sex differences in coagulation and fibrinolysis in relation to coronary stenosis in patients with coronary heart disease. They found elevated levels of circulating plasminogen activator inhibitor-1 (PAI-1), von Willebrand factor (vWF), fibrinogen, and factor VII:C (FVII:C) in women with angiographically proven CAD with respect to men.

Even when submitted to the same treatment, it appears that women and men with CAD differ in their reactions. A study conducted among patients subjected to coronary artery bypass graft (60 men, 30 women), who completed a battery of psychological questionnaires on or after the third day after surgery, showed that women reported significantly more depressive symptoms than men (Con et al. 1999). For women, pain was positively correlated with depressive symptoms and functional impairment. According to the authors, the results support the notion that psychosocial variables play different roles in the recovery paths of men and women. Another example is found in the study by Westin et al. (1999), who reported that female patients with ischemic heart disease had poorer quality of life than men both one month and one year after a cardiac event (acute myocardial infarction, coronary artery bypass grafting, or percutaneous transluminal coronary angioplasty).

In summary, the global picture of clinical investigations in the field of cardiac pain from CAD does show differences in both prevalence and clinical presentation of symptoms between women and men, but the reason for this gender difference, probably multifactorial, remains to be clarified (Swahn 1998). It is hoped that, in addition to clinical studies, experimental animal research will be conducted with the specific aim of addressing the issue of gender differences in this visceral domain. While numerous animal studies have concentrated on pain transmission from the heart (see references in Cervero 1996; Foreman 1999), to the best of our knowledge none of them has been devoted to identifying the possible mechanisms underlying differences in pain perception between the two sexes.

Pain from the digestive system. A number of painful pathologies from the digestive system are expressed differently in the two sexes (Merskey and Bogduk 1994). Biliary colics, for instance, are more frequent in women than in men, mostly due to the higher prevalence of calculosis in women (Caroli-Bosc et al. 1999), while pancreatic pain is more common in men (Bonica 1990; Berkley 1997). The most striking sex difference in this domain regards prevalence and perception of pain in the so-called functional gastrointestinal disorders, of which *irritable bowel syndrome* (IBS) is the most paradigmatic example (Mayer and Gebhart 1993; Naliboff et al. 1999). These disorders are thoroughly reviewed by Naliboff and colleagues in Chapter 16 of this volume.

Pain from the urinary tract. One of the most common and clinically prominent forms of pain from the urinary tract is *colic pain from calculosis* (see Vecchiet et al 1989; Giamberardino et al. 1994). Reports of differences between the two sexes for this condition are, however, scarce. Worth noting is a recent study by Robert et al. (1999) on patients submitted to extracorporeal shock-wave lithotripsy (SWL). SWL tolerance was significantly lower for women with renal stones than for men (i.e., women had more pain and thus required more sedation during treatment), which suggests a higher susceptibility of females to pain from the urinary tract.

Clearer differences between the two sexes are reported for other painful conditions of the lower urinary tract. *Interstitial cystitis* (IC) is a diagnostic entity that has come under increased study over the past decade. This condition predominantly affects women and is clinically diagnosed by the presence of frequency, urgency, nocturia, and pain (especially affecting the suprapubic region) in the absence of bacterial contamination of the urine (see Jaggar et al. 1998a; Doggweiler-Wiygul et al. 2000). The initial description of IC in *Campbell's Urology* (Pontari and Hanno 1995), i.e., "a symptom complex classically characterized by urgency, frequency and bladder pain that is generally relieved by voiding," runs parallel to the description of diarrhea-predominant IBS, which is classically characterized by urgency, frequency, and abdominal pain that is generally relieved by defecation. In a recent scientific survey of 2405 people with IC, IBS was the second most commonly associated medical condition (after allergies) found in this population (having been diagnosed in over 30% of patients). In Silverman's opinion (1999), many people with chronic bladder pain or urinary urgency without identified structural origin suffer from visceral hyperalgesia or allodynia, rooted in CNS dysfunction, as is the case for patients with abdominal or chest pain associated with IBS, nonulcer dyspepsia, or noncardiac chest pain. Viewed in this context, the overlap in symptomatology between IC and IBS is not unexpected, particularly considering the overlap in afferent neural pathways from the urinary and gastrointestinal tracts at the spinal and supraspinal levels (see references in Silverman 1999).

Clauw et al. (1997) have recently investigated the relationship between interstitial cystitis and fibromyalgia, the well-known syndrome characterized by chronic, diffuse musculoskeletal pain and tenderness (McCain 1993). Although genitourinary and musculoskeletal symptoms predominate in IC and fibromyalgia, respectively, both disorders share a number of features, including similar demographics, "allied conditions" (e.g., irritable bowel syndrome, headaches), natural history, aggravating factors, and effective therapies. Clauw and colleagues suspected a substantial clinical overlap between fibromyalgia and IC and examined cohorts of individuals with these two disorders to compare the spectrum of symptoms. Patients were questioned about current symptoms and underwent dolorimeter examination. The frequency of current symptoms was very similar for the fibromyalgia and IC groups. Both fibromyalgia and IC patients displayed increased pain sensitivity when compared to healthy individuals, at both tender and control points. According to the authors, these data suggest that fibromyalgia and IC have significant overlap in symptomatology and that IC patients display diffusely increased peripheral nociception, as is seen in fibromyalgia. Central mechanisms are suspected to contribute to the pathogenesis of fibromyalgia (see Giamberardino 1999); Clauw and colleagues speculate that the same types of mechanisms may be operative in IC, which has traditionally been regarded as a bladder disorder. Giamberardino et al. (1997b) reported that women affected with primary dysmenorrhea display increased sensitivity to painful stimuli at the muscle level, not only within the uterine viscerotomes (i.e., the abdomen, which can be interpreted as a sign of referred hyperalgesia of visceral origin), but also outside them (i.e., in the muscles of the upper and lower limbs), similar to the pattern observed in fibromyalgia patients. Although the women examined in this study did not meet the diagnostic criteria for fibromyalgia, the authors hypothesized that the generalized muscle hyperalgesia they found is the expression of some pathophysiologic mechanism common to both dysmenorrhea and fibromyalgia; the women evaluated in their study might be in a preclinical phase of fibromyalgia and thus eventually develop the syndrome later in life. Of course, only long-term prospective studies can answer this question.

A number of studies on the pathophysiology of visceral hyperalgesia at the urinary level have been conducted in animals. Such studies could lead to mechanism-based therapeutic interventions for the clinical expression of visceral hyperalgesia. One animal model relevant to IC is turpentine inflammation of the bladder in the rat (McMahon and Abel 1987). Although this inflammation truly models acute cystitis, it also mirrors some of the features of IC. Turpentine-induced inflammation gives rise to bladder hyper-reflexia (BHR); it is associated with intense afferent barrage to dorsal horn neurons and there is evidence for a slowly developing and maintained increase in the excitability of dorsal neurons following inflammation (see references in Jaggar et al. 1998a).

Spinal NMDA receptors are likely involved in central sensitization in this model, since NMDA-receptor antagonists (such as AP-5) proved able to prevent BHR (Rice and McMahon 1994). Spinal nitric oxide synthase (NOS) probably also plays a role in modulating bladder reflexes during inflammation; turpentine-induced BHR was prevented by spinal application of L-napna, a selective NOS inhibitor (Rice 1995).

Studies by Jaggar et al. (1998a) using the same model suggest that the hyper-reflexia is at least partially mediated by bradykinin (BK) receptors (B1 and B2), in particular by the B2 receptor in the early phase, with the B1 receptor only becoming important later. In another study, Jaggar et al. (1998b) showed that the cannabinoid anandamide and the putative CB2-receptor agonist palmitoylethanolamide were able to attenuate BHR. Their results confirm the analgesic potential of endogenous ligands at cannabinoid receptor sites.

VISCERAL PAIN FLUCTUATIONS AS A FUNCTION OF THE FEMALE HORMONAL CYCLE

Menstrual cyclicity is a major biological process for women during their reproductive years and is associated with significant changes in hormonal status and behavior (see Giamberardino et al. 1997b). It is therefore not surprising that menstrual cyclicity has been found to be a source of response variability to painful stimuli at various levels (Fillingim and Maixner 1995; Berkley 1997).

Most clinical studies examining variability of pain perception in relation to the monthly cycle in women refer, conventionally, to four specific phases, which are associated with different hormonal conditions (Ferin et al. 1993; see Chapter 10 of this volume for a detailed summary of menstrual cycle physiology).

Numerous pain conditions in women, including visceral pains, are reported to change in relation to the phases of the menstrual cycle (reviewed by Berkley 1997). Although the direction of these variations does not always correspond, the general tendency is for painful symptoms to accentuate as the premenstrual/menstrual period approaches. An example is pain from urinary calculosis, which is more easily triggered perimenstrually (either premenstrually or menstrually) than in other phases of the cycle in nondysmenorrheic women. This tendency is even more pronounced in dysmenorrheic women, who also have greater urinary pain around ovulation (Giamberardino et al. 1998b, 1999b). Although hormonal factors are likely to play a role, in the specific example it is probable that other mechanisms (phenomena of central sensitization) are responsible for the variation of ureteral pain perception with the phases of the menstrual cycle. As will be discussed in more detail below (see section "Are Women More Prone Than Men to Develop Chronic Visceral Pain Conditions?"), a specific viscero-visceral interaction could occur between the female reproductive system and the urinary tract, two visceral domains that share, in part, their central sensory projection (Giamberardino 1999, 2000).

In addition to clinical studies, numerous experimental studies in human volunteers have been performed to address the issue of variability of pain perception during the menstrual cycle. The vast majority of these investigations, however, have employed various stimuli at the somatic rather than the visceral level, due to the more difficult access to internal organs than to structures like the skin or muscles. The nature of the variations found at the somatic level has been inconsistent, with some authors reporting increased nociceptive sensitivity during the luteal or follicular phases, others during menses or premenstrually, others during both the perifollicular phase and menses, and still others finding no changes across the menstrual cycle (see references in Giamberardino et al. 1997b).

In the field of animal experiments, mostly in rats, numerous studies have evaluated possible changes in pain sensitivity as a function of the estrous cycle. Most female rats have a 4-day estrous cycle consisting of four sequential stages called, respectively, proestrus (P), estrus (E), metestrus (M), and diestrus (D) (Freeman 1994), the fertile period being P and the early morning of E, with M and D approximately corresponding to the perimenstrual period in women. Regarding evaluation of somatic sensitivity, similarly to what has been found for the menstrual pattern in human experimental studies, the estrous patterns observed in the different studies were inconsistent (see references in Bradshaw et al. 1999). Likewise, contradictory results were also found in rat studies addressing the issue of visceral sensitivity.

Pain behaviors occurring in response to the formation of an artificial stone in one upper ureter in female rats (repeated ureteric "crises" recorded over 4 days post-stone induction) (Giamberardino et al. 1995) are significantly greater when the rats are in M and D than when they are in P and E (Giamberardino et al. 1997a). This outcome provides the experimental counterpart of the phenomenon described in humans, i.e., urinary colics preferentially triggered in the perimenstrual period in women. Similar to findings in the ureter model, the results of Berkley et al. (1995), Bradshaw and Berkley (1996), and Bradshaw et al. (1999) employing vaginal and uterine distension in the rat suggest that under pathophysiological conditions, stimulation of the uterine horn and vaginal canal would be more likely to provoke escape behaviors in M and D than in P and E.

However, the amount of colonic distension necessary to provoke visceromotor and intracolonic responses in anesthetized rats is lowest in P (Sapsed-Byrne et al. 1996), while pain behaviors subsequent to bladder inflammation induced by cyclophosphamide vary little with estrous stage, being reduced only in a subset of rats tested on the morning of E (Bon et al. 1996).

The reasons for these inconsistencies remain unclear, and more studies are needed on animal models of pain from other internal organs to clarify this issue. As reviewed by Bradshaw et al. (1999), most of the estrous changes that occur in the rat's behavioral responses to noxious stimulation of visceral (but also somatic) structures take place as the rat moves from D through P and into E. This situation has raised the question of hormonal involvement in these changes, because P is the stage during which estradiol and then progesterone levels rise to their highest values (determining ovulation during the early morning of estrus), immediately after which hormonal levels fall precipitously (Freeman 1994). Studies in which ovariectomized rats have been given replacement hormones (estradiol or progesterone or combinations) show that the supplemental hormones clearly cause behavioral and electrophysiological changes; however, the direction of these changes is far from being consistent, with either increased or decreased sensitivity to pain in response to the same hormone in different experimental protocols (see references in Bradshaw et al. 1999). It is thus clear that hormonal levels alone cannot account for the changes in pain perception observed, and future studies must consider other variables.

ARE WOMEN MORE PRONE THAN MEN TO DEVELOP CHRONIC VISCERAL PAIN CONDITIONS?

An interesting point raised by Berkley (1997), based on discussion by Slocum (1984), is that one possible contributing factor to sex differences in pain perception is the ready access to internal pelvic structures provided by the vagina and cervix, which although necessary for physiological functions linked to reproduction, also provides access to infectious agents such as viruses and bacteria. Women thus have a greater propensity to develop a number of pelvic inflammatory conditions that deeply affect the visceral pain reactivity of the pelvic domain in the area. According to Berkley, the vaginal canal and cervix increase the vulnerability in women of the T10–L1 (innervating uterus and cervix) and S2–S4 segments (innervating vagina and cervix) to morbidity (Bonica 1990). The consequences of a persistent input from the periphery can be very important and long-lasting. Animal experiments have, in fact, documented lasting changes in the activity of spinal cells (central sensitization) subsequent to chronic infection, inflammation, and peripheral injury. This central increase in excitability of neurons is probably the mechanism of some forms of chronic pain whose organic cause is difficult to identify (Woolf 1984; McMahon 1992; Coderre et al. 1993; McMahon et al. 1993). Berkley's hypothesis is that some forms of diffuse, widespread pain, much more common in women than in men, develop from a persistent noxious stimulation via the vaginal/cervical canal. Also, input from C fibers (which are the predominant type of fiber innervating the vaginal canal and cervix; Berkley et al. 1993a,b) is particularly efficient at producing such states of central hyperexcitability (see Berkley 1997 for further discussion of this hypothesis).

Another important issue that needs to be raised when talking about the apparently higher susceptibility of women than men to chronic visceral pain conditions regards phenomena of viscero-visceral hyperalgesia. An increasing body of clinical evidence documents that a painful pathology of one visceral domain can affect the reactivity to painful stimuli of another viscus with partially overlapping innervation (see Vecchiet and Giamberardino 1998).

Although systematic studies have not yet been conducted, it is not unusual to observe in the clinical setting that patients with ischemic heart disease who are also affected with gallbladder calculosis complain of a higher number of anginal attacks than do those with a normal gallbladder (an interaction particularly evident in women, who are more prone to painful gallbladder pathologies). And, in fact, the gallbladder and heart have a partially overlapping central projection (at the T5 level) (see Giamberardino 1999).

Another example is the interaction between pathologies of the urinary tract and female reproductive organs, such as dysmenorrhea and urinary calculosis (Giamberardino 2000). As noted above, a recent epidemiologic study by our group (Giamberardino et al. 1998b, 1999b), conducted via an ad hoc questionnaire in fertile women, both nondysmenorrheic and dysmenorrheic, found a viscero-visceral interaction between the female reproductive organs and the urinary tract (common spinal segments: T10–L1). Fertile women affected with urinary calculosis (and a tendency to repeated colic episodes) who were also dysmenorrheic experienced a higher number of colics than did nondysmenorrheic women with urinary calculosis of comparable characteristics, when examined in a retrospective study over 3 years.

In a 2-year prospective evaluation, the same women manifested their urinary colic preferentially in one specific phase of their monthly cycle; this tendency was more pronounced if they also suffered from dysmenorrhea. In particular, the group of dysmenorrheic women could typically be divided into two subpopulations: in the first, the colics always occurred premenstrually, while in the second they always occurred at midcycle, i.e., around ovulation. These data indicate that colic pain from the urinary tract in the fertile women examined tended to occur in periods of the cycle when the input from the female reproductive organs was greatly enhanced by pelvic congestion (around either menstruation or ovulation). In addition to a higher number of urinary colics, dysmenorrheic women also presented a much greater degree of referred muscle hyperalgesia at the lumbar level, that is in the area of pain referral from the urinary tract, than did nondysmenorrheic women who had experienced a comparable number of colics. Thus, referred hyperalgesia from the urinary tract was notably enhanced by the concomitant presence of an inflammatory condition of the reproductive organs.

Viscero-visceral hyperalgesia is a complex form of hypersensitivity that is likely to be subserved by more than one mechanism (Giamberardino 2000). Since this phenomenon takes place preferentially between visceral organs that share, at least in part, their central projection, processes of central sensitization may play an important role. Hyperactivity and hyperexcitability could involve viscero-visceral convergent neurons at the central level. As reported above in the section on pathophysiological aspects of visceral pain, viscero-visceral convergences have, in fact, been documented in electrophysiological studies in animals, for instance between the gallbladder and heart (Foreman 1999) (which would explain the frequent interaction between pathologies of these two organs), and between the colon/rectum, urinary bladder, vagina, and uterine cervix (Berkley et al. 1993a,b; see also Ness et al. 1990) (which would explain the clinical interaction between female reproductive organs and the urinary tract). The increased input from one visceral domain could trigger changes in the excitability of these neurons and thus enhance the central effect of the input from the second visceral domain.

This hypothesis, however, must be verified experimentally, and other possible mechanisms could also be implicated. It would be of great importance to have a reliable animal model of the condition of viscero-visceral hyperalgesia observed in patients.

One such model has recently been set up that reproduces the characteristics of the viscero-visceral interaction between the female reproductive organs and the urinary tract. Our group combined the model of urinary calculosis in rats with the above-mentioned model of experimental endometriosis established by Wood et al. (1995) and Bradshaw and Berkley (1996). Endometriosis was chosen because it is a very frequent cause of secondary dysmenorrhea in women (Bonica 1990). Preliminary data in this model have shown that rats with experimental endometriosis plus urinary stones display a significantly higher number and longer duration of typical ureteral crises than do rats with sham endometriosis plus urinary stones. In addition, rats with endometriosis show a much higher degree of referred muscle hyperalgesia (Giamberardino et al. 1998a; 1999b,c). This model appears to be the experimental counterpart of the clinical condition, and may be a useful tool for further investigation of underlying mechanisms.

CONCLUSIONS

Clinical and experimental research points to the existence of sex- and sex-hormonal-related differences in pain from internal organs. The direction of these differences, however, is often inconsistent among various studies, and interpretation of the results remains difficult. Nevertheless, some important generalizations can be made on the basis of the available data.

First, when we consider sex-specific internal organs (i.e., the reproductive organs), women appear more subject than men in the course of their life to manifest a number of visceral pains, whether acute, recurrent, or chronic. This phenomenon is partly linked to "paraphysiological" factors, i.e., the more complicated hormonal array and more complex nature of the reproductive function in females than in males. Women are thus subject to mild to severe recurrent pain from the uterus (depending on whether they are dysmenorrheic) with the ovarian cycle during their fertile years and may eventually undergo labor pain as well as several forms of visceral "after pains" of the post-partum period. This different impact, however, is also due to frank pathological events such as ascending genital infections, which, for anatomical reasons, can give rise more frequently in women than in men to states of persistent pain from the pelvic area.

Second, when we consider internal organs other than those of the reproductive area, many painful pathologies display a different prevalence while others show a different clinical profile of painful symptoms in the two sexes. As regards prevalence, some conditions—mostly organic—predominantly affect men (e.g., coronary heart disease, at least before age 55), while others prevail in women (e.g., gallbladder pathologies), mainly because of differences in risk factors between the two sexes (e.g., for atherosclerosis or biliary calculosis) linked to both hormonal status and lifestyle. Other conditions—mostly dysfunctional or without identifiable organic cause, such as irritable bowel syndrome or interstitial cystitis—are largely prevalent in women because of a supposed higher susceptibility of the female sex to have "visceral hyperalgesia," a phenomenon whose pathophysiological bases are actively been investigated.

As regards the clinical profile of painful symptoms for the same visceral pathological entity, sex differences are not always consistent across studies; reported differences include the intensity, location, and quality of pain as well as the nature of other accompanying symptoms. Visceral pain appears less predictive in women than in men of a specific visceral disease and is thus more difficult to identify and treat. According to most authors, a crucial role in these symptom diversities is played by sociocultural factors, which would affect the way women and men (both patients and physicians) approach the pain problem.

Third, whether we consider sex-specific or non-sex-specific internal organs, visceral algogenic conditions in women appear to be exacerbated at specific periods of the menstrual cycle during the fertile years, while men normally experience a more stable profile of painful symptoms over comparable periods of time. Animal studies also point to variations of behavioral expressions of visceral pain in relation to the female reproductive cycle. However, both clinical and experimental studies show variable outcomes as to which phase of the cycle is linked to enhanced pain perception; this variability suggests that fluctuations of sex hormones are not the only factor underlying the phenomenon, and that they may have a different impact in diverse visceral domains.

Fourth, women appear more prone than men to present phenomena of viscero-visceral hyperalgesia between organs with partially overlapping innervation. An example is the interaction between the female reproductive organs and urinary tract, two visceral domains that frequently are the site of potentially painful conditions throughout the course of a woman's life. These phenomena are likely to predispose women to more intricate and often more long-lasting painful experiences from internal organs compared to men, especially in the abdominal/pelvic area. In addition, since visceral pain is referred to somatic areas of the body, where hyperalgesia most often develops, women are more likely than men to have extended areas of somatic (especially muscle) hyperalgesia as a consequence of multiple, concurrent, and recurrent visceral pains.

In conclusion, although the field of sex-related and hormonal variation of visceral pain perception is far from being completely explored, current research data suggest not only more frequent and persistent clinical conditions in women, but also a female tendency to more insidious and complicated complaints. In contrast, visceral pain in men tends to manifest with a more clear-cut profile (e.g., chest pain), which is much more easily traced back to a specific pathology. As a result, visceral painful conditions often are more difficult to diagnose correctly in women than in men. In addition, many physicians underestimate algogenic processes of the female reproductive organs simply because pain from this area is regarded as "normal." The net result is that visceral pain is often undertreated in women relative to men, or is given symptomatic rather than mechanism-based therapy. It is hoped that greater and earlier clinical attention to even mild algogenic processes from internal organs, together with further development of animal models adequate for investigating sex differences in visceral pain, will ultimately lead to improved management of this important symptom in the future.

REFERENCES

Adams MG, Pelter MM, Wung SF, et al. Frequency of silent myocardial ischemia with 12-lead ST segment monitoring in the coronary care unit: are there sex-related differences? *Heart Lung* 1999; 28:81–86.

Aloisi AM. Sex differences in pain-induced effects on the septo-hippocampal system. *Brain Res Rev* 1997; 25:39–406.

Aral SO, Mosher WD, Cates W Jr. Self-reported pelvic inflammatory diseases in the United States, 1988. *JAMA* 1991; 266:2570–2573.

Arendt-Nielsen L. Induction and assessment of experimental pain from human skin, muscle and viscera. In: Jensen TS, Turner JA, Wiesenfeld-Hallin Z (Eds). *Proceedings of the 8th World Congress on Pain*, Progress in Pain Research and Management, Vol. 8. Seattle: IASP Press, 1997, pp 393–425.

Ashcroft GS, Dodsworth J, van Boxtel E, et al. Estrogen accelerates cutaneous wound healing associated with an increase in TGF-beta 1 levels. *Nat Med* 1997; 3:1209–1215.

Bates MS. Ethnicity and pain: a bio-cultural model. *Soc Sci Med* 1987; 24:47–50.

Behar S, Halabi M, Reicher-Reiss H, et al. Circadian variation and possible external triggers of onset of myocardial infarctions. SPRINT Study Group. *Am J Med* 1993; 94:395–400.

Berkley KJ. Sex and chronobiology: opportunities for a focus on the positive. *IASP Newsletter*, Jan–Feb 1993; pp 2–5.

Berkley KJ. Sex differences in pain. *Behav Brain Sci* 1997; 20:371–380.

Berkley KJ, Holdcroft A. Sex and gender differences in pain. In: Wall PD, Melzack R (Eds). *Textbook of Pain*, 4th ed. Edinburgh: Churchill Livingstone, 1999, pp 951–965.

Berkley KJ, Guilbaud G, Benoist JM, et al. Responses of neurons in and near the thalamic ventrobasal complex of the rat to stimulation of uterus, cervix, vagina, colon and skin. *J Neurophysiol* 1993a; 69:557–568.

Berkley KJ, Hubscher CH, Wall PD. Neuronal responses to stimulation of the cervix, uterus, colon and skin in the rat spinal cord. *J Neurophysiol* 1993b; 69:533–544.

Berkley KJ, Wood E, Scofield SL, et al. Behavioral responses to uterine or vaginal distension in the rat. *Pain* 1995; 61:121–131.

Bon K, Lantéri-Minet D, Menétrey D, et al. Sex, time of day, and estrus variations in the behavioral consequences of cyclophosphamide-induced cystitis in rats. *Abstracts: 8th World Congress on Pain.* Seattle: IASP Press, 1996, p 248.

Bonica JJ (Ed). *The Management of Pain,* 2nd ed. Philadephia: Lea & Febiger, 1990.

Bradshaw HB, Berkley KJ. Effects of estrous stage and endometriosis on escape response to vaginal distention and vaginal tone in the awake rat. *Abstracts: 8th World Congress on Pain.* Seattle: IASP Press, 1996, p 247.

Bradshaw HB, Temple JL, Wood E, et al. Estrous variations in behavioral responses to vaginal and uterine distention in the rat. *Pain* 1999; 82:187–197.

Caroli-Bosc FX, Deveau C, Harris A, et al. Prevalence of cholelithiasis: results of an epidemiologic investigation in Vidauban, southeast France. General Practitioner's Group of Vidauban. *Dig Dis Sci* 1999; 44:1322–1329.

Cervero F. Pathophysiology of referred pain and hyperalgesia from viscera. In: Vecchiet L, Albe-Fessard D, Lindblom U, Giamberardino MA (Eds). *New Trends in Referred Pain and Hyperalgesia,* Pain Research and Clinical Management, Vol. 7. Amsterdam: Elsevier, 1993, pp 35–46.

Cervero F. Sensory innervation of the viscera: peripheral basis of visceral pain. *Physiol Rev* 1994; 74(1):95–138.

Cervero F. Mechanisms of visceral pain: past and present. In: Gebhart GF (Ed). *Visceral Pain,* Progress in Pain Research and Management, Vol. 5. Seattle: IASP Press, 1995a, pp 25–40.

Cervero F. Visceral pain: mechanisms of peripheral and central sensitization. *Ann Med* 1995b; 2:235–239.

Cervero F. Visceral nociceptors. In: Belmonte C, Cervero F (Eds). *Neurobiology of Nociceptors.* Oxford: Oxford University Press, 1996, pp 220–240.

Chiamvimonvat V, Sternberg L. Coronary artery disease in women. *Can Fam Physician* 1998; 44:2709–2717.

Clauw DJ, Schmidt M, Radulovic D, et al. The relationship between fibromyalgia and interstitial cystitis. *J Psychiatr Res* 1997; 31:125–131.

Coderre TJ, Katz J, Vaccarino AL, et al. Contribution of central neuroplasticity to pathological pain. Review of clinical and experimental evidence. *Pain* 1993; 52:259–285.

Con A, Linden W, Thompson JM, et al. The psychology of men and women recovering from coronary artery bypass surgery. *J Cardiopulm Rehabil* 1999; 19:152–161.

Costabile RA, Hahn M, McLeod DG. Chronic orchialgia in the pain prone patient: the clinical perspective. *Am Urol Assoc* 1991; 146:1571–1574.

Davis DM, Noble MJ, Weigel JW, et al. Analysis and management of chronic testicular pain. *J Urol* 1990; 143:936–939.

Doggweiler-Wiygul R, Blankenship J, MacDiarmid SA. Interstitial cystitis, the painful bladder syndrome. *Curr Rev Pain* 2000; in press.

Douglas PS, Ginsberg GS. The evaluation of chest pain in women. *N Engl J Med* 1996; 334:1311–1315.

Ferin M, Jewelewicz R, Warren M. *The Menstrual Cycle.* New York: Oxford University Press, 1993.

Fillingim RB, Maixner W. Gender differences in the responses to noxious stimuli. *Pain Forum* 1995; 4:209–221.

Fillingim RB, Maixner W, Kincaid S, et al. Sex differences in temporal summation but not sensory-discriminative processing of thermal pain. *Pain* 1998; 75:121–127.
Foreman RD. Mechanisms of cardiac pain. *Ann Rev Physiol* 1999; 61:143–147.
Forslund L, Hjemdahl P, Held C, et al. Ischaemia during exercise and ambulatory monitoring in patients with stable angina pectoris and healthy controls. Gender differences and relationships to catecholamines. *Eur Heart J* 1998; 19:578–587.
Foster S, Mallik M. A comparative study of differences in the referral behaviour patterns of men and women who have experienced cardiac-related chest pain. Intensive. *Crit Care Nurs* 1998; 14:192–202.
Foussas SG, Adamopoulou EN, Kafaltis NA, et al. Clinical characteristics and follow-up of patients with chest pain and normal coronary arteries. *Angiology* 1998; 49:349–354.
Fox HS. Sex steroids and the immune system. In: Bock GR, Goode JA (Eds). *Non-Reproductive Actions of Sex Steroids*. Chichester: John Wiley, 1995; pp 203–217.
Freeman ME. The neuroendocrine control of the ovarian cycle of the rat. In: Knobil E, Neill JD (Eds). *The Physiology of Reproduction,* 2nd ed. New York: Raven Press, 1994.
Frye CA, Duncan JE. Progesterone metabolites, effective at the GABA receptor complex, attenuate pain sensitivity in rats. *Brain Res* 1994; 642:194–203.
Garber CE, Carelton, RA, Heller GV. Comparison of rose questionnaire angina to exercise thallium scintigraphy: different findings in males and females. *J Clin Epidemiol* 1992; 45:715–720.
Gebhart GF (Ed). *Visceral Pain,* Progress in Pain Research and Management, Vol. 5. Seattle: IASP Press, 1995a.
Gebhart GF. Visceral nociception: consequences, modulation and the future. *Eur J Anaesthesiol* 1995b; 12(10):24–27.
Giamberardino MA. Recent and forgotten aspects of visceral pain. *Eur J Pain* 1999; 3:77–92.
Giamberardino MA. Visceral hyperalgesia. In: Devor M, Rowbotham MC, Wiesenfeld-Hallin Z (Eds). *Proceedings of the 9th World Congress on Pain,* Progress in Pain Research and Management, Vol. 16. Seattle: IASP Press, 2000, pp 523–550.
Giamberardino MA, Vecchiet L. Experimental studies on pelvic pain. *Pain Rev* 1994; 1:102–115.
Giamberardino MA, Vecchiet L. Pathophysiology of visceral pain. *Curr Rev Pain* 1996; 1:23–33.
Giamberardino MA, de Bigontina P, Martegiani C, et al. Effects of extracorporeal shock-wave lithotripsy on referred hyperalgesia from renal/ureteral calculosis. *Pain* 1994; 56:77–83.
Giamberardino MA, Valente R, de Bigontina P, et al. Artificial ureteral calculosis in rats: behavioural characterization of visceral pain episodes and their relationship with referred lumbar muscle hyperalgesia. *Pain* 1995; 61:459–469.
Giamberardino MA, Dalal A, Valente R, et al. Changes in activity of spinal cells with muscular input in rats with referred muscular hyperalgesia from ureteral calculosis. *Neurosci Lett* 1996; 203:89–92.
Giamberardino MA, Affaitati G, Valente R, et al. Changes in visceral pain reactivity as a function of estrous cycle in female rats with artificial ureteral calculosis. *Brain Res* 1997a; 74:234–238.
Giamberardino MA, Berkley KJ, Iezzi S, et al. Pain threshold variations in somatic wall tissues as a function of menstrual cycle, segmental site and tissue depth in non-dysmenorrheic women, dysmenorrheic women and men. *Pain* 1997b; 71:187–197.
Giamberardino MA, Valente R, Affaitati G, et al. Central neuronal changes in recurrent visceral pain. *Int J Clin Pharmacol Res* 1997c; 17(2/3):63–66.
Giamberardino MA, Affaitati G, Vecchiet L, et al. Effects of endometriosis on pain behaviours induced by ureteral calculosis in female rats. *J Musculoskeletal Pain* 1998a; 6(2):172.
Giamberardino MA, de Laurentis S, Affaitati G, et al. The impact of menstrual cycle upon pain perception from urinary calculosis. *Dolor* 1998b; 13:32.
Giamberardino MA, Affaitati G, Iezzi S, et al. Referred muscle pain and hyperalgesia from viscera. In: Vecchiet L, Giamberardino MA (Eds). Muscle Pain, Myofascial Pain, and Fibromyalgia: Recent Advances. *J Musculoskeletal Pain* 1999a; 7:61–69.

Giamberardino MA, Affaitati G, Lerza R, et al. The impact of painful gynecological conditions on pain of urological origin. *Soc Neurosci Abstracts* 1999b; 25:143.

Giamberardino MA, Berkley KJ, Affaitati G, et al. The influence of endometriosis on pain behaviors induced by ureteral calculosis in female rats. *Abstracts: 9th World Congress on Pain*. Seattle: IASP Press, 1999c, p 392.

Goldberg RJ, O'Donnell C, Yarzebski J, et al. Sex differences in symptom presentation associated with acute myocardial infarction: a population-based perspective. *Am Heart J* 1998; 136(2):189–95.

Goodman HM. *Basic Medical Endocrinology,* 2nd ed. New York: Raven Press, 1994.

Holdcroft A. Postpartum lower abdominal pain. *Curr Rev Pain* 1999; 2:137–143.

Hsia J. Gender differences in diagnosis and management of coronary disease. *J Womens Health* 1993; 2:349–352.

Jaggar SI, Habib S, Rice ASC. The modulatory effects of bradykinin B1 and B2 receptor antagonists upon viscero-visceral hyper-reflexia in a rat model of visceral hyperalgesia. *Pain* 1998a; 75:169–176.

Jaggar SI, Hasnie FS, Sellaturay S, et al. The anti-hyperalgesic actions of the cannabinoid anandamide and the putative CB2 receptor agonist palmitoylethanolamide in visceral and somatic inflammatory pain. *Pain* 1998b; 76:189–199.

Kanui TI. Responses of spinal cord neurones to noxious and non-noxious stimulation of the skin and testicle of the rat. *Neurosci Lett* 1985: 58:315–319.

LeResche L. Gender considerations in the epidemiology of chronic pain. In: Crombie IK, Croft PR, Linton SJ, LeResche L, Von Korff M (Eds). *Epidemiology of Pain*. Seattle: IASP Press, 1999, pp 43–52.

Lipscomb GH, Ling FW. Relationship of pelvic infection and chronic pelvic pain. *Obstet Gynecol Clin North Am* 1993, 20:699–708.

Majewska MD. Sex differences in brain morphology and pharmacodynamics. In: Jensvold MF, Halbreich U, Hamilton JA (Eds). *Psychopharmacology and Women: Sex, Gender and Hormones.* Washington, DC: American Psychiatry Press, 1996, pp 73–83.

Marcus DA. Interrelationships of neurochemical, estrogen, and recurring headache. *Pain* 1995; 62:129–141.

Margaria E, Gollo E, Castelletti I. Gynecological and obstetrical pain. In: Vecchiet L, Albe-Fessard D, Lindblom U, Giamberardino MA (Eds). *New Trends in Referred Pain and Hyperalgesia,* Pain Research and Clinical Management, Vol. 7. Amsterdam: Elsevier, 1993, pp 299–307.

Mayer EA, Gebhart G. Functional bowel disorders and the visceral hyperalgesia hypothesis. In: Mayer EA, Raybould HE (Eds). *Basic and Clinical Aspects of Chronic Abdominal Pain,* Pain Research and Clinical Management, Vol. 9. Amsterdam: Elsevier, 1993, pp 3–28.

McCain GA. The clinical features of the fibromyalgic syndrome. In: Voeroy H, Merskey H (Eds). *Progress in Fibromyalgia and Myofascial Pain*, Pain Research and Clinical Management, Vol. 6. Amsterdam: Elsevier, 1993, pp 195–215.

McMahon SB. Plasticity of central terminations of primary sensory neurons in the adult animal. In: Scott SA (Ed). *Sensory Neurons: Diversity, Development, and Plasticity*. Oxford: Oxford University Press, 1992.

McMahon SB, Abel C. A model for the study of visceral pain states: chronic inflammation of the chronic decerebrate rat urinary bladder by irritant chemicals. *Pain* 1987; 28:109–127.

McMahon SB, Lewin GR, Wall PD. Central excitability triggered by noxious inputs. *Curr Opin Neurobiol* 1993; 3:602–610.

Meischke H, Larsen MP, Eisenberg MS. Gender differences in reported symptoms for acute myocardial infarction: impact on prehospital delay time interval. *Am J Emerg Med* 1998; 16(4):363–366.

Melzack R, Taenzer P, Feldman P, et al. Labor is still painful after prepared childbirth. *CMAJ* 1981; 125:357–363.

Mendelson G. Psychological and social factors predicting responses to pain treatment. In: Bond MR, Charlton JE, Woolf CJ (Eds). *Proceedings of the 6th World Congress on Pain.* Amsterdam: Elsevier, 1991.

Merskey H, Bogduk N (Eds). *Classification of Chronic Pain: Descriptions of Chronic Pain Syndromes and Definitions of Pain Terms,* 2nd ed. Seattle: IASP Press, 1994.

Milner KA, Funk M, Richards S, et al. Gender differences in symptom presentation associated with coronary heart disease. *Am J Cardiol* 1999; 15:396–399.

Moser DK, Dracup K. Gender differences in treatment-seeking delay in acute myocardial infarction. *Prog Cardiovasc Nurs* 1993; 8:6–12.

Murabito JM, Evans JC, Larson MG, et al. Prognosis after the onset of coronary heart disease. An investigation of differences in outcome between the sexes according to initial coronary disease presentation. *Circulation* 1993; 88:2548–2555.

Murray A, Holdcroft A. Incidence and intensity of postpartum lower abdominal pain. *BMJ* 1989; 298:1619.

Naliboff B, Lembo A, Mayer EA. Abdominal pain in irritable bowel syndrome. *Curr Rev Pain* 1999; 3:144–152.

Ness TJ, Metcalf AM, Gebhart GF. A psychophysiological study in humans using phasic colonic distension as a noxious visceral stimulus. *Pain* 1990; 43:377–386.

Orencia A, Bailey K, Yawn BP, et al. Effect of gender on long-term outcome of angina pectoris and myocardial infarction/sudden unexpected death. *JAMA* 1993; 269:2392–2397.

Ossei-Gerning N, Wilson IJ, Grant PJ. Sex difference in coagulation and fibrinolysis in subjects with coronary artery disease. *Thromb Haemost* 1998; 7:36–40.

Penque S, Halm M, Smith M, et al. Women and coronary heart disease: relationship between descriptors of signs and symptoms and diagnostic and treatment course. *Am J Crit Care* 1998; 7:175–182.

Pontari MA, Hanno PM. Interstitial cystitis. In Walsh PC, et al (Eds). *Campbell's Urology,* update 14. Philadelphia: WB Saunders, 1995, pp 1–19.

Procacci P, Zoppi M, Maresca M. Clinical approach to visceral sensation. In: Cervero F, Morrison JFB (Eds). *Visceral Sensation,* Progress in Brain Research, Vol. 67. Amsterdam: Elsevier, 1986, pp 21–28.

Redberg RF. Coronary artery disease in women: understanding the diagnostic and management pitfalls. *Medscape Womens Health* 1998; 3(5):1.

Rice AS. Topical spinal administration of a nitric oxide synthase inhibitor prevents the hyper-reflexia associated with a rat model of persistent visceral pain. *Neurosci Lett* 1995; 187:111–114.

Rice ASC, McMahon SB. Pre-emptive intrathecal administration of an NMDA receptor antagonist (AP-5) prevents hyper-reflexia in a model of persistent visceral pain. *Pain* 1994; 57:335–340.

Riley III JL, Robinson ME, Wise EA, et al. Sex differences in the perception of noxious experimental stimuli: a meta-analysis. *Pain* 1998; 74:181–187.

Robert M, Lanfrey P, Rey G, et al. Analgesia in piezoelectric SWL: comparative study of kidney and upper ureter treatments. *J Endourol* 1999; 13:391–395.

Roger VVL, Jacobsen SJ, Weston SA, et al. Sex differences in the epidemiology and outcomes of heart disease: population based trends. *Lupus* 1999; 8:346–350.

Roof RL, Hoffman SW, Stein DG. Progesterone protects against lipid peroxidation following traumatic brain injury in rats. *Mol Chem Neuropathol* 1997; 31:1–11.

Roza C, Laird JMA, Cervero F. Spinal mechanisms underlying persistent pain and referred hyperalgesia in rats with an experimental ureteric stone. *J Neurophysiol* 1998; 79:1603–1612.

Ryder RM. Chronic pelvic pain. *Am Fam Physician* 1996; 54:2225–2232.

Sapsed-Byrne S, Ridout D, Ma D, et al. Responses to colonic distension during estrous cycle. *Abstracts: 8th World Congress on Pain.* Seattle: IASP Press, 1996, p 248.

Scheuermann W, Ladwig KH. Sex-specific differences in risks and management of coronary heart disease. *Z Kardiol* 1998; 87:528–536.

Seeman T, Mendes de Leon C, Berkman L, et al. Risk factors for coronary heart disease among older men and women: a prospective study of community-dwelling elderly. *Am J Epidemiol* 1993; 15:1037–1049.

Silverman DHS. Cerebral activity in the perception of visceral pain. *Curr Rev Pain* 1999; 3(4):291–299.

Slocum JC. Neurological factors in chronic pelvic pain: trigger points and the abdominal pelvic syndrome. *Am J Obstet Gynecol* 1984; 149:536–543.

Strong J, Ashton R, Chant D. The measurement of attitudes towards and beliefs about pain. *Pain* 1992; 48:227–236.

Sullivan AK, Holdright DR, Wright CA, et al. Chest pain in women: clinical, investigative, and prognostic features. *BMJ* 1994; 308:883–836.

Swahn E. The care of patients with ischaemic heart disease from a gender perspective. *Eur Heart J* 1998; 19:1758–1765.

Vecchiet L, Giamberardino MA. Clinical and pathophysiological aspects of visceral hyperalgesia. In: De Vera JA, Parris W, Erdine S (Eds). *Management of Pain. A World Perspective III*. Bologna: Monduzzi, 1998, pp 214–230.

Vecchiet L, Giamberardino MA, Dragani L, et al. Pain from renal/ureteral calculosis: evaluation of sensory thresholds in the lumbar area. *Pain* 1989; 36:289–295.

Vecchiet L, Giamberardino MA, Dragani L, et al. Referred muscular hyperalgesia from viscera: clinical approach. *Adv Pain Res Ther* 1990; 13:175–182.

Vecchiet L, Giamberardino MA, de Bigontina P. Referred pain from viscera: when the symptom persists despite the extinction of the visceral focus. *Adv Pain Res Ther* 1992; 20:101–110.

Vecchiet L, Giamberardino MA, de Bigontina P et al. Comparative sensory evaluation of parietal tissues in painful and nonpainful areas in fibromyalgia and myofascial pain syndrome. In: Gebhart GF, Hammond DL, Jensen TS (Eds). *Proceedings of the 7th World Congress on Pain*, Progress in Pain Research and Management, Vol. 2. Seattle: IASP Press, 1994, pp 177–185.

Vecchiet L, Iezzi S, Giamberardino MA. Relationship between occurrence of biliary colics and sensory/trophic changes in abdominal parietal tissues in patients with gallbladder calculosis. *Abstracts: 8th World Congress on Pain*. Seattle: IASP Press, 1996, pp 255–256.

Wenger NK. An update on coronary heart disease in women. *Int J Fertil Womens Med* 1998; 43:84–90.

Wesselmann W, Lai J. Mechanisms of referred visceral pain: uterine inflammation in the adult virgin rat results in neurogenic plasma extravasation in the skin. *Pain* 1997; 73:309–317.

Wesselmann U, Czakanski PP, Affaitati G, et al. Uterine inflammation as a noxious visceral stimulus: behavioral characterization in the rat. *Neurosci Lett* 1998; 246:73–76.

Wesselmann U, Burnett AL, Heinberg LJ. The urogenital and rectal pain syndromes. *Pain* 1999; 73:269–294.

Westin L, Carlsson R, Erardt L, et al. Differences in quality of life in men and women with ischemic heart disease. A prospective controlled study. *Scand Cardiovasc J* 1999; 33:160–165.

Wood E, Pauley S, Bradshaw H, et al. Vaginal allodynia and hyperalgesia in rats with endometriosis and after pre-senescent ovariectomy. *Soc Neurosci Abstr* 1995; 21:388.

Woolf CJ. Long term alterations in the excitability of the flexion reflex produced by peripheral tissue injury in the chronic decerebrate rat. *Pain* 1984; 18:325–343.

Ylikorkala O, Dawood MY. New concepts in dysmenorrhea. *Am J Obstet Gynecol* 1978; 130:833–847.

Correspondence to: Maria Adele Giamberardino, MD, via Carlo de Tocco n. 3, 66100 Chieti, Italy. Tel/Fax: (laboratory): 0871-565286; email: mag@unich.it.

Sex, Gender, and Pain, Progress in Pain Research and Management, Vol. 17, edited by R.B. Fillingim, IASP Press, Seattle, © 2000.

9

Sex and Gender Differences in Responses to Experimentally Induced Pain in Humans

Gary B. Rollman,[a] Stefan Lautenbacher,[b,c] and Kevin S. Jones[a]

[a]*Department of Psychology, University of Western Ontario, London, Ontario, Canada;* [b]*Department of Psychiatry and Psychotherapy, University of Marburg, Marburg, Germany;* [c]*Department of Physiological Psychology, University of Bamberg, Bamberg, Germany*

Sex differences have long interested scientific and medical researchers, and the pain literature is replete with laboratory and clinical studies comparing the reactions of men and women. Often, these studies are based on small samples of convenience, but sufficient evidence has accumulated for us to conclude that males and females often show divergent responses to noxious stimuli. Still, the biological and psychological mechanisms underlying these differences or, for that matter, the experimental conditions giving rise to such differences, are poorly understood.

Several lengthy review and meta-analytic papers have carefully documented the literature on sex differences. Berkley (1997) noted that "when differences are observed under these carefully controlled experimental circumstances, it is often the case that women have lower thresholds, rate similar stimuli as more painful, or have less tolerance for intense stimuli." However, she also indicated that the "differences are inconsistently observed, relatively minor, exist only for certain forms of stimulation, and can be affected by numerous situation variables in daily life such as the presence of disease, the setting of the experiment, the characteristics of the experimenter, and even nutritive status."

Fillingim and Maixner (1995) examined 34 human experimental studies of sex and pain and found sex differences in about two-thirds of them. They concluded that "females exhibit greater sensitivity to laboratory pain compared to males," that "these gender differences do not appear to be site specific," that "some forms have produced more consistent findings than others (e.g., pressure vs. thermal)," and that "pain responses are characterized by great interindividual variability."

Riley and colleagues (1998) used meta-analytic techniques to extend the evaluation of the studies reviewed by Fillingim and Maixner. They calculated effect sizes for 22 studies of sex differences that had used a variety of stimuli, body sites, measures, sample sizes, populations, and age groups. For pain threshold and pain tolerance, male subjects had higher values than females for all types of noxious stimuli, although the largest effect sizes were obtained when pressure pain was compared across the sexes, followed by electrical pulses and then by thermal stimuli. Statistical analysis suggested that about 40 subjects per group are necessary to provide adequate power to test a sex difference, although only 7 of the 34 studies reviewed by Fillingim and Maixner met this criterion.

In speculating why females are more responsive than males to pain, Riley and colleagues touched on a number of earlier suggestions including sociocultural factors, hormonal influences, body size, and anxiety, concluding that "the conflicting evidence for causal mechanisms only serves to emphasize the complexity of these differences, which, as with most psychological phenomena, are likely to be multidetermined."

Given the ready availability of reviews of the experimental data, this chapter will focus on the mechanisms underlying sex differences in pain responsiveness, paying particular attention to developmental, biological, and psychological factors. Our aim is to bring a broad perspective to the understanding of an issue that is scientifically perplexing and yet highly significant.

Each of these explanatory mechanisms contributes to our understanding of the variables underlying sex differences in pain. Many of the biological data suggest that critical differences arise in early stages of nociceptive processing, while the psychological studies emphasize factors related to pain perception, evaluation, and expression.

DEVELOPMENTAL FACTORS

It would be informative to learn whether there is a particular developmental stage at which sex differences in pain sensitivity begin to appear. An understanding of when biological or psychological correlates of sex differences become operative would allow us to develop more thorough explanatory models. The literature in this area is sparse, yet some experimental studies have attempted to shed light on this issue. Meier et al. (1999) presented the results of a comprehensive study on a group of children and adolescents (54 girls and 52 boys, ranging in age from 6 to 17 years). The authors measured somatosensory sensitivity to warmth, cold, and vibration and pain sensitivity to heat and cold in the subjects' hands and feet. Even in this relatively large sample, they observed no sex differences in pain sensitivity, although girls had lower thresholds for nonpainful temperatures (warmth and cold) than did boys.

In a study with more clinical content, Bournaki (1997) investigated the responses to venipuncture in 51 girls and 43 boys, ranging in age from 8 to 12 years. Various measures of subjective pain experience as well as heart rate responses failed to reveal a difference between girls and boys. The only difference found was a behavioral measure: girls cried more than boys. Fowler-Kerry and Lander (1991) examined venipuncture pain and anxiety among 90 male and 90 female children and adolescents (aged 5–17 years) and determined that males and females were alike regarding how much they expected the procedure to hurt and how much it did hurt. Overgaard and Knudsen (1999), measuring crying time in neonates during heel prick, also found no sex difference, although Grunau and Craig (1987), for the same procedure, observed that boys were quicker to cry and to display facial expressions of pain.

Particularly interesting is a group of studies that dealt with the pressure pain thresholds of girls and boys, since this experimental pain induction method has yielded especially stable sex differences in adults (Fillingim and Maixner 1995; Berkley 1997; Riley et al. 1998). Hogeweg et al. (1996) used a variable pressure algometer to assess pressure pain thresholds at various body sites in 36 girls and 33 boys, ranging from 6 to 17 years of age. No sex differences were observed, despite findings in the adult literature that male subjects have significantly higher pressure pain thresholds than females (Hogeweg et al. 1992).

Likewise, Pothmann (1993) reported no sex differences in the pressure pain thresholds of 27 children aged 7–15 years, assessed by pressing an algometer against the tip of the index finger. In contrast, Buskila et al. (1993), who determined pressure pain thresholds at various body sites in a sizable sample of schoolchildren (n = 338), found that girls had significantly lower pressure pain thresholds than boys at both fibromyalgia tender points and control sites.

In summary, evidence is mixed as to whether sex differences in pain sensitivity occur in childhood and adolescence. Whereas pressure pain induction almost guarantees sex differences in adults, such differences are rarely demonstrated in studies involving children and adolescents. It is tempting to suggest that at least some important causes of sex differences in pain sensitivity might first become active after puberty.

BIOLOGICAL FACTORS

BLOOD PRESSURE

Given the well-established differences between men and women in many cardiovascular parameters and the documented interaction of blood pressure and reactions to pain, blood pressure regulation must be considered in any attempt to explain sex differences in pain sensitivity (Bruehl et al. 1992; Sheps et al. 1992; McCubbin and Bruehl 1994; Guasti et al. 1999).

Fillingim and Maixner (1996) assessed the impact of resting blood pressure on sex differences in pain reactivity in 23 female and 25 male subjects. They measured pain and tolerance thresholds for contact heat and ischemia and obtained ratings of the intensity and unpleasantness of those stressors. Sex differences occurred only in the ratings of pain intensity for suprathreshold heat stimuli and in ischemic pain tolerance thresholds, with women appearing more sensitive to pain. However, the men had higher blood pressure than the women; the significant differences in male versus female pain reactivity disappeared when blood pressure was used as a covariate. Consequently, blood pressure could be a powerful influence on sex differences in pain sensitivity. A subsequent correlational analysis, however, indicated that blood pressure is inversely related to pain sensitivity only in men, suggesting that this pain-modulatory system may be sex-specific.

To further investigate the hypothesis that higher resting blood pressure does not suppress pain sensitivity in women, Fillingim et al. (1998a) applied contact heat stimuli to the volar forearm and to the face of 21 female subjects. In accordance with the earlier findings, resting blood pressure did not affect pain threshold or pain tolerance threshold. Verbal descriptor pain ratings of suprathreshold stimuli were also unaffected. However, a median split of the blood pressure values indicated that women with higher blood pressure rated thermal pain as less unpleasant than did women whose blood pressure was lower. The relationship between resting blood pressure and pain sensitivity thus appears to depend on the pain dimension under investigation.

A related question concerns whether stress-related changes in blood pressure influence pain sensitivity in a gender-dependent manner. Bragdon et al. (1997) compared 38 men and 36 women for links between stress-evoked cardiovascular responses and changes in pain sensitivity. Contact heat stimuli were administered to the volar forearm to assess pain and tolerance thresholds, both before and after recall of a stressful situation. At baseline, no sex differences in thermal pain sensitivity were present. The stressful situation diminished pain sensitivity only in women with a low resting blood pressure, suggesting that an interaction of stress-induced analgesia and resting blood pressure modulates pain reactivity only in women.

Findings of an earlier study by the same research group seemingly contradict these observations. Maixner and Humphrey (1993) assessed both subjective and cardiovascular responses to tonic ischemic pain produced by a submaximal effort tourniquet technique in 33 women and 34 men. There were no sex differences in pain and tolerance thresholds, but ratings of pain intensity and unpleasantness were higher in women than in men. A blood pressure increase was observed among men during pain stimulation, but no comparable trend was apparent in women. The pain-related changes in blood pressure correlated substantially with the degree of pain experienced by men. Bragdon et al. (1997), however, found that situation-related changes in blood pressure influenced pain sensitivity only in women, although these authors assessed blood pressure responses at rest and during a nonpainful stressor, and then correlated those measures with pain sensitivity (finding that both were positively correlated with pain tolerance among women), while Maixner and Humphrey evaluated changes in blood pressure during the painful task itself (observing that pressure was positively related to the amount of pain experienced).

A predisposition for hypertension may be as important as current blood pressure in accounting for the relationship between cardiovascular reactions and pain responsiveness, since normotensive males with a parental history of hypertension were found to have reduced pain sensitivity (Stewart and France 1996). To discover whether this relationship holds for both sexes, al'Absi et al. (1999) investigated 46 women and 82 men either with or without a parental history of hypertension. The responses to cold-pressor pain were assessed by using concurrent numerical ratings and the McGill Pain Questionnaire. Men with a positive parental history of hypertension differed from the other three groups by showing stronger cardiovascular reactions and lower pain responses to the stressor, but these effects were not found for women. However, D'Antono et al. (1999) did find that women with a parental history of hypertension and/or normatively high resting systolic blood pressure experienced significantly less pain during finger pressure and cold-pressor tests compared to normotensive females.

These relationships are clearly complex and are likely to be clarified in coming years. While current blood pressure and a predisposition for hypertension may contribute to the explanation of sex differences in pain sensitivity, they probably do so only to a moderate degree. It is still far from clear whether the interactions between blood pressure and pain sensitivity, on the one hand, and hypertension risk and pain sensitivity, on the other, are themselves gender-dependent.

BODY SIZE

It has been argued that women are more pain sensitive than men because biological features such as thinner skin, greater density of nociceptive fibers, and shorter length of the afferent pathways accompany their typically smaller body size. Larkin et al. (1986) found that sex differences in electrocutaneous detection and "annoyance" thresholds were eliminated when they covaried the thresholds for body weight or surface area. However, Rollman et al. (1990) found a sex difference in electrical detection, pain, and tolerance thresholds that remained even after statistical correction for body size.

Analyses based on covariance techniques are potentially very instructive, but they are also prone to misinterpretation. To provide evidence for a relationship between body size and pain responsiveness, substantial correlations between these factors must be uncovered both across and within the two sexes. To this end, Lautenbacher and Strian (1991) investigated warmth, cold, phasic pain, and tonic pain thresholds at the hands and feet of 32 women and 32 men. Sex differences occurred only for warmth thresholds, with women being more sensitive than men. As in the study by Larkin et al. (1986), these differences could be removed by using body height and body weight as covariates. Furthermore, multiple correlations between height, weight, and warmth sensitivity were substantial both within and across genders. Hence, individual differences in body size helped to account for sex differences in warmth sensitivity. However, the correlations between body size and pain thresholds were much lower and were barely significant. The lack of a relationship between pain sensitivity and body size within separate male or female groups was corroborated by two later studies (Lautenbacher and Rollman 1993; Lautenbacher and Strian 1993). Consequently, while some evidence has accumulated to suggest that sex differences in sensitivity to nonpainful somatosensory stimuli can be partially attributed to individual differences in body size, the same has not held true for pain sensitivity.

MENSTRUAL CYCLE

Variation of pain sensitivity during the menstrual cycle is reviewed in Chapter 10 of this volume, but we will present a brief overview here. Knowledge regarding the role of the hormonal milieu can enrich our understanding of sex differences in two ways: (1) It is possible that women differ from men in pain sensitivity during certain phases of the menstrual cycle but not during others. If so, studies on sex differences should control for the effect of the menstrual cycle and for the use of oral contraceptives. (2) Variations in pain sensitivity during the menstrual cycle would indicate a relationship between pain sensitivity and sexual hormones, with the latter, of course, being inherently different between the two sexes.

Unfortunately, the available data on the associations between pain responsiveness and menstrual phase are far from clear (Riley et al. 1999). The results of the various studies diverge more than they converge, perhaps because of methodological differences such as variations in the sampling procedure, the experimental pain induction technique, and the determination of menstrual phase, as well as the fact that cyclic variations are only a minor source of variance in pain sensitivity (see Chapter 10 for a detailed discussion). Some studies show that pain sensitivity is higher in the luteal or premenstrual phases than in the follicular or postmenstrual phases (Procacci et al. 1974; Goolkasian 1980, 1983; Hapidou and De Catanzaro 1988; Fillingim et al. 1997), but others have shown no effects or another pattern of cyclic changes (Tedford et al. 1977; Veith et al. 1984; Giamberardino et al. 1997; Hapidou and Rollman 1998). Thus, as Riley et al. (1999) concluded, menstrual cycle phase may influence pain responses among females, but these effects are generally moderate and do not completely explain sex differences in pain sensitivity.

TEMPORAL AND SPATIAL SUMMATION

Clear evidence shows that the method of pain induction is of critical relevance in establishing whether sex differences in pain sensitivity occur in the laboratory. For example, whereas women have reliably appeared to be more pain sensitive than men when pressure pain was applied, results have been inconsistent in the case of thermal stimuli (Fillingim and Maixner 1995; Berkley 1997; Riley et al. 1998). Besides the nature of the physical stimulus, pain induction methods also differ with respect to the temporal aspects (frequency and duration) and spatial characteristics (size and location) of the noxious stimulation. An examination of these factors may help to explain the inconsistency of the findings regarding sex differences within a single pain induction method (Lautenbacher and Rollman 1993).

Only recently have a few studies begun to address this issue. Fillingim et al. (1998b) measured temporal summation of heat pain as well as heat pain threshold, heat tolerance threshold, thermal discrimination ability, and magnitude estimation of heat stimuli in 27 female and 22 male subjects. The women exhibited lower pain thresholds and pain tolerance thresholds than men, but did not differ from men in their discrimination ability or magnitude estimation. Of greatest interest, when tested with a paradigm involving repeated stimulation at noxious temperature levels (designed for measuring temporal summation and "wind-up" of C-fiber-mediated pain; Price et al. 1977), women increased their ratings of pain intensity significantly more than men. This enhancement occurred during the first few trials, suggesting that in women, only a short series of stimuli is required for an augmentation of the pain response.

Fillingim et al. (1998b) suggested that gender differences in thermal pain perception may be more robust for sustained thermal stimuli with a strong C-fiber component, perhaps due to differentially enhanced central wind-up of pain-signaling neurons. Tentative support for this idea came from Fillingim et al. (1999a), who demonstrated that a slow rise time to a painful peak temperature, which also prolongs the time of noxious stimulation, produces slightly greater sex differences in pain threshold than does a fast rise time. Consequently, there is some evidence that women integrate pain signals over time more effectively than men.

A similar hypothesis regarding spatial integration was not supported by the results of a study conducted by Lautenbacher et al. (1999). In 20 women and 20 men, pain thresholds and ratings of suprathreshold stimuli applied to the volar forearm were assessed for four different sizes of thermode ranging from 1 to 10 cm^2. The hypothesis was that women possess a more efficient spatial integration system than men, leading to a robust pain response from smaller areas of stimulation. However, women did not differ from men in any pain measures at any size of thermode. This study indicated that the two sexes have a similar capacity for integrating spatially distinct pain signals.

DIFFUSE NOXIOUS INHIBITORY CONTROLS (DNIC)

"Diffuse noxious inhibitory controls" (DNIC) is the term applied to the finding, first identified in animal-based neurophysiological studies conducted by Le Bars et al. (1979), that noxious stimulation produces antinociceptive effects in an anatomically heterotopic fashion even in far-removed sites. Put more simply, painful stimulation at one body site can suppress pain at more distant loci. DNIC effects are believed to be caused by a descending inhibitory control system that includes supraspinal links in the brainstem. The associated phenomena have also been repeatedly observed in humans (Willer et al. 1984, 1990).

Since the experimental paradigms developed for studying DNIC use two concurrently applied pain stimuli, one for eliciting pain inhibition (the conditioning stimulus) and one for assessing pain inhibition (the test stimulus), the bulk of the laboratory findings on sex differences obtained in single-stimulus procedures cannot be explained by DNIC-like mechanisms. Nevertheless, it is of great interest to determine whether women differ from men in this endogenous pain-inhibitory system.

France and Suchowiecki (1999) investigated sex differences in DNIC effects among 44 women and 39 men. They used ischemic pain on the forearm, produced by a modification of the submaximal effort tourniquet test, as the conditioning stimulus, which activated DNIC and evoked pain inhibition. The inhibitory effect was tested by assessing the amplitude of the R-III nocifensive reflex before and during concurrent ischemic forearm pain. In both males and females, the reflex amplitude was reduced by the concurrent ischemic pain stimulation without any indication of a sex difference. As such, DNIC appeared to be similarly effective in both sexes.

S. Lautenbacher and G.B. Rollman (unpublished data) used a very different methodological approach. We presented concurrent tonic (contact heat to the thigh) and phasic (electrical current to the forearm) pain stimuli at levels above and below pain threshold. The perceptual interaction between the two pain types was assessed in 20 women and 20 men by asking them for combined visual analogue scale ratings of the two pains. Our findings demonstrated, in accord with a DNIC-like phenomenon, that tonic painful heat suppresses the perceived intensity of the phasic stimulus, but that tonic nonpainful heat does not. However, there were no differences between women and men in this respect. Hence, it appears unlikely that DNIC can account for sex differences in pain processing.

PSYCHOLOGICAL FACTORS

ANXIETY

Lautenbacher and Rollman (1993), testing a single group of men and women, found no sex differences in heat pain thresholds, but significant sex differences in pain and tolerance thresholds for electrical pulses applied to the skin (with lower thresholds in women). Likewise, magnitude estimates were similar in women and men for thermal stimuli, but women rated electrical stimuli from 2.5 mA on as more intense than did men. A biological interpretation might suggest that the difference is due to differential activation in men and women of receptors, afferent fibers, spinal pathways, or central regions. It is also plausible to suggest that the differential activation of anxiety could play an important role.

Perhaps women are less familiar with certain noxious stimuli such as electrical pulses or are more likely to catastrophize about dreadful outcomes. In the Lautenbacher and Rollman (1993) study, women had higher state anxiety scores than men (although the differences did not achieve statistical significance). Rollman et al. (1990), however, did find a significant sex difference in anxiety about electrical pulses. So, too, did Robin et al. (1987), who also found a significant correlation between anxiety scores and pain tolerance threshold.

Much has been published on the relationship between anxiety and pain. Cornwall and Donderi (1988) found that anxiety-evoking instructions increased pain ratings, stress intensity ratings, and heart rate compared to standard control instructions when painful pressure was applied to the skin. von Graffenried et al. (1978) indicated that anxiety had a marked effect on experimental pain thresholds.

Women show greater dental anxiety (Liddell and Locker 1997) and greater fear of stimuli associated with dental care (e.g., "feeling the drill in the mouth") (Holtzman et al. 1997). Women have more fear than men of coronary angiography (Heikkila et al. 1999), and girls have more fear than boys about medical procedures (Aho and Erickson 1985). Girls give higher fear ratings for lightning, enclosed spaces, darkness, flying, heights, spiders, snakes, injections, dentists, and injuries (Fredrikson et al. 1996), and they generally report significantly higher levels of fearfulness of objects and situations than do boys (Gullone and King 1993).

Rollman (1995) reviewed a series of studies in which anxiety enhanced pain responsivity and disrupted self-control strategies for dealing with pain. He cited a number of animal studies in which female rats or mice showed more defensive behaviors to threat, had lower levels of analgesia mediated by endogenous opioids after exposure to a predator, and exhibited significantly less opioid and non-opioid stress-induced analgesia than did males. Detailed information about animal studies is found in Chapters 3 and 5 of this volume and in recent articles (e.g., Cicero et al. 1997, 2000; Craft et al. 1999; Kest et al. 1999).

Anxiety sensitivity (fear of anxiety-related bodily sensations) predicts pain sensitivity and anxiety in the cold-pressor task (Schmidt and Cook 1999). Keogh and Birkby (1999) recently reported, for the same test, that high anxiety sensitivity was associated with enhanced pain sensitivity in females, but not males. Asmundson and Taylor (1996) suggested that anxiety sensitivity may act as a risk factor for chronic pain. Indeed, women are at greater risk for a multitude of pain syndromes (Unruh 1996), and interference due to pain has a greater impact on threat appraisal of pain for women and leads to greater health care utilization (Unruh et al. 1999). Clearly, the findings obtained from laboratory studies with induced pain provide provocative proposals regarding clinical pain perception and coping patterns in men and women.

The issue of differential engagement of neural mechanisms associated with emotion and pain appraisal is made all the more germane by the results of a neuroimaging study conducted by Paulson et al. (1998). The authors used positron emission tomography to detect increases in regional cerebral blood flow in normal male and female subjects as they discriminated differences in the intensity of innocuous and noxious heat stimuli applied to the forearm. Females rated the 50°C stimuli as significantly more intense than did males and had significantly greater activation of the contralateral prefrontal cortex, a region seen as particularly salient in encoding anxiety (Wedzony et al. 1996; Kimbrell et al. 1999).

We still have much to learn about the relation between anxiety and pain. Recently, Rhudy and Meagher (2000) examined the effects of experimentally induced fear and anxiety on radiant heat pain thresholds. Fear was induced by exposure to three brief shocks and anxiety by the threat of shock. While fear resulted in decreased pain reactivity, anxiety had the opposite effect. It would be interesting to see whether there are interactions among the nature of the affective stimulus, pain responsiveness, and sex. We also need to look carefully at measures of pain-specific anxiety and fear that are focused on the experimental stressors rather than simply assessing the more wide-ranging state anxiety.

STRESS RESPONSES

Curiously, while the animal literature contains much evidence of sex differences in stress reactions, little is known about stress as a candidate for accounting in sex differences in human pain responsiveness. Among mice, a sexual dimorphism in the pituitary-adrenal function is evidenced by higher corticosterone levels in females (Gaillard and Spinedi 1998). Exposure to mild electrofoot shocks caused female rats to secrete significantly more adrenocorticotropic hormone, a stress hormone, than did male animals (Rivier 1999). Romero and Bodnar (1986) discovered that female rats show significantly less stress-induced analgesia than males following both continuous cold-water (non-opioid) and intermittent cold-water (opioid) swims, and others have demonstrated sex-dependent alterations in the neurochemical mediation of stress and pain in mice and rats (e.g., Mogil and Belknap 1997; Aloisi et al. 1998; Sternberg 1999).

Jones et al. (1997) showed that women who suffer temporomandibular dysfunction (TMD) (a disorder in which the prevalence rate for women is much greater than that for men) showed a significantly higher cortisol response to experimental stress than did a control group. The patient data indicated the presence of two subgroups, one of which was particularly reactive to stress. The findings suggest a biological predisposition to TMD; the epidemiologic data (e.g., LeResche 1997), suggest a differential effect on women. Given the overrepresentation of women in other disorders such as fibromyalgia and chronic fatigue syndrome, researchers ought to conduct more laboratory-based studies of sex differences in stress perception, stress response, stress-induced analgesia, and the elicitation of hormones and neuropeptides. Derangements in the stress axis and accompanying neuroendocrine modifications may render women particularly vulnerable to numerous complex pain syndromes (Rollman and Lautenbacher 1993; Clauw 1995; Clauw and Chrousos 1997; Demitrack 1997).

The literature on the relationship between stress and the organism's sex has largely looked at stress-induced analgesia elicited by environmental stressors. Both animal and human studies are needed that carefully examine sex differences in the behavioral and neuroendocrinological correlates of the stress induced by exposure to the pain laboratory itself (Dworkin and Chen 1982) and to the trial-by-trial discomfort of various noxious stimuli. We must explore the implications of any resulting differences in accounting for disproportionate incidence of chronic pain disorders (Winfield 1999).

CRITERION EFFECTS

Perhaps because of anxiety, perhaps because of greater wisdom, women may choose not to play the same game as men. That is, women and men may perceive experimentally induced pain to be equally painful, but women prefer not to go to higher levels. Some data might counter that argument. In studies using electrical pulses (Rollman and Harris 1987; Rollman et al. 1990; Lautenbacher and Rollman 1993), women had a significantly lower detection threshold than men (even in experiments that used forced-choice adaptive techniques that eliminated response bias). Also, compared to men, women gave higher pain ratings to equally intense stimuli, for both thermal pulses (Feine et al. 1991) and electrical pulses (Lautenbacher and Rollman 1993).

Still, data indicate that at least part of the sex difference in pain responsiveness is related to willingness rather than ability to endure discomfort. Rollman (1995) describes an experiment in which male and female observers were tested for pain threshold and tolerance with three different noxious stimuli: electric shock, cold-pressor pain, and a constant-pressure algometer. When subjects felt that they had reached the appropriate level, they were asked to use a 10-point scale to describe the painfulness of their experience. There were interesting differences across induction methods (the mean rating when subjects had reached the maximum level they were willing to endure was 5.9 for shock but 7.9 for cold and 7.1 for pressure). Moreover, women stopped the presentation of electrical pulses at a level of about 5 (moderate), whereas men went to nearly 7. It appears that women knew that this was not truly their tolerance; rather, they preferred to call a halt at a level far below maximum tolerance. The same tendency was observed for cold and pressure, but the difference was considerably smaller. Rollman (1995) suggested that the sex difference in self-described tolerance, particularly for electrical shock, was due to differential anxiety to the stimuli, an interpretation supported by the results of an experiment in which electrical pain tolerance levels increased over repeated testing sessions for women but remained constant for men.

A more recent study by Rollman and Hervieux (1999) had a somewhat different outcome. Recognizing that numerous earlier studies that looked at the scaling of noxious stimuli at different intensities were obliged to drop potential subjects who were unable to tolerate the stimuli at the upper end of the range (thereby obtaining a nonrepresentative sample of women), Rollman and Hervieux measured each subject's pain threshold and tolerance for electrical shocks and tailored the range for the scaling experiment to span that range. Large sex differences in pain threshold and tolerance were found. The power functions that related perceived intensity or unpleasantness to current were essentially parallel, with those for women shifted to the left of those for men. Moreover, although members of both sexes reached tolerance at a self-admittedly low level of pain, the average ratings for threshold and tolerance were much the same across sexes. These data suggest that an important biological component may underlie the sex difference in electrically induced pain. A corresponding study with thermal heat stimuli is in progress (G.B. Rollman and L. Parlea, unpublished data).

Related evidence for a low-level contribution to sex differences comes from a study by Ellermeier and Westphal (1995) on responses to tonic finger pressure. Female subjects reported greater pain than males at high levels of stimulation and showed greater pupil dilations. Since pupil response is seen as an autonomic indicator of pain that is beyond voluntary control, these sex differences should reflect fundamental sensory or affective components of pain. The R-III reflex, a spinal nociceptive reflex recorded from the biceps femoris and typically considered to be outside conscious control, also occurs at a lower level of electrical stimulation for females relative to males (France and Suchowiecki 1999).

Signal detection theory methods have been proposed as a way to learn about criterion effects in pain. While there are questions about the unambiguous interpretation of the resulting data (Rollman 1977), Clark and Mehl (1971) stated that women had a lower criterion than men for reporting pain. Likewise, Ellermeier (1997), in a re-analysis of scaling data (Ellermeier and Westphal 1995) showing that women rate various levels of pressure on the finger as more painful than men, suggested that the two sexes are equal in sensory discrimination but that women have a greater bias to assign higher ratings, particularly as stimulus intensity approaches tolerance.

HYPERVIGILANCE

Numerous disorders (e.g., fibromyalgia, temporomandibular disorders, irritable bowel syndrome) have a large preponderance of women among the patients (Dworkin et al. 1990; Wolfe et al. 1995; Toner and Akman 2000). In these syndromes, patients generally have lower pain thresholds and tolerance levels than do pain-free controls (e.g., Scudds et al. 1987; Rollman 1989; Gibson et al. 1994; Lautenbacher et al. 1994; Maixner et al. 1995; Fillingim et al. 1996; Naliboff et al. 1997; Kashima et al. 1999). Might these factors be related?

Gender imbalance in prevalence for painful disorders and enhanced pain sensitivity may be linked through the concept of hypervigilance (Rollman and Lautenbacher 1993). Hypervigilance reflects a generalized pattern of hyper-responsiveness to internal and external discomfort which, because it is also seen for response to other sensory inputs such as noise (McDermid et al. 1996), extends beyond the traditional pain domain. The hyper-responsiveness in fibromyalgia patients may account for their report of a wide range of bodily symptoms and complaints including headache, irritable bowel, dysmenorrhea, light sensitivity, temporomandibular dysfunction, and paresthesias (Yunus et al. 1991; Waylonis and Heck 1992). Even certain forms of the DNIC paradigm, discussed above, may reflect an attentional disorder in which individuals concentrate on all noxious inputs while others channel their attentional capacity to the longest and most intense input.

Further research must determine whether the heightened responsiveness seen in these patients, and perhaps more generally in women, reflects a widespread disturbance of sensory processing (Dohrenbusch et al. 1997), a localized or generalized hyperalgesia (Okifuji et al. 1999), a neural sensitization (Bell et al. 1998), or a more comprehensive alteration in pain detection, interpretation, and response.

Rollman and Lautenbacher have proposed that hypervigilance is a more focused hypothesis than hypochondriasis, emphasizing perceptual and cognitive processes rather than psychopathological ones (Rollman and Lautenbacher 1993; Lautenbacher and Rollman 1999). As applied to sex differences, the concept goes beyond differences in sensory transduction and transmission to include a series of affective and cognitive states (Rollman 1998). Women may be more likely than men to monitor internal and external events (Miller 1987), to attribute bodily signs to physiological causes rather than to environmental or psychological factors (Robbins and Kirmayer 1991; van Wijk and Kolk 1997), to demonstrate a maladaptive pattern of coping in attempting to deal with their situation (Unruh et al. 1999), and to react to negative events and cognitions with increased pain responsiveness. Additionally, women may respond to noxious events with one or more bodily reactions such as localized or widespread muscle tension, altered gastric motility, and marked autonomic or cardiovascular function.

van Wijk and Kolk (1997) noted that health surveys, studies on symptom reporting, and examination of medical records all reveal consistent sex differences in the description of physical symptoms, with women having higher rates independent of morbidity. The authors' symptom perception model, an expansion of the symptom sensitivity hypothesis (Gijsbers van Wijk et al. 1991), emphasizes sex differences in selection of information about one's body, attribution of somatic sensations, and the personality factors of somatization and negative affectivity.

Further research is needed to relate individual differences in symptom perception, symptom appraisal, symptom reporting, illness behavior, and negative mood (e.g., Verbrugge 1980; van Vliet et al. 1994; Katon and Walker 1998; Almeida et al. 1999; Gijsbers van Wijk et al. 1999; Wolfe and Hawley 1999). Corresponding differences in the sensory, affective, and cognitive response to experimentally induced pain (e.g., Fillingim et al. 1999b) must be investigated, with particular attention paid to the role of sex.

PSYCHOSOCIAL INFLUENCES

Thoughts, attitudes, and behaviors are all generated within a social context (Jacklin 1989). Individuals are likely to think about and react to painful events in a manner consistent with socially accepted, gender-based expectations. However, the influence of gender on the sensory, affective, and cognitive components of pain has only recently begun to be explored.

Gender has been defined as "a scheme for the social categorization of individuals" (Sherif 1982), and has been proposed as a term that allows us to distinguish between the biological and social components of sex (Unger 1979). As opposed to the study of more biologically oriented sex differences, research on gender seeks to view differences between men and women through a culturally defined lens, one that provides an image of appropriate traits and behaviors for men and women. Gender (or sex) roles have been characterized as scripts that men and women follow in specific situations; they contain information relating to socially expected and encouraged patterns of masculine or feminine behavior (Bem 1981).

Gender-based psychosocial factors may predispose men and women to respond to pain in different ways. For instance, several studies have demonstrated that sex differences in health behavior can be partially explained by role obligations (Verbrugge 1985; Unruh 1996). By means of cognitive appraisal, men and women may come to develop different interpretations of the meaning of a painful experience.

Unruh (1996) argues that some pain experienced by women is associated with normal biological events related to the reproductive cycle; women must therefore make more distinctions than men between the kinds of pain that originate from normal and abnormal processes. Other authors have noted that the consequences of pain, especially in its more chronic manifestations, are linked to gender-based self-perceptions. In a study looking at women with musculoskeletal pain, Johansson et al. (1999) found that many described such discomfort as having negative consequences for their everyday life, challenging their self-perceptions as women. These findings highlight the corollaries of pain that operate on social and interpersonal levels.

The role of sex in pain-coping strategies figured prominently in a recent paper by Affleck et al. (1999). Patients with osteoarthritis or rheumatoid arthritis completed daily diaries, over a 30-day period, rating their pain, mood, and ability to cope. The average pain of women patients was 72% greater than that of men; women tended to emphasize emotion-focused strategies (venting emotions, redefinition, seeking spiritual comfort, and seeking emotional support) rather than problem-focused coping (attempted pain reduction, relaxation, and distraction).

Several studies have determined that the choice of coping strategies is mediated not only by sex but also by gender-role orientation (Evans 1982; Nezu and Nezu 1987; Long 1989). Bendelow (1993) postulated that while women may be expected to possess superior capacities for coping with pain because it is linked to their biological and reproductive systems, cultural role expectations and socialization processes undermine these potential strengths because both women and men are taught that high tolerance of pain is a "masculine" trait. Women tend to be more worried and irritated about pain (Bendelow 1993), and men to be more embarrassed by lapses of stoicism (Klonoff and Landrine 1992).

Research suggests that male and female reactions to stressors relate to whether the situations elicit an appraisal process based on perceived sex-role expectations. Lash et al. (1991) found that sex differences in cardiovascular reactivity to a stressor were strongly related to the participants' cognitive appraisals of the stressor as involving masculine or feminine components. When confronted with a cold-pressor task, men showed greater cardiovascular response when they had been given instructions that were framed in a masculine way (emphasizing perseverance or endurance) as opposed to a gender-neutral manner. Wright et al. (1997) found that physiological responsivity in a stressful task was linked to expectations about differential sex-linked performance. However, further research is needed to determine the extent to which such attributions and beliefs underlie the experimental pain experience.

As discussed in detail above (see "Criterion Effects" section), Rollman (1995) noted that women called for the cessation of aversive electrical shock when it had reached only a moderate degree of painfulness, whereas men waited until the stimulus train was more painful before they stopped the trial. In essence, the women were aware that their true tolerance levels were higher than those they reported. Perhaps these results can be ascribed to the influence of gender-role expectations regarding the pain experience.

Some evidence supports this claim. Otto and Dougher (1985) uncovered a significant interaction between masculinity-femininity scores and sex for pain thresholds. High masculinity scores on the Bem Sex Role Inventory (Bem 1974) were linked to higher pain threshold and tolerance, indicating that men and women may base their perceptions of the appropriateness of a particular pain response on their affiliation with traditional masculine or feminine roles.

A recent study by Jones and Rollman (1999) attempted to determine the relative influence of gender role and gender-based appraisal on the pain experience. Significant sex differences existed for a number of traditionally gender-based variables (e.g., masculinity-femininity, instrumentality-expressiveness, attitudes toward women), but their ability to predict pain responsivity in a cold-pressor task was overshadowed by the influence of sex as a predictor variable in subsequent regression analyses. The relationship between sex and pain, on the one hand, and sex and gender identity, on the other, are each so strong that it is fruitless to try to argue for a purely biological or purely psychosocial explanation of male-female differences in pain response.

Higher scores on the Bem femininity subscale were linked with lower pain threshold scores in female participants, while a negligible relationship was observed between these variables for the male group. Additional results indicated that increased femininity scores were associated with higher pain intensity ratings in women, while increased masculinity scores were associated with lower pain ratings in men. This tendency may directly reflect differences in early socialization practices relating to pain behavior. Bendelow (1993) found that men indicated that as boys they already felt an obligation, when faced with pain, to display stoicism, while women reported that as children they were permitted to be much more expressive. Fearon et al. (1996) found no sex differences among a group of 3- to 7-year-old children in the incidence of everyday pain from mishaps such as bumps, cuts, and scrapes, but that girls engaged more often in distress responses and received more physical comfort from adult caregivers.

Jones and Rollman (1999) found that male participants, when asked to report their own pain tolerance on a 0–100 scale, gave a significantly higher value than that given by females. The majority of both male and female participants endorsed the notion that the laboratory pain tolerance of men is higher than that of women. Interestingly, the women's concession that men were more tolerant of experimental pain did not necessarily imply that they believed men were less sensitive to pain in general.

These various cognitive-evaluative judgments relating to expectations and beliefs concerning pain demonstrate gender differences along several interesting lines. Further investigation into the pain-related beliefs of men and women would help to determine which factors influence the formation of such beliefs and how they are implicated in interpretations of and coping reactions to pain. Research must determine whether gender-based beliefs and attributions (Unruh et al. 1999) apply equally to experimentally induced and clinical pain, since the former is brief and voluntary while the latter is often extended and outside the individual's control. As Morris (1999) noted, pain is infused with meaning, and our beliefs concerning pain (its cause, control, and duration) are determinants of our reactions to it. The relationship between gender-dependent beliefs concerning sex differences in pain and responses to both experimental and clinical pain situations is an area worthy of further investigation.

CONCLUDING REMARKS

Psychologists are fond of saying that behavior is multiply determined. Perhaps nowhere is that as evident as in the literature on sex differences in pain. An argument can be made for the importance of each of the factors reviewed in this chapter and for many more. None of them alone can explain sex differences. Research on sex differences, whether in the laboratory or in the clinic, validates the biopsychosocial model with respect to all aspects of pain: etiology, pathogenesis, suffering, and management.

This chapter has illustrated the interplay of developmental, biological, and psychological variables in accounting for pain behavior. While some may question the validity of studies conducted in the pain laboratory, the robust findings reported here suggest that such experiments have direct and immediate applicability to our understanding of "real world" pain experiences. Clearly, there are differences in the outcomes of seemingly similar experiments. Investigators are faced with the need to carefully identify the stimulus, situational, and response variables that distinguish those studies and to develop models that permit us to specify, with greater precision, the role of direct and moderating influences.

To take just one example, that of experimental pain induction, the evidence suggests that mechanical, electrical, thermal, and chemical stimulation techniques differ in terms of neural mechanisms, central integration, affective responses, and cognitive evaluations. Given that sex differences are seen most often when pressure is used as the noxious input (Fillingim and Maixner 1995; Berkley 1997; Riley et al. 1998), and given the clinical relevance of that form of stimulation, efforts should be made to develop and use precisely controlled mechanical stimuli in explanatory studies.

Even simple situational variables deserve more attention. Researchers rarely ask subjects about recent nicotine consumption, yet Jamner et al. (1998) demonstrated in 44 female and 30 male smokers that nicotine increased the pain threshold and tolerance ratings for electrocutaneous stimuli in men but had no effect on the pain parameters of women. Similarly, the consumption of high-sugar snacks, a frequent behavior that differs across the sexes (e.g., Millen et al. 1996; Hoglund et al. 1998) is largely overlooked in pain research, yet women were more likely than men to exhibit a decrease of pain sensitivity after consuming sugar (Mercer and Holder 1997). Accordingly, common behaviors that affect pain sensitivity in a gender-dependent manner and are likely to take place shortly before laboratory experiments need to be considered in the design of future studies.

Electrophysiological and brain imaging studies indicate that sex differences occur at many stages of pain processing (Paulson et al. 1998; Chapman et al. 1999). Numerous biological factors are candidates to account for sex differences in pain sensitivity, including blood pressure, body size, menstrual cycle, temporal and spatial summation, and dysregulation of central nervous system structures involved in pain inhibition and stress responses. These reports indicate that the variables associated with sex differences start with the onset of nociceptive processing and extend to late affective and cognitive components of pain. Given that men and women differ in many biological and psychological domains, the next step is to develop a scientific framework for understanding these differences and for generating accurate predictions about sex differences that have not yet been fully uncovered.

The influence of gender roles, attitudes, and self-beliefs concerning the ability of men and women to withstand experimental pain situations requires further investigation. Since any sex differences are likely to be tightly intertwined with being male or female, the ability to successfully define such influences will ultimately depend on the nature of the empirical questions asked and the strength of the associated research designs. Indeed, as argued by Spence and Buckner (1995), the notion of gender includes within it a huge collection of characteristics. Future research should attempt to delineate the specific traits, tendencies, or beliefs more commonly associated with one gender versus the other that help to determine how men and women perceive, feel, and react in a pain situation.

This need was summarized concisely by Leventhal (1994), who stated that as the various factors that distinguish men and women are identified, incorporated, and sequenced in a multifactorial model of gender and health, the confusion created by the often divergent responses made by men and women will vanish. Instead, these differences will come to be seen as consequences of diverse antecedent factors, driving mechanisms that are somewhat overlapping and somewhat independent.

People endow many objects and events with gender significance (Spence and Buckner 1995). Pre-existing beliefs concerning sex differences in pain may largely result from the differential socialization of males and females into masculine and feminine roles. Given the need for rehabilitative strategies that target the different behaviors and strengths exhibited by men and women in response to pain, research focusing on the effects of sex and gender on reactions to pain is both scientifically justified and clinically relevant. While the measurement of gender-based differences may tap into only one of the complex multidimensional components involved in the human experience of pain, it represents a quest that continues to be both timely and appropriate.

ACKNOWLEDGMENT

This contribution was assisted by a grant from the TransCoop Program of the German-American Academic Council Foundation to S. Lautenbacher and G.B. Rollman and by a grant from the Natural Sciences and Engineering Research Council of Canada to G.B. Rollman.

REFERENCES

Affleck G, Tennen H, Keefe FJ, et al. Everyday life with osteoarthritis or rheumatoid arthritis: independent effects of disease and gender on daily pain, mood, and coping. *Pain* 1999; 83:601–609.

Aho AC, Erickson MT. Effects of grade, gender, and hospitalization on children's medical fears. *J Dev Behav Pediatr* 1985; 6:146–153.

al'Absi M, Buchanan TW, Marrero A, Lovallo WR. Sex differences in pain perception and cardiovascular responses in persons with parental history for hypertension. *Pain* 1999; 83:331–338.

Almeida SA, Trone DW, Leone DM, et al. Gender differences in musculoskeletal injury rates: a function of symptom reporting? *Med Sci Sports Exerc* 1999; 31:1807–1812.

Aloisi AM, Ceccarelli I, Lupo C. Behavioural and hormonal effects of restraint stress and formalin test in male and female rats. *Brain Res Bull* 1998; 47:57–62.

Asmundson GJ, Taylor S. Role of anxiety sensitivity in pain-related fear and avoidance. *J Behav Med* 1996; 19:577–586.

Bell IR, Baldwin CM, Russek LG, Schwartz GE, Hardin EE. Early life stress, negative paternal relationships, and chemical intolerance in middle-aged women: support for a neural sensitization model. *J Womens Health* 1998; 7:1135–1147.

Bem SL. The measurement of psychological androgyny. *J Consult Clin Psychol* 1974; 42:155–162.

Bem SL. Gender schema theory: a cognitive account of sex-typing. *Psychol Rev* 1981; 88:354–364.

Bendelow G. Pain perceptions, emotions and gender. *Sociol Health Ill* 1993; 15:273–293.

Berkley KJ. Sex differences in pain. *Behav Brain Sci* 1997; 20:371–380.

Bournaki MC. Correlates of pain-related responses to venipunctures in school-age children. *Nurs Res* 1997; 46:147–154.

Bragdon EE, Light KC, Girdler SS, Maixner W. Blood pressure, gender, and parental hypertension are factors in baseline and poststress pain sensitivity in normotensive adults. *Int J Behav Med* 1997; 4:17–38.

Bruehl S, Carlson CR, McCubbin JA. The relationship between pain sensitivity and blood pressure in normotensives. *Pain* 1992; 48:463–467.

Buskila D, Press J, Gedalia A, et al. Assessment of nonarticular tenderness and prevalence of fibromyalgia in children. *J Rheumatol* 1993; 20:368–370.

Chapman CR, Oka S, Bradshaw DH, Jacobson RC, Donaldson GW. Phasic pupil dilation response to noxious stimulation in normal volunteers: relationship to brain evoked potentials and pain report. *Psychophysiology* 1999; 36:44–52.

Cicero TJ, Nock B, Meyer ER. Sex-related differences in morphine's antinociceptive activity: relationship to serum and brain morphine concentrations. *J Pharmacol Exp Ther* 1997; 282:939–944.

Cicero TJ, Ennis T, Ogden J, Meyer ER. Gender differences in the reinforcing properties of morphine. *Pharmacol Biochem Behav* 2000; 65:91–96.

Clark WC, Mehl L. Thermal pain: a sensory decision theory analysis of the effect of age and sex on d′, various response criteria, and 50 per cent pain threshold. *J Abnorm Psychol* 1971; 78:202–212.

Clauw DJ. The pathogenesis of chronic pain and fatigue syndromes, with special reference to fibromyalgia. *Med Hypotheses* 1995; 44:369–378.

Clauw DJ, Chrousos GP. Chronic pain and fatigue syndromes: overlapping clinical and neuroendocrine features and potential pathogenic mechanisms. *Neuroimmunomodulation* 1997; 4:134–153.

Cornwall A, Donderi DC. The effect of experimentally induced anxiety on the experience of pressure pain. *Pain* 1988; 35:105–113.

Craft RM, Stratmann JA, Bartok RE, Walpole TI, King SJ. Sex differences in development of morphine tolerance and dependence in the rat. *Psychopharmacology (Berl)* 1999; 143:1–7.

D'Antono B, Ditto B, Rios N, Moskowitz DS. Risk for hypertension and diminished pain sensitivity in women: autonomic and daily correlates. *Int J Psychophysiol* 1999; 31:175–187.

Demitrack MA. Neuroendocrine correlates of chronic fatigue syndrome: a brief review. *J Psychiatr Res* 1997; 31:69–82.

Dohrenbusch R, Sodhi H, Lamprecht J, Genth E. Fibromyalgia as a disorder of perceptual organization? An analysis of acoustic stimulus processing in patients with widespread pain. *Z Rheumatol* 1997; 56:334–341.

Dworkin SF, Chen AC. Pain in clinical and laboratory contexts. *J Dent Res* 1982; 61:772–774.

Dworkin SF, Huggins KH, LeResche L, et al. Epidemiology of signs and symptoms in temporomandibular disorders: clinical signs in cases and controls. *J Am Dent Assoc* 1990; 120:273–281.

Ellermeier W. On separating pain from the willingness to report it. *Behav Brain Sci* 1997; 20:448–449.

Ellermeier W, Westphal W. Gender differences in pain ratings and pupil reactions to painful pressure stimuli. *Pain* 1995; 61:435–439.

Evans RG. Defense mechanisms in females as a function of sex-role orientation. *J Clin Psychol* 1982; 38:816–817.

Fearon I, McGrath PJ, Achat H. 'Booboos': the study of everyday pain among young children. *Pain* 1996; 68:55–62.

Feine JS, Bushnell MC, Miron D, Duncan GH. Sex differences in the perception of noxious heat stimuli. *Pain* 1991; 44:255–262.

Fillingim RB, Maixner W. Gender differences in the responses to noxious stimuli. *Pain Forum* 1995; 4:209–221.

Fillingim RB, Maixner W. The influence of resting blood pressure and gender on pain responses. *Psychosom Med* 1996; 58:326–332.

Fillingim RB, Maixner W, Kincaid S, Sigurdsson A, Harris MB. Pain sensitivity in patients with temporomandibular disorders: relationship to clinical and psychosocial factors. *Clin J Pain* 1996; 12:260–269.

Fillingim RB, Maixner W, Girdler SS, et al. Ischemic but not thermal pain sensitivity varies across the menstrual cycle. *Psychosom Med* 1997; 59:512–520.

Fillingim RB, Maixner W, Bunting S, Silva S. Resting blood pressure and thermal pain responses among females: effects on pain unpleasantness but not pain intensity. *Int J Psychophysiol* 1998a; 30:313–318.

Fillingim RB, Maixner W, Kincaid S, Silva S. Sex differences in temporal summation but not sensory-discriminative processing of thermal pain. *Pain* 1998b; 75:121–127.

Fillingim RB, Maddux V, Shackelford JA. Sex differences in heat pain thresholds as a function of assessment method and rate of rise. *Somatosens Mot Res* 1999a; 16:57–62.

Fillingim RB, Edwards RR, Powell T. The relationship of sex and clinical pain to experimental pain responses. *Pain* 1999b; 83:419–425.

Fowler-Kerry S, Lander J. Assessment of sex differences in children's and adolescents' self-reported pain from venipuncture. *J Pediatr Psychol* 1991; 16:783–793.

France CR, Suchowiecki S. A comparison of diffuse noxious inhibitory controls in men and women. *Pain* 1999; 81:77–84.

Fredrikson M, Annas P, Fischer H, Wik G. Gender and age differences in the prevalence of specific fears and phobias. *Behav Res Ther* 1996; 34:33–39.

Gaillard RC, Spinedi E. Sex- and stress-steroids interactions and the immune system: evidence for a neuroendocrine-immunological sexual dimorphism. *Domest Anim Endocrinol* 1998; 15:345–352.

Giamberardino MA, Berkley KJ, Iezzi S, de Bigontina P, Vecchiet L. Pain threshold variations in somatic wall tissues as a function of menstrual cycle, segmental site and tissue depth in non-dysmenorrheic women, dysmenorrheic women and men. *Pain* 1997; 71:187–197.

Gibson SJ, Littlejohn GO, Gorman MM, Helme RD, Granges G. Altered heat pain thresholds and cerebral event-related potentials following painful CO_2 laser stimulation in subjects with fibromyalgia syndrome. *Pain* 1994; 58:185–193.

Gijsbers van Wijk CM, van Vliet KP, Kolk AM, Everaerd WT. Symptom sensitivity and sex differences in physical morbidity: a review of health surveys in the United States and The Netherlands. *Womens Health* 1991; 17:91–124.

Gijsbers van Wijk CM, Huisman H, Kolk AM. Gender differences in physical symptoms and illness behavior: a health diary study. *Soc Sci Med* 1999; 49:1061–1074.

Goolkasian P. Cyclic changes in pain perception: an ROC analysis. *Percept Psychophys* 1980; 27:499–504.

Goolkasian P. An ROC analysis of pain reactions in dysmenorrheic and nondysmenorrheic women. *Percept Psychophys* 1983; 34:381–386.

Grunau RV, Craig KD. Pain expression in neonates: facial action and cry. *Pain* 1987; 28:395–410.

Guasti L, Gaudio G, Zanotta D, et al. Relationship between a genetic predisposition to hypertension, blood pressure levels and pain sensitivity. *Pain* 1999; 82:311–317.

Gullone E, King NJ. The fears of youth in the 1990s: contemporary normative data. *J Genet Psychol* 1993; 154:137–153.

Hapidou EG, De Catanzaro D. Sensitivity to cold pressor pain in dysmenorrheic and non-dysmenorrheic women as a function of menstrual cycle phase. *Pain* 1988; 34:277–283.

Hapidou EG, Rollman GB. Menstrual cycle modulation of tender points. *Pain* 1998; 77:151–161.

Heikkila J, Paunonen M, Virtanen V, Laippala P. Gender differences in fears related to coronary arteriography. *Heart Lung* 1999; 28:20–30.

Hogeweg JA, Langereis MJ, Bernards AT, Faber JA, Helders PJ. Algometry. Measuring pain threshold, method and characteristics in healthy subjects. *Scand J Rehabil Med* 1992; 24:99–103.

Hogeweg JA, Kuis W, Oostendorp RA, Helders PJ. The influence of site of stimulation, age, and gender on pain threshold in healthy children. *Phys Ther* 1996; 76:1331–1339.

Hoglund D, Samuelson G, Mark A. Food habits in Swedish adolescents in relation to socioeconomic conditions. *Eur J Clin Nutr* 1998; 52:784–789.

Holtzman JM, Berg RG, Mann J, Berkey DB. The relationship of age and gender to fear and anxiety in response to dental care. *Spec Care Dentist* 1997; 17:82–87.

Jacklin CN. Female and male: issues of gender. *Am Psychol* 1989; 44:127–133.

Jamner LD, Girdler SS, Shapiro D, Jarvik ME. Pain inhibition, nicotine, and gender. *Exp Clin Psychopharmacol* 1998; 6:96–106.

Johansson EE, Hamberg K, Westman G, Lindgren G. The meanings of pain: an exploration of women's descriptions of symptoms. *Soc Sci Med* 1999; 48:1791–1802.

Jones DA, Rollman GB, Brooke RI. The cortisol response to psychological stress in temporomandibular dysfunction. *Pain* 1997; 72:171–182.

Jones KS, Rollman GB. Gender-related differences in response to experimentally-induced pain: the influence of psychosocial variables. *Abstracts of the 18th Annual Meeting of the American Pain Society*. American Pain Society, 1999, p 127.

Kashima K, Rahman OI, Sakoda S, Shiba R. Increased pain sensitivity of the upper extremities of TMD patients with myalgia to experimentally-evoked noxious stimulation: possibility of worsened endogenous opioid systems. *Cranio* 1999; 17:241–246.

Katon WJ, Walker EA. Medically unexplained symptoms in primary care. *J Clin Psychiatry* 1998; 59 (Suppl 20):15–21.

Keogh E, Birkby J. The effect of anxiety sensitivity and gender on the experience of pain. *Cognition Emotion* 1999; 13:813–829.

Kest B, Wilson SG, Mogil JS. Sex differences in supraspinal morphine analgesia are dependent on genotype. *J Pharmacol Exp Ther* 1999; 289:1370–1375.

Kimbrell TA, George MS, Parekh PI, et al. Regional brain activity during transient self-induced anxiety and anger in healthy adults. *Biol Psychiatry* 1999; 46:454–465.

Klonoff EA, Landrine H. Sex roles, occupational roles, and symptom-reporting: a test of competing hypotheses on sex differences. *J Behav Med* 1992; 15:355–364.

Larkin WD, Reilly JP, Kittler LB. Individual differences in sensitivity to transient electrocutaneous stimulation. *IEEE Trans Biomed Eng* 1986; 33:495–504.

Lash SJ, Gillespie BL, Eisler RM, Southard DR. Sex differences in cardiovascular reactivity: effects of the gender relevance of the stressor. *Health Psychol* 1991; 10:392–398.

Lautenbacher S, Rollman GB. Sex differences in responsiveness to painful and non-painful stimuli are dependent upon the stimulation method. *Pain* 1993; 53:255–264.

Lautenbacher S, Rollman GB. Somatization, hypochondriasis, and related conditions. In: Block AR, Kremer EF, Fernandez E (Eds). *Handbook of Pain Syndromes: Biopsychosocial Perspectives*. Mahwah, NJ: Lawrence Erlbaum Associates, 1999, pp 613–632.

Lautenbacher S, Strian F. Sex differences in pain and thermal sensitivity: the role of body size. *Percept Psychophys* 1991; 50:179–183.

Lautenbacher S, Strian F. The role of body size in somatosensory testing. *Electromyogr Clin Neurophysiol* 1993; 33:113–118.

Lautenbacher S, Rollman GB, McCain GA. Multi-method assessment of experimental and clinical pain in patients with fibromyalgia. *Pain* 1994; 59:45–53.

Lautenbacher S, Nielsen J, Andersen T, Arendt-Nielsen L. Spatial summation of heat pain in males and females. *Abstracts: 9th World Congress on Pain*. Seattle: IASP Press, 1999, p 409.

Le Bars D, Dickenson AH, Besson JM. Diffuse noxious inhibitory controls (DNIC). I. Effects on dorsal horn convergent neurones in the rat. *Pain* 1979; 6:283–304.

LeResche L. Epidemiology of temporomandibular disorders: implications for the investigation of etiologic factors. *Crit Rev Oral Biol Med* 1997; 8:291–305.

Leventhal EA. Gender and aging: women and their aging. In: Adesso VJ, Reddy DM, Fleming R (Eds). *Psychological Perspectives on Women's Health*. Washington, DC: Taylor and Francis, 1994, pp 11–35.

Liddell A, Locker D. Gender and age differences in attitudes to dental pain and dental control. *Community Dent Oral Epidemiol* 1997; 25:314–318.

Long BC. Sex-role orientation, coping strategies, and self-efficacy of women in traditional and nontraditional occupations. *Psychol Women Quart* 1989; 13:307–324.

Maixner W, Humphrey C. Gender differences in pain and cardiovascular responses to forearm ischemia. *Clin J Pain* 1993; 9:16–25.

Maixner W, Fillingim R, Booker D, Sigurdsson A. Sensitivity of patients with painful temporomandibular disorders to experimentally evoked pain. *Pain* 1995; 63:341–351.

McCubbin JA, Bruehl S. Do endogenous opioids mediate the relationship between blood pressure and pain sensitivity in normotensives? *Pain* 1994; 57:63–67.

McDermid AJ, Rollman GB, McCain GA. Generalized hypervigilance in fibromyalgia: evidence of perceptual amplification. *Pain* 1996; 66:133–144.

Meier P, Berde C, Di Canzio J, Zurakowski D, Sethna N. Thermal and vibratory perception and pain thresholds in children. *Abstracts: 9th World Congress on Pain*. Seattle: IASP Press, 1999, p 406.

Mercer ME, Holder MD. Antinociceptive effects of palatable sweet ingesta on human responsivity to pressure pain. *Physiol Behav* 1997; 61:311–318.

Millen BE, Quatromoni PA, Gagnon DR, et al. Dietary patterns of men and women suggest targets for health promotion: the Framingham Nutrition Studies. *Am J Health Promot* 1996; 11:42–52.

Miller SM. Monitoring and blunting: validation of a questionnaire to assess styles of information seeking under threat. *J Pers Soc Psychol* 1987; 52:345–353.

Mogil JS, Belknap JK. Sex and genotype determine the selective activation of neurochemically-distinct mechanisms of swim stress-induced analgesia. *Pharmacol Biochem Behav* 1997; 56:61–66.

Morris DB. Sociocultural and religious meanings of pain. In: Gatchel RJ, Turk DC (Eds). *Psychosocial Factors in Pain: Critical Perspectives*. New York: Guilford Press, 1999, 118–131.

Naliboff BD, Munakata J, Fullerton S, et al. Evidence for two distinct perceptual alterations in irritable bowel syndrome. *Gut* 1997; 41:505–512.

Nezu AM, Nezu CM. Psychological distress, problem solving, and coping reactions: sex role differences. *Sex Roles* 1987; 16:205–214.

Okifuji A, Turk DC, Marcus DA. Comparison of generalized and localized hyperalgesia in patients with recurrent headache and fibromyalgia. *Psychosom Med* 1999; 61:771–780.

Otto MW, Dougher MJ. Sex differences and personality factors in responsivity to pain. *Percept Mot Skills* 1985; 61:383–390.

Overgaard C, Knudsen A. Pain-relieving effect of sucrose in newborns during heel prick. *Biol Neonate* 1999; 75:279–284.

Paulson PE, Minoshima S, Morrow TJ, Casey KL. Gender differences in pain perception and patterns of cerebral activation during noxious heat stimulation in humans. *Pain* 1998; 76:223–229.

Pothmann R. Pressure algesimetry in children: normal values and clinical evaluation in headaches. In: Oleson J, Schoenen J (Eds). *Tension-Type Headache: Classification, Mechanisms, and Treatment.* New York: Raven Press, 1993:225–230.

Price DD, Hu JW, Dubner R, Gracely RH. Peripheral suppression of first pain and central summation of second pain evoked by noxious heat pulses. *Pain* 1977; 3:57–68.

Procacci P, Zoppi M, Maresca M, Romano S. Studies on the pain threshold in man. In: Bonica JJ (Eds). *Advances in Neurology.* New York: Raven Press, 1974, pp 107–113.

Rhudy JL, Meagher MW. Fear and anxiety: divergent effects on human pain thresholds. *Pain* 2000; 84:65–75.

Riley JL III, Robinson ME, Wise EA, Myers CD, Fillingim RB. Sex differences in the perception of noxious experimental stimuli: a meta-analysis. *Pain* 1998; 74:181–187.

Riley JL III, Robinson ME, Wise EA, Price DD. A meta-analytic review of pain perception across the menstrual cycle. *Pain* 1999; 81:225–235.

Rivier C. Gender, sex steroids, corticotropin-releasing factor, nitric oxide, and the HPA response to stress. *Pharmacol Biochem Behav* 1999; 64:739–751.

Robbins JM, Kirmayer LJ. Attributions of common somatic symptoms. *Psychol Med* 1991; 21:1029–1045.

Robin O, Vinard H, Vernet-Maury E, Saumet JL. Influence of sex and anxiety on pain threshold and tolerance. *Funct Neurol* 1987; 2:173–179.

Rollman GB. Signal detection theory measurement of pain: a review and critique. *Pain* 1977; 3:187–211.

Rollman GB. Measurement of pain in fibromyalgia in the clinic and laboratory. *J Rheumatol Suppl* 1989; 19:113–119.

Rollman GB. Gender differences in pain: role of anxiety. *Pain Forum* 1995; 4:231–234.

Rollman GB. Culture and pain. In: Kazarian SS, Evans DR (Eds). *Cultural Clinical Psychology: Theory, Research, and Practice.* New York: Oxford University Press, 1998, pp 267–286.

Rollman GB, Harris G. The detectability, discriminability, and perceived magnitude of painful electrical shock. *Percept Psychophys* 1987; 42:257–268.

Rollman GB, Hervieux M. Psychophysical scaling of noxious electrical pulses: Gender differences. *Abstracts: 9th World Congress on Pain.* Seattle: IASP Press, 1999, 356–357.

Rollman GB, Lautenbacher S. Hypervigilance effects in fibromyalgia: pain experience and pain perception. In: Vaeroy H, Merskey H (Eds). *Progress in Fibromyalgia and Myofascial Pain.* Amsterdam: Elsevier, 1993, pp 149–159.

Rollman GB, Hapidou EG, Jarmain SH. Gender differences in pain responsiveness: contributing factors. *Pain* 1990; Suppl 5:314.

Romero MT, Bodnar RJ. Gender differences in two forms of cold-water swim analgesia. *Physiol Behav* 1986; 37:893–897.

Schmidt NB, Cook JH. Effects of anxiety sensitivity on anxiety and pain during a cold pressor challenge in patients with panic disorder. *Behav Res Ther* 1999; 37:313–323.

Scudds RA, Rollman GB, Harth M, McCain GA. Pain perception and personality measures as discriminators in the classification of fibrositis. *J Rheumatol* 1987; 14:563–569.

Sheps DS, Bragdon EE, Gray TF III, et al. Relation between systemic hypertension and pain perception. *Am J Cardiol* 1992; 70:3F–5F.

Sherif CW. Needed concepts in the study of gender identity. *Psychol Women Quart* 1982; 6:375–398.

Spence JT, Buckner C. Masculinity and femininity: defining the undefinable. In: Kalbfleish PJ, Cody MJ (Eds). *Gender, Power, and Communication in Human Relationships.* Hillsdale, NJ: Lawrence Erlbaum Associates, 1995, pp 105–138.

Sternberg WF. Sex differences in the effects of prenatal stress on stress-induced analgesia. *Physiol Behav* 1999; 68:63–72.

Stewart KM, France CR. Resting systolic blood pressure, parental history of hypertension, and sensitivity to noxious stimuli. *Pain* 1996; 68:369–374.

Tedford WH, Warren DE, Flynn WE. Alteration of shock aversion thresholds during menstrual cycle. *Percept Psychophys* 1977; 21:193–196.

Toner BB, Akman D. Gender role and irritable bowel syndrome: literature review and hypothesis. *Am J Gastroenterol* 2000; 95:11–16.

Unger RK. Toward a redefinition of sex and gender. *Am Psychol* 1979; 34:1085–1094.

Unruh AM. Gender variations in clinical pain experience. *Pain* 1996; 65:123–167.

Unruh AM, Ritchie J, Merskey H. Does gender affect appraisal of pain and pain coping strategies? *Clin J Pain* 1999; 15:31–40.

van Vliet KP, Everaerd W, van Zuuren FJ, et al. Symptom perception: psychological correlates of symptom reporting and illness behavior of women with medically unexplained gynecological symptoms. *J Psychosom Obstet Gynaecol* 1994; 15:171–181.

van Wijk CM, Kolk AM. Sex differences in physical symptoms: the contribution of symptom perception theory. *Soc Sci Med* 1997; 45:231–246.

Veith JL, Anderson J, Slade SA, et al. Plasma beta-endorphin, pain thresholds and anxiety levels across the human menstrual cycle. *Physiol Behav* 1984; 32:31–34.

Verbrugge LM. Sex differences in complaints and diagnoses. *J Behav Med* 1980; 3:327–355.

Verbrugge LM. Gender and health: an update on hypotheses and evidence. *J Health Soc Behav* 1985; 26:156–182.

von Graffenried B, Adler R, Abt K, Nuesch E, Spiegel R. The influence of anxiety and pain sensitivity on experimental pain in man. *Pain* 1978; 4:253–263.

Waylonis GW, Heck W. Fibromyalgia syndrome. New associations. *Am J Phys Med Rehabil* 1992; 71:343–348.

Wedzony K, Mackowiak M, Fijal K, Golembiowska K. Evidence that conditioned stress enhances outflow of dopamine in rat prefrontal cortex: a search for the influence of diazepam and 5-HT1A agonists. *Synapse* 1996; 24:240–247.

Willer JC, Roby A, Le Bars D. Psychophysical and electrophysiological approaches to the pain-relieving effects of heterotopic nociceptive stimuli. *Brain* 1984; 107(Pt 4):1095–1112.

Willer JC, Le Bars D, De Broucker T. Diffuse noxious inhibitory controls in man: involvement of an opioidergic link. *Eur J Pharmacol* 1990; 182:347–355.

Winfield JB. Pain in fibromyalgia. *Rheum Dis Clin North Am* 1999; 25:55–79.

Wolfe F, Hawley DJ. Evidence of disordered symptom appraisal in fibromyalgia: increased rates of reported comorbidity and comorbidity severity. *Clin Exp Rheumatol* 1999; 17:297–303.

Wolfe F, Ross K, Anderson J, Russell IJ. Aspects of fibromyalgia in the general population: sex, pain threshold, and fibromyalgia symptoms. *J Rheumatol* 1995; 22:151–156.

Wright RA, Murray JB, Storey PL, Williams BJ. Ability analysis of gender relevance and sex differences in cardiovascular response to behavioral challenge. *J Person Soc Psychol* 1997; 73:417.

Yunus MB, Ahles TA, Aldag JC, Masi AT. Relationship of clinical features with psychological status in primary fibromyalgia. *Arthritis Rheum* 1991; 34:15–21.

Correspondence to: Gary B. Rollman, PhD, Department of Psychology, University of Western Ontario, Social Science Centre, London, Ontario, Canada, N6A 5C2. Tel: 519-661-3677; Fax: 519-661-3961; email: rollman@ julian.uwo.ca.

Sex, Gender, and Pain, Progress in Pain Research and Management, Vol. 17, edited by R.B. Fillingim, IASP Press, Seattle, © 2000.

10

The Influence of Menstrual Cycle and Sex Hormones on Pain Responses in Humans

Roger B. Fillingim[a,b] and Timothy J. Ness[c]

Departments of [a]Psychology, [b]Orthodontics, and [c]Anesthesiology, University of Alabama at Birmingham, Birmingham, Alabama, USA

Females and males differ in their experience of both clinical and experimental pain, and these sex-related differences are undoubtedly produced by complex interactions among multiple biopsychosocial factors. One obvious reason for sex differences in pain responses is the influence of gonadal hormones. Ample literature from nonhuman animal research demonstrates clear hormonal influences on nociceptive responses (see Chapter 5). However, experimental findings are at times inconsistent, and the picture presented by research on hormonal effects in humans is even less clear. This chapter reviews the human literature relating gonadal hormones to pain responses in both the experimental and clinical setting, presenting first a brief review of human menstrual cycle physiology.

PHYSIOLOGY OF THE HUMAN MENSTRUAL CYCLE

The human menstrual cycle is characterized by various hormonal alterations (see Fig. 1) that influence the structure and function of both the peripheral and central nervous systems. Two gonadotropic hormones, follicle-stimulating hormone (FSH) and luteinizing hormone (LH), secreted by the pituitary gland, control the menstrual cycle. The cycle is typically divided into four functional phases: follicular, ovulatory, luteal, and menstrual. The first half of the cycle constitutes the follicular phase, when both FSH and LH are secreted at relatively steady, low-to-moderate levels. During this phase, estradiol gradually increases, peaking just prior to ovulation, and progesterone remains at a steady low level, rising slightly before midcycle. The midcycle ovulatory phase represents the transition from

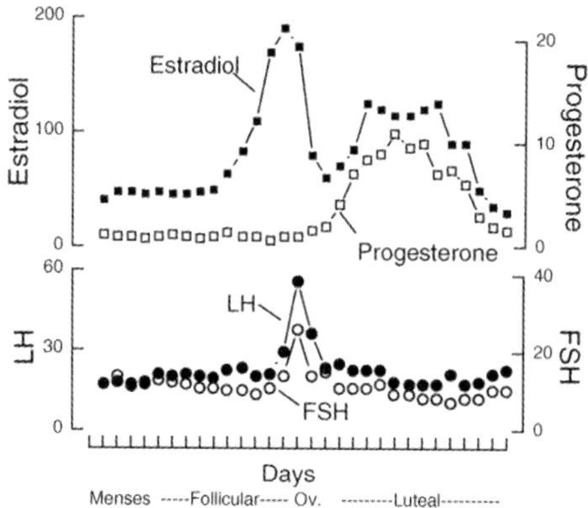

Fig. 1. Levels of gonadal hormones at different phases of the human menstrual cycle (menses, follicular, ovulation [ov.], and luteal). Estradiol and progesterone are shown in the top panel, and luteinizing hormone (LH) and follicle-stimulating hormone (FSH) in the bottom panel. Adapted from Yen (1998).

follicular to luteal phases. Approximately 1 day before ovulation, both LH and FSH increase substantially, and peak for roughly 48 hours (Yen 1998). A cascade of events follows the LH surge, starting with the release of follicular steroid hormones containing small amounts of progesterone. Ultimately, the follicle ruptures, resulting in ovulation, after which the luteal phase begins. In contrast to the follicular phase, the majority of the luteal phase is characterized by greater levels of progesterone than estrogen. Progesterone peaks during the mid-luteal phase, and estrogen increases slightly; however, estrogen levels remain well below their preovulatory peak. These increasing levels of estrogen, and to some degree progesterone, provide negative feedback to the pituitary, resulting in decreased secretion of LH and FSH across the luteal phase, which causes the corpus luteum to degenerate. This, in turn, decreases secretion of estrogen and progesterone, which has two effects: (1) the negative feedback to the pituitary ceases, permitting increased secretion of FSH and LH and starting a new ovarian cycle, and (2) menstruation begins. During the menstrual phase—the transition from luteal to follicular phases—levels of estrogen, progesterone, LH, and FSH all remain low.

METHODOLOGICAL ISSUES

Researchers examining menstrual cycle effects on pain responses must attend to numerous methodological issues. First, accurate determination of menstrual cycle phase is imperative. The most commonly used method is self-report based on a menstrual cycle calendar; however, this method is highly susceptible to problems associated with variable cycle lengths, and it fails to confirm ovulation, which is important given that up to 20% of cycles can be anovulatory (Girdler et al. 1993). Assessment of basal body temperature is often used to document the time of ovulation; however, compliance can be problematic, and this method is less accurate than hormonal measurement (Luciano et al. 1990; Kesner et al. 1992). The ideal methodology would include hormonal assays at the time of testing combined with LH surge detection kits (e.g., ClearPlan by Unipath) to confirm ovulation and facilitate scheduling of postovulatory visits. Unfortunately, these methods require considerable resources and therefore have not been used in most studies examining menstrual cycle effects on pain. Another issue related to timing of menstrual cycle phase is that researchers often have chosen different time points within the same cycle phase for testing subjects. Because the hormonal milieu changes considerably within phases, results may differ for subjects tested in the early versus late luteal phase, and likewise for the follicular phase.

In addition to issues specific to the menstrual cycle, other important methodological variables include the choice of pain tasks and pain assessment methods, the effects of repeated testing, and the inclusion/exclusion criteria for subjects. Studies of experimental pain have used several pain induction stimuli, including heat pain, cold pressor pain, electrical pain, pressure pain, and ischemic pain. These stimuli differ along multiple dimensions, including time course (phasic versus tonic), site of stimulation, depth of stimulation (e.g., cutaneous versus deep), area of stimulation, ratio of pain intensity to pain unpleasantness, and classes of afferents recruited. Previous research has shown low correlations between different forms of painful stimulation (Janal et al. 1994; Lautenbacher and Rollman 1997); studies using highly divergent pain induction techniques thus may yield discrepant results. The assessment method is also important. Pain threshold is the most common measure, but many studies also include various suprathreshold scaling procedures. One important design consideration is whether to study cycle phase within or between subjects. Between-subject designs, in which different women are studied at various cycle phases, provide far less experimental power and require much larger numbers of subjects. Most experimental studies employ a within-subject design, which requires consideration of the effects of repeated testing. Counterbalancing the cycle phase in which subjects undergo their first session is one way to address this issue; however, because an order by cycle phase interaction is possible, a better approach involves combining counterbalancing with an introductory session to reduce novelty effects. The characteristics of the subject population can also vary widely across studies. Important factors to consider include age, ethnic diversity, and educational level. Methods for identifying and possibly excluding subjects with menstrual-cycle-related disorders (e.g., dysmenorrhea, premenstrual syndrome) should be specified. When studies include subjects using oral contraceptives (OC), the class and doses of their specific formulations should be reported.

MENSTRUAL CYCLE AND HORMONAL INFLUENCES ON EXPERIMENTAL PAIN

Numerous studies have examined changes in perceptual responses to noxious stimuli across the menstrual cycle in humans; these studies vary widely in both methodology and results, as summarized in Table I. Several authors have examined pressure pain sensitivity across the menstrual cycle. In one of the earliest studies of menstrual cycle effects on sensory perception, Herren (1933) found lower thresholds for two-point discrimination for painful and nonpainful stimuli during the premenstrual period, compared to postmenstrual and midcycle time points. Robinson and Short (1977) examined sensitivity to pressure pain applied to the breast in a small group of women across several menstrual cycles. Pain thresholds varied with the cycle, with 75% of subjects demonstrating greatest sensitivity during the menstrual or premenstrual phases; however, the pattern varied considerably across cycles. Another study compared pressure pain threshold in women with premenstrual syndrome (PMS) and non-PMS controls, and reported no menstrual cycle effects (Kuczmierczyk and Adams 1986). A subsequent study using the same painful stimulus found no menstrual cycle effects in dysmenorrheic or healthy women (Amodei and Nelson Gray 1989). Higher pain thresholds to a mechanical stimulus have also been reported during the midmenstrual phase (days 15–18) in normally cycling women, but not in OC users (Rao et al. 1987b). More recently, Hapidou and Rollman (1998) investigated pressure pain sensitivity as a function of cycle phase in healthy women using two measures, number of tender points based on manual palpation and pressure pain threshold using a pressure algometer. These authors reported no menstrual cycle effects on pressure pain thresholds, but the number of tender points was higher during the follicular compared to the luteal phase. This cycle effect was absent in women taking oral contraceptives. However, none of these studies used hormonal measures to verify cycle phase or confirm ovulation. A recent study using a different form of mechanical pain evaluated menstrual cycle influences on responses to esophageal distension (Nguyen et al. 1995). These authors used serum progesterone levels to verify cycle phase; they found no difference in sensory or pain thresholds during the follicular (days 5–7) versus the luteal phase (days 20–22).

Thermal pain responses have also been evaluated at different menstrual cycle phases. In two studies employing signal detection methods, Goolkasian (1980, 1983) reported increased discrimination of painful stimuli during the "ovulation" phase (between days 8 and 14 of the menstrual cycle), but no menstrual cycle changes in response criteria emerged. Using a similar stimulus but a different assessment method, Procacci et al. (1974) noted a lower pain threshold during the premenstrual phase. Recently, we (Fillingim et al. 1997) examined thermal pain threshold and tolerance as well as suprathreshold ratings of thermal pain at three points during the menstrual cycle, the mid-follicular phase (days 5–8), the mid-to-late luteal phase (approximately 5 days before menses), and the ovulatory phase (within 24 hours of a positive ovulation test). All cycle phases were confirmed through plasma hormone levels. The results indicated no significant effect of cycle phase on any of the thermal pain responses; however, regardless of cycle phase, higher estrogen levels were associated with enhanced thermal pain sensitivity. This is the only study of thermal pain responses that has confirmed ovulation and cycle phase using hormone assays.

Several investigators have determined menstrual cycle effects on electrically induced pain. Tedford et al. (1977) applied electrical stimuli to the middle and index fingers of the nondominant hand and found the lowest pain threshold 1 week postmenses and the highest threshold between days 15 and 21 of the cycle. Another study of electrical pain applied to the wrist reported no menstrual cycle effects on pain threshold (Veith et al. 1984). These authors asked subjects to monitor basal body temperature to determine cycle phase and confirm ovulation. More recently, Giamberardino and colleagues (1997) investigated menstrual cycle effects on electrical pain thresholds in women with dysmenorrhea and pain-free controls. Electrical stimuli were applied to different body sites (abdomen, leg, and arm) and at different tissue depths (skin, subcutis, and muscle). Regardless of group or site tested, the highest thresholds occurred for the luteal phase (days 17–22). Lowest thresholds for skin sites occurred during the periovulatory phase (days 12–16), while for subcutis and muscle stimulation, thresholds were lowest perimenstrually (days 25–28 and days 2–6). Again, while one of these studies used basal body temperature for cycle timing and ovulation detection, none of them performed hormone assays to confirm cycle phases.

Several investigators have used tonic pain procedures that produce pain of greater duration than the procedures described above. The most common of these procedures is ischemic arm pain using a tourniquet and the cold pressor task. One study examining responses to ischemic arm pain in women with dysmenorrhea and pain-free controls determined each subject's menstrual cycle phase based on one item on a medical screening questionnaire (Aberger et al. 1983). The authors state that pain thresholds and tolerances were higher in women tested during the premenstrual phase; however, they present no data to substantiate this statement and provide no information regarding determination of cycle phase. More recently, we (Fillingim et al. 1997) examined responses to ischemic arm pain in 11 healthy women during

Table I
Summary of human studies investigating menstrual cycle effects on baseline pain responses

Reference	Subjects	Pain Measure	Hormonal Manipulation	Results	Comments
Aberger et al. 1983	56 DYS F, 18 non-DYS F	Ischemic pain	One question to determine cycle phase of each woman (menstrual, pre- and postmenstrual)	Higher threshold and tolerance for subjects in premenstrual phase	No data presented, no definition of cycle phases; no hormonal measures
Amodei and Nelson-Gray 1989	35 DYS F, 12 non-DYS F	Pressure pain (Forgione-Barber)	Menstrual cycle (premenstrual, menstrual, "intermenstrual")	No menstrual cycle effects	No verification of ovulation or cycle phase.
Fillingim et al. 1997	11 normal F	Thermal and ischemic pain	Menstrual cycle (follicular, ovulatory, luteal)	Greater ischemic pain sensitivity in luteal vs. follicular phase; no effects on thermal pain	Cycle phases verified hormonally
Giamberardino et al. 1997	10 DYS F, 10 normal F, 10 normal M	Electrical pain	Menstrual cycle (menstrual, periovulatory, luteal, premenstrual)	Higher pain threshold in luteal phase	Effects of cycle phase depended on tissue depth; no verification of ovulation or cycle phase
Goolkasian 1980	24 normal F, 12 normal M	Thermal pain (signal detection)	Menstrual cycle (menstrual, postmenstrual, ovulatory, premenstrual); OC use	Greater pain discrimination at ovulation in cycling women; no cyclic effects in OC users	Ovulation pinpointed using basal body temperatures; no cycle effects on nonpainful stimuli
Goolkasian 1983	12 DYS F, 12 non-DYS F	Thermal pain (signal detection)	Menstrual cycle (menstrual, pre- and postmenstrual, ovulatory)	Greater pain discrimination at ovulation in non-DYS F; no cycle effects in DYS F	Basal body temperature to verify ovulation; no cycle effects on nonpainful stimuli
Hapidou and De Catanzaro 1988	27 DYS F, 19 non-DYS F	Cold pressor pain	Menstrual cycle (follicular, luteal)	Lower pain threshold in luteal vs. follicular phase in both groups; lower pain rating in follicular phase in DYS F	No cycle effects among OC users; no verification of cycle phases or ovulation
Hapidou and Rollman 1998	66 normal F	Pressure pain (palpation and algometer)	Menstrual cycle (menstrual, follicular, luteal, premenstrual); OC use	Higher tender point count in follicular vs. luteal phase in non-OC users only	No cycle effect in OC users; no effects for pain threshold

Herren 1933	5 normal F	Two-point threshold (pain and touch)	Menstrual cycle (pre-, post- and intermenstrual)	Lower two-point discrimination for pain and touch	No verification of cycle phase or ovulation
Kuczmierczyk and Adams 1986	11 PMS F, 10 normal F	Pressure pain (Forgione-Barber)	Menstrual cycle (menstrual, intermenstrual, and premenstrual)	No cycle effects	No verification of cycle phase or ovulation
Nguyen et al. 1995	10 healthy F	Esophageal balloon distension	Menstrual cycle (follicular, premenstrual)	No cycle effects	Serum progesterone to confirm luteal phase timing
Procacci et al. 1974	Unknown	Thermal pain	Menstrual cycle	Lower pain threshold in premenstrual vs. postmenstrual phase	Original source not obtainable; based on data presented in review article
Pfleeger et al. 1997	11 normal F	Ischemic pain	Menstrual cycle (follicular, luteal)	Lower pain tolerance in luteal vs. follicular phase	Ovulation verified with ovulation test
Rao et al. 1987a	40 normal F, 20 post-OVX F, 25 F taking OC	Mechanical pain	Menstrual cycle (menstrual, mid- and premenstrual); OVX; OC use	Pain threshold higher midmenstrual in normal F; lower in menstrual phase in OC users; lower in post-OVX F vs. controls	No verification of cycle phase or ovulation
Robinson and Short 1977	6 normal F	Pressure pain on the breast	Menstrual cycle	Lower pain threshold in premenstrual and menstrual phases	Wide variability across cycles; no verification of cycle phase or ovulation
Tedford et al. 1977	18 normal F, 5 normal M	Electrical pain threshold	Menstrual cycle (menstrual, ovulatory, pre- and postmenstrual); OC use	Higher pain threshold in pre- vs. postmenstrual phase; no cycle effect in OC users	No verification of cycle phase or ovulation
Veith et al. 1984	16 normal F	Electrical pain threshold, cold pressor	Menstrual cycle (menstrual, follicular, ovulatory, luteal, premenstrual); OC use	No cycle or OC effects	Basal body temperature to verify ovulation

Note: DYS = dysmenorrheic; F = female; M = male; non-DYS = nondysmenorrheic; OC = oral contraceptives; post-OVX = post-ovariectomy.

the follicular phase (days 5–8), the ovulatory phase (within 24 hours of the LH surge), and the luteal phase (2–5 days premenses). We also used ovulation tests and hormone assays to confirm cycle phases and ovulation. The results indicated significantly lower pain tolerance during the luteal versus the follicular phase of the cycle. Pain threshold was marginally lower during the luteal phase, and both threshold and tolerance were marginally lower during the ovulatory compared to the follicular phase. We later replicated these findings in another sample, and showed that both ischemic pain threshold and tolerance were higher during the follicular (days 4–9) versus the luteal phase (5–10 days after ovulation) (Pfleeger et al. 1997). Two studies have examined cold pressor pain, with one reporting no significant effects of menstrual cycle (Veith et al. 1984), and the other finding lower pain thresholds during the luteal (days 15–21) compared to the follicular phase (days 8–14) (Hapidou and De Catanzaro 1988).

When considered individually, these studies present an inconsistent picture of menstrual cycle effects on pain sensitivity. However, small sample sizes are the norm in this area of research, and considering the other methodological shortcomings mentioned above, the conflicting results are understandable. One method that overcomes the small sample sizes inherent in this literature is meta-analysis, which amounts to combining the data from multiple studies and using statistical analysis to determine overall effects. Riley and colleagues (1999) recently conducted a meta-analysis on studies examining menstrual cycle effects on pain threshold and tolerance. This analysis revealed that for all pain stimuli other than electrical, pain threshold and tolerance were highest during the follicular compared to the periovulatory and luteal phases. Conversely, electrical pain thresholds were highest during the luteal phase. Overall, effect sizes were in the small to moderate range. The reasons for the different pattern of results with electrical pain are unclear; however, electrical pain has been criticized as an experimental pain induction procedure because it activates all subclasses of afferents, producing both painful and nonpainful sensations that can feel less natural than those produced by other forms of stimulation and may be difficult for subjects to distinguish (Gracely 1994). Also, because electrical pain directly activates primary afferents, any menstrual-cycle-related effects on the transducer component of the primary afferent neuron may be bypassed.

The influence of exogenous hormones on experimental pain responses in humans has received relatively little attention. A few studies have examined the effects of oral contraceptives on pain perception. One study reported lower electrical pain thresholds postmenstrually among normally cycling women, but no menstrual cycle effects among women taking oral contraceptives (OC) (Tedford et al. 1977). Goolkasian (1980) reported that women not using OC evinced greater thermal pain sensitivity than men and were more sensitive to such pain at ovulation, but women using OC did not differ from men and showed no menstrual cycle changes in their pain responses. Thompson et al. (1997) recently reported that women taking OC reported less exercise-induced muscle soreness than did women not taking OC when tested during the luteal phase. Hapidou and Rollman (1998), using manual palpation, detected a greater number of tender points during the follicular versus the luteal phase in normally cycling women, but not in women using OC. These experimental studies suggest that OC use obviates menstrual cycle influences on pain perception and may be associated with diminished pain sensitivity. Unfortunately, the effects of hormone replacement therapy on pain responses in postmenopausal women have not been investigated.

MENSTRUAL CYCLE AND HORMONAL INFLUENCES ON CLINICAL PAIN

In addition to their effects on experimental pain, gonadal hormones appear to influence the experience of clinical pain. Menstrual-cycle-related symptoms are a clinically significant phenomenon. Epidemiologic studies demonstrate that pain and other symptoms are greater during the premenstrual (luteal) phase among healthy women (Boyle et al. 1987; Huerta-Franco and Malacara 1993). Premenstrual pain and other symptoms are associated with increased use of nonprescription analgesics (Hart and Hill 1997). Numerous disorders related to the menstrual cycle include pain as a common symptom, including PMS (Korzekwa and Steiner 1997), dysmenorrhea (Ylikorkala and Dawood 1978), and menstrual migraines (Facchinetti et al. 1990). We have previously reported that women with PMS demonstrate greater ischemic pain sensitivity during their symptomatic phase than non-PMS controls (Fillingim et al. 1995).

Several female-predominant pain disorders also are characterized by increased symptomatology at certain menstrual cycle phases. Patients with irritable bowel syndrome (Heitkemper et al. 1995), other gastrointestinal disorders (Kane et al. 1998), and headache (Keenan and Lindamer 1992) report increased pain and other symptoms during the late luteal phase of the cycle. Also, hormonal fluctuations have been implicated in symptom severity among women with rheumatoid arthritis (Da Silva and Hall 1992). One retrospective study of fibromyalgia (FM) patients indicated that 72% of patients reported increased symptoms during the premenstrual phase

(Ostensen et al. 1997), and a more recent prospective report indicated greater pain and other symptoms during the perimenstrual versus the ovulatory phase in FM patients (Anderberg et al. 1998). In another study, temporomandibular disorder patients not using OC demonstrated slightly more variance in pain reports across the menstrual cycle compared to those using OC, with peak pain occurring during the menstrual and premenstrual phases (Dao et al. 1998). Several authors have stated that the symptoms of interstitial cystitis, a predominantly female painful bladder condition, are influenced by the menstrual cycle (Webster and Brennan 1995; Elbadawi 1997; Theoharides et al. 1998); however, data to support this contention have not been reported.

A few studies have explored the influence of exogenous hormones on clinical pain responses. For example, LeResche et al. (1997; see also Chapter 15, this volume) reported that use of oral contraceptives and estrogen replacement therapy in pre- and postmenopausal women, respectively, was associated with significantly increased risk for temporomandibular disorders (TMD). Dao et al. (1998) reported slightly, but not significantly, higher pain levels in TMD patients using OC versus normally cycling patients. Women using hormone replacement therapy were at increased risk for low back pain (Brynhildsen et al. 1998). Also, among postmenopausal women with orofacial pain, use of hormone replacement therapy has been associated with increased reports of clinical pain (Wise et al. 2000). Conversely, treatment with combined estrogen-progestin reduced back pain and disability in premenopausal women with low bone density in the lumbar spine; however, this effect was more likely due to improvements in bone density rather than to direct effects on pain (Kyllonen et al. 1999).

MECHANISMS UNDERLYING HORMONAL EFFECTS ON PAIN PERCEPTION

We have recently reviewed the mechanisms whereby gonadal hormones may influence nociceptive processing (Fillingim and Ness 2000). Briefly, gonadal hormones can influence nociceptive pathways at multiple levels, including at primary afferent nerves and the spinal cord, and through complex actions in the brain. The obvious first step at which gonadal hormones affect nociception is at the level of the primary afferent nerve fiber. In nonhuman animals, estrogen administration has been shown to alter receptive field properties of primary afferents in the trigeminal (Bereiter et al. 1980) and pudendal nerves (Komisaruk et al. 1972). Also, certain afferents arising from the uterus appear to be mechanically insensitive at some points during the estrous cycle and mechanically sensitive at others (Berkley et al.

1988; Robbins et al. 1990, 1992). One mechanism by which hormones may affect primary afferents could be related to nerve growth factor (NGF) and one of its high-affinity receptors, trkA. The trkA receptor is involved in sensitization of primary afferents, and gonadal hormones influence expression of trkA receptors (Sohrabji et al. 1994; Liuzzi et al. 1999). Hormonal effects on primary afferents may also be mediated by other mechanisms. Levine and colleagues demonstrated sex differences in plasma extravasation following bradykinin injections, and considered these differences to be dependent on sex steroids (Green et al. 1999).

In addition to their effects on primary afferents, gonadal hormones clearly influence multiple central nervous system pathways involved in pain transmission (see Chapter 2). For example, sex steroids alter levels of multiple neuromodulators involved in spinal nociceptive processing, including substance P (Kerdelhue et al. 1985; Duval et al. 1996), amino acids such as GABA and glutamate, and other neurotransmitters (e.g., dopamine, serotonin, and norepinephrine) (Smith 1994). In addition, LH desensitizes brain opioid receptors (Berglund et al. 1988a; Berglund and Simpkins 1988b); the preovulatory LH surge is followed by diminished opioid tone and increased pain sensitivity persisting into the mid- to late luteal phase (Berglund et al. 1988a; Ratka and Simpkins 1990). Indeed, abnormal luteal phase opioid function has been implicated in menstrual cycle disorders such as PMS and menstrual migraine (Facchinetti et al. 1988). Nonhuman animal research has revealed colocalization of endogenous opioid peptides and estrogen in some hypothalamic nuclei (Morrell et al. 1985) as well as estrogen-mediated increases in μ-opioid receptor mRNA levels in the ventromedial hypothalamus (Quinones-Jenab et al. 1997). In contrast, a negative correlation between circulating estradiol and μ-opioid receptor binding in the hypothalamus and amygdala in humans has recently been reported (Smith et al. 1998). Gonadal hormones also affect central cholinergic systems (McEwen et al. 1998), which could help explain sex differences in cholinergic analgesia (Eisenach and Hood 1998; Lavand'homme et al. 1998).

In addition, there may be indirect effects of gonadal hormones on nociceptive responses. For instance, decreased sensorimotor inhibition has been reported in healthy women during the luteal as compared to the follicular phase of the menstrual cycle (Swerdlow et al. 1997), and such decreased inhibitory influence could potentiate pain transmission. In the luteal phase, sleep disturbances (Driver et al. 1996; Manber and Bootzin 1997), and changes in behavioral and affective states (Priest and Pfaff 1995; Backstrom 1995; Klaiber et al. 1996) may enhance pain sensitivity. These findings indicate widespread effects of gonadal hormones in the peripheral and central nervous systems that could affect nociceptive processing. Interactions between gonadal hormones and peripheral and central nociceptive pathways could influence baseline pain sensitivity, which in turn may enhance the perception of clinical pain.

In addition to their effects on nociceptive processing, sex hormones can influence pain through their effects on underlying disease processes. For instance, estrogen replacement prevents decreases in bone mineral density, which can reduce the pain associated with decreased bone density, as in the study described above of low back pain in osteopenic women (Kyllonen et al. 1999). Also, progesterone slows gastric emptying and reduces esophageal sphincter tone, which may in part explain menstrual cycle influences on irritable bowel symptoms (Case and Reid 1998). Thus, hormonal effects on pain responses most likely result from complex actions at multiple sites of the peripheral and central nervous systems.

IMPLICATIONS AND FUTURE DIRECTIONS

The literature reviewed above suggests that the menstrual cycle and exogenous hormonal manipulations can influence pain sensitivity and clinical pain responses. The results, however, are inconsistent, especially for studies of experimental pain. This inconsistency is probably due to widely varying methodologies combined with small to moderate effect sizes, as demonstrated by the meta-analysis (Riley et al. 1999). Given these modest effect sizes, it seems unlikely that menstrual cycle effects alone can account for previously observed sex differences in laboratory pain sensitivity, which have larger effect sizes (Riley et al. 1998). Nonetheless, these findings have important neurophysiological, methodological, and clinical implications. Further investigation of hormonal effects on nociceptive processing may provide new insights regarding nociceptive transmission and modulation. Such information may enhance our understanding not only of sex-related pain conditions, but of pain disorders in general. From a methodological perspective, attention to menstrual cycle phase is imperative in pain research to reduce error variability and to detect important menstrual-cycle-related effects. Determining whether subjects and patients are using exogenous hormones is equally important.

The clinical implications of menstrual cycle effects on pain are not yet clear. It is possible, of course, that the effects of sex steroids on pain transmission could prove to be minimal compared to the influence of other factors, but we contend that their potential clinical impact is substantial. Indeed, Case and Reid (1998) have recently noted that the menstrual cycle influences the symptoms of a variety of medical disorders, both pain-related and nonpainful. As reviewed above, many clinical conditions are characterized by enhanced symptoms perimenstrually, and recent findings indicate that exogenous hormone use may increase risk for pain (LeResche et al. 1997; Brynhildsen et al. 1998; Wise et al. 2000). Understanding these effects may ultimately facilitate pain prevention and treatment. To the extent that reproductive hormones influence clinical pain, novel treatment applications are possible. For example, antiestrogenic agents such as tamoxifen appear to be effective in treating cyclical mastalgia in women (Messinis and Lolis 1988; Kontostolis et al. 1997) and gynecomastia in men (McDermott et al. 1990). It is plausible that anti-estrogen therapies could be effective in treating other chronic pain conditions that are hormonally influenced (e.g., rheumatoid arthritis, temporomandibular disorder, and fibromyalgia). Further, such hormonal therapies could potentiate the effects of other analgesic agents, providing a more optimal therapeutic profile. The application of various sex-steroid compounds to the management of clinical pain remains an important yet unexplored area of investigation.

SUMMARY

Taken together, the studies discussed above indicate potentially important influences of sex steroids on nociceptive responses. Women's sensitivity to experimental pain varies across the menstrual cycle, with greatest sensitivity to most forms of painful stimulation occurring during the luteal phase. In addition, many pain conditions demonstrate menstrual cyclicity, although the patterns may vary across disorders. Women using oral contraceptives generally do not show menstrual cycle effects on experimental pain perception, but exogenous hormone use has been associated with increased clinical pain in certain populations. These results highlight the importance of incorporating menstrual cycle assessment and determining use of exogenous hormones in both experimental and clinical pain research. Additional research is needed to determine the mechanisms underlying these hormonal effects on pain and to clarify their implications for clinical practice.

ACKNOWLEDGMENTS

This work was supported in part by NIH grants DE12261 and DK57257 (R.B. Fillingim) and DK51314 (T.J. Ness).

REFERENCES

Aberger E, Denney D, Hutchings DF. Pain sensitivity and coping strategies among dysmenorrheic women: much ado about nothing. *Behav Res Ther* 1983; 21:119–127.

Amodei N, Nelson Gray RO. Reactions of dysmenorrheic and nondysmenorrheic women to experimentally induced pain throughout the menstrual cycle. *J Behav Med* 1989; 12:373–385.

Anderberg UM, Marteinsdottir I, Hallman J, Backstrom T. Variability in cyclicity affects pain and other symptoms in female fibromyalgia syndrome patients. *J Musculoskel Pain* 1998; 6:5–22.

Backstrom T. Symptoms related to the menopause and sex steroid treatments. *Ciba Found Symp* 1995; 191:171–180.

Bereiter DA, Stanford LR, Barker DJ. Hormone-induced enlargement of receptive fields in trigeminal mechano-receptive neurons. II. Possible mechanisms. *Brain Res* 1980; 184:411–423.

Berglund LA, Simpkins JW. Alterations in brain opiate receptor mechanisms on proestrous afternoon. *Neuroendocrinology* 1988b; 48:394–400.

Berglund LA, Derendorf H, Simpkins JW. Desensitization of brain opiate receptor mechanisms by gonadal steroid treatments that stimulate luteinizing hormone secretion. *Endocrinology* 1988a; 122:2718–2726.

Berkley KJ, Robbins A, Sato Y. Afferent fibres supplying the uterus in the rat. *J Neurophysiol* 1988; 59:142–163.

Boyle CA, Berkowitz GS, Kelsey JL. Epidemiology of premenstrual symptoms. *Am J Public Health* 1987; 77:349–350.

Brynhildsen JO, Bjors E, Skarsgard C, Hammar ML. Is hormone replacement therapy a risk factor for low back pain among postmenopausal women? *Spine* 1998; 23:809–813.

Case AM, Reid RL. Effects of the menstrual cycle on medical disorders. *Arch Int Med* 1998; 158:1405–1412.

Da Silva JA, Hall GM. The effects of gender and sex hormones on outcome in rheumatoid arthritis. *Baillieres Clin Rheum* 1992; 6:196–219.

Dao TT, Knight K, Ton-That V. Modulation of myofascial pain by the reproductive hormones: a preliminary report. *J Prosthet Dent* 1998; 79:663–670.

Driver HS, Dijk DJ, Werth E, Biedermann K, Borbely AA. Sleep and the sleep electroencephalogram across the menstrual cycle in young healthy women. *J Clin Endocrinol Metab* 1996; 81:728–735.

Duval P, Lenoir V, Moussaoui S, Garret C, Kerdelhue B. Substance P and neurokinin A variations throughout the rat estrous cycle; comparison with ovariectomized and male rats: II. Trigeminal nucleus and cervical spinal cord. *J Neurosci Res* 1996; 45:610–616.

Eisenach JC, Hood DD. Sex differences in analgesia from intrathecal neostigmine in humans. *Anesthesiology* 1998; 89:A1106.

Elbadawi A. Interstitial cystitis: a critique of current concepts with a new proposal for pathologic diagnosis and pathogenesis. *Urology* 1997; 49(Suppl 5A):14–40.

Facchinetti F, Marti gnoni E, Sola D, et al. Transient failure of central opioid tonus and premenstrual symptoms. *J Reprod Med* 1988; 33:633–638.

Facchinetti F, Martignoni E, Fioroni L, Sances G, Genazzani AR. Opioid control of the hypothalamus-pituitary-adrenal axis cyclically fails in menstrual migraine. *Cephalalgia* 1990; 10:51–56.

Fillingim RB, Ness TJ. Sex-related hormonal influences on pain and analgesic responses. *Neurosci Biobehav Rev;* 24:485–501.

Fillingim RB, Girdler SS, Booker DK, et al. Pain sensitivity in females with premenstrual dysphoric disorder: a preliminary report. *J Women's Health* 1995; 4:367–374.

Fillingim RB, Maixner W, Girdler SS, et al. Ischemic but not thermal pain sensitivity varies across the menstrual cycle. *Psychosom Med* 1997; 59:512–520.

Giamberardino MA, Berkley KJ, Iezzi S, Debigontina P, Vecchiet L. Pain threshold variations in somatic wall tissues as a function of menstrual cycle, segmental site and tissue depth in non-dysmenorrheic women, dysmenorrheic women and men. *Pain* 1997; 71:187–197.

Girdler SS, Pedersen CA, Stern RA, Light KC. Menstrual cycle and premenstrual syndrome: modifiers of cardiovascular reactivity in women. *Health Psychol* 1993; 12:180–192.

Goolkasian P. Cyclic changes in pain perception: an ROC analysis. *Percept Psychophys* 1980; 27:499–504.

Goolkasian P. An ROC analysis of pain reactions in dysmenorrheic and nondysmenorrheic women. *Percept Psychophys* 1983; 34:381–386.

Gracely RH. Studies of pain in normal man. In: Melzack R, Wall PD (Eds). *Textbook of Pain,* Vol. 3. London: Churchill Livingstone, 1994, pp 315–336.

Green PG, Dahlqvist SR, Isenberg WM, et al. Sex steroid regulation of the inflammatory response: sympathoadrenal dependence in the female rat. *J Neurosci* 1999; 19:4082–4089.

Hapidou EG, De Catanzaro D. Sensitivity to cold pressor pain in dysmenorrheic and non-dysmenorrheic women as a function of menstrual cycle phase. *Pain* 1988; 34:277–283.

Hapidou EG, Rollman GB. Menstrual cycle modulation of tender points. *Pain* 1998; 77:151–161.

Hart KE, Hill AL. Generalized use of over-the-counter analgesics: relationship to premenstrual symptoms. *J Clin Psychol* 1997; 53:197–200.

Heitkemper MM, Jarrett M, Cain KC. Daily gastrointestinal symptoms in women with and without a diagnosis of IBS. *Dig Dis Sci* 1995; 40:1511–1519.

Herren RY. The effect of high and low female sex hormone concentration on the two-point threshold of pain and touch and upon tactile sensitivity. *J Exp Psychol* 1933; 16:324–327.

Huerta-Franco MR, Malacara JM. Association of physical and emotional symptoms with the menstrual cycle and life-style. *J Reprod Med* 1993; 38:448–454.

Janal MN, Glusman M, Kuhl JP, Clark WC. On the absence of correlation between responses to noxious heat, cold, electrical and ischemic stimulation. *Pain* 1994; 58:403–411.

Kane SV, Sable K, Hanauer SB. The menstrual cycle and its effect on inflammatory bowel disease and irritable bowel syndrome: a prevalence study. *Am J Gastroenterol* 1998; 93:1867–1872.

Keenan PA, Lindamer LA. Non-migraine headache across the menstrual cycle in women with and without premenstrual syndrome. *Cephalalgia* 1992; 12:356–359.

Kerdelhue B, Tartar A, Lenoir V, et al. Binding studies of substance P anterior pituitary binding sites: changes in substance P binding sites during the rat estrous cycle. *Regul Pept* 1985; 10:133–143.

Kesner JS, Wright DM, Schrader SM, Chin NW, Krieg EF Jr. Methods of monitoring menstrual function in field studies: efficacy of methods. *Reprod Toxicol* 1992; 6:385–400.

Klaiber EL, Broverman DM, Vogel W, Peterson LG, Snyder MB. Individual differences in changes in mood and platelet monoamine oxidase (MAO) activity during hormonal replacement therapy in menopausal women. *Psychoneuroendocrinology* 1996; 21:575–592.

Komisaruk BR, Adler NT, Hutchison J. Genital sensory field: enlargement by estrogen treatment in female rats. *Science* 1972; 178:1295–1298.

Kontostolis E, Stefanidis K, Navrozoglou I, Lolis D. Comparison of tamoxifen with danazol for treatment of cyclical mastalgia. *Gynecol Endocrinol* 1997; 11:393–397.

Korzekwa MI, Steiner M. Premenstrual syndromes. *Clin Obstet Gynecol* 1997; 40:564–576.

Kuczmierczyk AR, Adams HE. Autonomic arousal and pain sensitivity in women with premenstrual syndrome at different phases of the menstrual cycle. *J Psychosom Res* 1986; 30:421–428.

Kyllonen ES, Vaananen HK, Vanharanta JV, Heikkinen JE. Influence of estrogen-progestin treatment on back pain and disability among slim premenopausal women with low lumbar spine bone mineral density: a 2-year placebo-controlled randomized trial. *Spine* 1999; 24:704–708.

Lautenbacher S, Rollman GB. Possible deficiencies of pain modulation in fibromyalgia. *Clin J Pain* 1997; 13:189–196.

Lavand'homme P M, Pan HL, Eisenach JC. Sex differences in spinal cholinergic analgesia following capsaicin. *Anesthesiology* 1998; 89:A1170.

LeResche L, Saunders K, Von Korff MR, Barlow W, Dworkin SF. Use of exogenous hormones and risk of temporomandibular disorder pain. *Pain* 1997; 69:153–160.

Liuzzi FJ, Scoville SA, Bufton SM. Long-term estrogen replacement coordinately decreases trkA and beta-PPT mRNA levels in dorsal root ganglion neurons. *Exp Neurol* 1999; 155:260–267.

Luciano AA, Peluso J, Koch EI, et al. Temporal relationship and reliability of the clinical, hormonal, and ultrasonographic indices of ovulation in infertile women. *Obstet Gynecol* 1990; 75:412–416.

Manber R, Bootzin RR. Sleep and the menstrual cycle. *Health Psychol* 1997; 16:209–214.

McDermott MT, Hofeldt FD, Kidd GS. Tamoxifen therapy for painful idiopathic gynecomastia. *South Med J* 1990; 83:1283–1285.

McEwen BS, Alves SE, Bulloch K, Weiland NG. Clinically relevant basic science studies of gender differences and sex hormone effects. *Psychopharmacol Bull* 1998; 34:251–259.

Messinis IE, Lolis D. Treatment of premenstrual mastalgia with tamoxifen. *Acta Obstet Gynecol Scand* 1988; 67:307–309.

Morrell JI, McGinty JF, Pfaff DW. A subset of beta-endorphin- or dynorphin-containing neurons in the medial basal hypothalamus accumulates estradiol. *Neuroendocrinology* 1985; 41:417–426.

Nguyen P, Lee SD, Castell DO. Evidence of gender differences in esophageal pain threshold. *Am J Gastroenterol* 1995; 90:901–905.

Ostensen M, Rugelsjoen A, Wigers SH. The effect of reproductive events and alterations of sex hormone levels on the symptoms of fibromyalgia. *Scand J Rheum* 1997; 26:355–360.

Pfleeger M, Stravena PA, Fillingim RB, Maixner W, Girdler SS. Menstrual cycle, blood pressure and ischemic pain sensitivity in women. *Int J Psychophysiol* 1997; 27:161–166.

Priest CA, Pfaff DW. Actions of sex steroids on behaviours beyond reproductive reflexes. *Ciba Found Symp* 1995; 191:74–84.

Procacci P, Zoppi M, Maresca M, Romano S. Studies of the pain threshold in man. In: Bonica JJ (Ed). *Advances in Neurology,* Vol. 4. New York: Raven Press, 1974, pp 107–113.

Quinones-Jenab V, Jenab S, Ogawa S, Inturrisi C, Pfaff DW. Estrogen regulation of mu-opioid receptor mRNA in the forebrain of female rats. *Brain Res Mol Brain Res* 1997; 47:134–138.

Rao SS, Ranganekar AG, Saifi AQ. Pain threshold in relation to sex hormones. *Indian J Physiol Pharmacol* 1987a; 31:250–254.

Ratka A, Simpkins JW. A modulatory role for luteinizing hormone-releasing hormone in nociceptive responses of female rats, *Endocrinology* 1990; 127:667–673.

Riley JL, Robinson ME, Wise EA, Myers CD, Fillingim RB. Sex differences in the perception of noxious experimental stimuli: a meta-analysis. *Pain* 1998; 74:181–187.

Riley JLI, Robinson ME, Wise EA, Price DD. A meta–analytic review of pain perception across the menstrual cycle. *Pain* 1999; 81:225–235.

Robbins A, Sato Y, Hotta H, Berkley KJ. Responses of hypogastric nerve afferent fibers to uterine distension in estrous or metestrous rats. *Neurosci Lett* 1990; 110:82–85.

Robbins A, Berkley KJ, Sato Y. Estrous cycle variation of afferent fibers supplying reproductive organs in the female rat. *Brain Res* 1992; 596:353–356.

Robinson JE, Short RV. Changes in breast sensitivity at puberty, during the menstrual cycle, and at parturition. *BMJ* 1977; 1:1188–1191.

Smith SS. Female sex steroid hormones: from receptors to networks to performance-actions on the sensorimotor system. *Prog Neurobiol* 1994; 44:55–86.

Smith YR, Zubieta JK, del Carmen MG, et al. Brain opioid receptor measurements by positron emission tomography in normal cycling women: relationship to luteinizing hormone pulsatility and gonadal steroid hormones. *J Clin Endocrinol Metab* 1998; 83:4498–4505.

Sohrabji F, Miranda RC, Toran-Allerand CD. Estrogen differentially regulates estrogen and nerve growth factor receptor mRNAs in adult sensory neurons. *J Neurosci* 1994; 14:459–471.

Swerdlow NR, Hartman PL, Auerbach PP. Changes in sensorimotor inhibition across the menstrual cycle: implications for neuropsychiatric disorders. *Biol Psychiatry* 1997; 41:452–460.

Tedford WH, Warren DE Jr, Flynn WE. Alteration of shock aversion thresholds during the menstrual cycle. *Percept Psychophys* 1977; 21:193–196.

Theoharides TC, Pang X, Letourneau R, Sant GR. Interstitial cystitis: a neuroimmunoendocrine disorder. *Ann NY Acad Sci* 1998; 840:619–634.

Thompson HS, Hyatt JP, De Souza MJ, Clarkson PM. The effects of oral contraceptives on delayed onset muscle soreness following exercise. *Contraception* 1997; 56:59–65.

Veith JL, Anderson J, Slade SA. Plasma beta-endorphin, pain thresholds and anxiety levels across the human menstrual cycle. *Physiol Behav* 1984; 32:31–34.

Webster DC, Brennan T. Use and effectiveness of psychological self-care strategies for interstitial cystitis. *Health Care Women Internat* 1995; 16:463–475.

Wise EA, Riley JL III, Robinson ME. Clinical pain perception and hormone replacement therapy in post-menopausal females experiencing orofacial pain. *Clin J Pain* 2000; in press.

Yen SSC. The human menstrual cycle: neuroendocrine regulation. In: Yen SSC, Jaffe RB, Barbieri RL (Eds). *Reproductive Endocrinology,* Vol. 4. Philadelphia: W.B. Saunders, 1998, pp 191–217.

Ylikorkala O, Dawood MY. New concepts in dysmenorrhea. *Am J Obstet Gynecol* 1978; 130:833–841.

Correspondence to: Roger B. Fillingim, PhD, Department of Operative Dentistry, Public Health Services and Research, University of Florida, P.O. Box 100404, 1600 SW Archer Road, D8-37, Gainesville, FL 32610-0404, USA. Email: RFillingim@ufl.edu.

Sex, Gender, and Pain, Progress in Pain Research and Management, Vol. 17, edited by R.B. Fillingim, IASP Press, Seattle, © 2000.

11

Sex-Related Differences in Analgesic Responses

Christine Miaskowski,[a] Robert W. Gear,[b] and Jon D. Levine[b]

Departments of [a]Physiological Nursing and [b]Oral and Maxillofacial Surgery, University of California, San Francisco, California, USA

In a recent review of gender differences in pharmacokinetics and pharmacodynamics, Beierle and colleagues (1999) point out that until 1993, women were excluded from clinical phase I and early phase II trials due to the potential risks of studying women with child-bearing potential. Therefore, for most drugs, including analgesics, there is a real paucity of information on sex differences in the pharmacokinetics as well as in the dose-response relationship and adverse effects of these drugs. However, in 1993, the U.S. Food and Drug Administration (FDA) recognized the need to include women in the early phases of drug studies and developed new guidelines for drug research. These guidelines emphasize that clinical trials of new drugs should address three pharmacological issues: the effects of menstrual cycle and menopausal status on the pharmacokinetics of a drug, the effects of estrogens and oral contraceptives on the pharmacokinetics of a drug, and the influence of oral contraceptives on the effectiveness of a drug (Merkatz et al. 1993; Kando et al. 1995). Clinical drug trials, conducted under the new FDA guidelines, will provide us with much-needed information on sex differences in drug pharmacokinetics and pharmacodynamics that should have a significant clinical impact.

While human studies of sex differences in responses to pharmacological agents will increase, it should be noted that for reasons that are unclear, there is also a paucity of animal research on sex differences in the pharmacological actions and effects of various drugs. We hope that the new FDA guidelines for clinical drug research will also prompt an expansion of investigations using animal models to test for sex differences in pharmacokinetics and pharmacodynamics.

This chapter provides a summary and critique of the animal and human studies that have evaluated sex differences in responses to analgesic medications. Some of the studies examined both pharmacokinetic and pharmacodynamic differences in responses, while others evaluated only one aspect. We will address some of the discrepancies in the findings from studies conducted in animals and humans.

ANIMAL STUDIES OF SEX-RELATED DIFFERENCES IN ANALGESIC RESPONSES

Table I summarizes 10 rodent studies that evaluated sex differences in response to analgesic medications. The table lists antinociceptive effects observed using various types of opioid agonists and different kinds of noxious stimuli, and summarizes the effects in relationship to the phases of the estrous cycle in female rats, and the effects in gonadectomized rodents. Other chapters in this volume describe the results of experimental studies of sex-related factors that influence nociceptive responses in animals (Chapter 5) and discuss research on female-specific antinociceptive mechanisms (e.g., pregnancy-induced analgesia; Chapter 6).

SEX DIFFERENCES IN ANTINOCICEPTIVE EFFECTS OBSERVED WITH DIFFERENT OPIOID AGONISTS

Eight of the 10 papers reviewed (Table I) evaluated sex differences using opioid agonists with activity at the μ receptor (morphine, fentanyl, alfentanil, buprenorphine, and DAMGO; Kepler et al. 1989, 1991; Islam et al. 1993; Ali et al. 1995; Cicero et al. 1996, 1997; Bartok and Craft 1997; Boyer et al. 1998). In five of the six experiments that used morphine as the μ-opioid agonist (83.3%), male rats demonstrated significantly greater antinociceptive effects to morphine than did female rats. Ali et al. (1995) detected no sex differences in the antinociceptive effects of morphine. Alfentanil, used in one study (Cicero et al. 1997), showed a similar sexual dimorphism to morphine. No sex differences were reported with the μ-opioid agonists fentanyl and buprenorphine (Bartok and Craft 1997). The only selective μ-opioid agonist tested was DAMGO (Kepler et al. 1991). Male rats that received an intracerebroventricular (i.c.v.) injection of DAMGO demonstrated significantly greater antinociceptive effects than females on the tail-flick test (a thermal nociceptive stimulus), but not on the jump test (an electrical nociceptive stimulus).

Only two studies (Kepler et al. 1991; Bartok and Craft 1997) evaluated for sex differences using selective δ-opioid agonists (DSLET, DPDPE, and deltorphin). Sex differences in antinociceptive effects were not observed for DSLET in either the tail-flick test or the jump test (Kepler et al. 1991). With DPDPE, peak antinociceptive effects tended to occur earlier in female rats than in males when the hot-plate test was used (Bartok and Craft 1997). However, at the highest dose used in these experiments, both DPDPE and deltorphin produced greater antinociceptive effects on the hot-plate test in males compared to females. No sex differences were observed with DPDPE or deltorphin when the tail-withdrawal test was used (Bartok and Craft 1997).

Sex differences in the antinociceptive effects of κ opioids (U69,593, bremazocine, PNU50488H, and asimadoline) were evaluated in three studies (Bartok and Craft 1997; Kavaliers and Choleris 1997; Binder et al. 2000). The studies that used rats (Bartok and Craft 1997; Binder et al. 2000), found that the κ opioids used had significantly greater antinociceptive effects in females than in males. However, these effects were dependent on the type of noxious stimulus used. The study that used mice (Kavaliers and Choleris 1997) found no sex differences in the antinociceptive effects of the κ-opioid agonist U69,593.

SEX DIFFERENCES IN THE ANTINOCICEPTIVE EFFECTS OF OPIOIDS BASED ON THE TYPE OF NOXIOUS STIMULUS

Several of the animal investigations on sex differences in antinociceptive responses noted that these differences depended on the type of noxious stimulus used (Kepler et al. 1991; Bartok and Craft 1997; Binder et al. 2000). These stimulus-specific responses occurred with μ-, δ-, and κ-opioid agonists. The μ agonist DAMGO showed sex-specific responses with the tail-flick test (antinociception was greater in males compared to females), but not in the jump test (Kepler et al. 1991). Both DPDPE and deltorphin had greater antinociceptive effects in male rats than in females in the hot-plate test but not in the tail-withdrawal test (Bartok and Craft 1997). When given the κ-opioid agonist asimadoline, female rats exhibited enhanced antinociceptive effects compared to male rats when tested with a thermal stimulus (i.e., paw-withdrawal latency). However, when a mechanical stimulus (i.e., paw-withdrawal test) was used, no sex differences were observed (Binder et al 2000).

ANTINOCICEPTIVE EFFECTS OF OPIOIDS BASED ON THE PHASES OF THE ESTROUS CYCLE

Only two studies (Banerjee et al. 1983; Kepler et al. 1989) evaluated for changes in antinociceptive responses during the phases of the estrous cycle

Table I
Animal studies that evaluated for sex-related differences in analgesic responses

Reference; Purpose of Study	Species; Test	Opioid Agonist; Route	EC Effects Rated?	GTX Effects Rated?	Results
Ali et al. (1995); to examine the role of sex in relation to morphine analgesia in rats and mice subjected to two noxious stimuli and to determine whether GTX alters the response to pain or to morphine-induced analgesia	Albino mice, Sprague Dawley rats; thermal HP test	Morphine, s.c.	No	Yes	No sex differences were found between sham-operated male and female rats in morphine-induced antinociception. GTX male and female rats and GTX male mice displayed sign. greater morphine analgesia than did sham-operated controls. OVX female rats demonstrated sign. greater analgesia than did GTX male rats.
Banerjee et al. (1983); to study the effects of ovarian steroids on antinociceptive responses of female rats to morphine	Charles Foster rats; thermal TF test	Morphine, s.c.	Yes	Yes	Increased efficacy of morphine was observed during days 3 and 4 of the EC. OVX attenuated the effects of morphine observed at days 3 and 4 of the EC.
Bartok and Craft (1997); to more fully characterize sex differences in thermal antinociception produced by a variety of opioids in the rat	Sprague Dawley rats; thermal HP test, TW test	Fentanyl, s.c.; buprenorphine, s.c.; U69,593, s.c.; bremazocine, s.c.; DPDPE, i.c.v.; deltorphin, i.c.v.	No	No	No sex differences were observed in the antinociceptive effects of fentanyl or buprenorphine in either nociceptive test. Sex differences in the antinociceptive effects of the κ and δ agonists were assay-, dose-, and/or time-dependent. No sex differences were found in the antinociceptive effects of U69,593 on the HP test. Peak effects of U69,593 on the TW test tended to occur earlier in females than in males. Bremazocine produced greater antinociceptive effects in females on the TW test, but no sex differences were observed using the HP test. Peak effects of DPDPE, on the HP test, tended to occur earlier in females. The highest dose of DPDPE and deltorphin produced greater antinociception in the HP test in males compared to females. No sex differences were observed with DPDPE or deltorphin on the TW test.

Binder et al. (2000); to investigate sex differences in the anti-inflammatory and analgesic actions of two κ-opioid agonists (PNU50488H, which acts on the CNS and at peripheral locations; and asimadoline, which has essentially peripheral actions).	Dark Agouti rats with adjuvant arthritis; mechanical PW test, thermal PW latency	PNU50488H, i.p.; asimadoline, i.p.	No	No	No sex differences were observed in the anti-inflammatory effects of PNU50488H and asimadoline. With a mechanical test, no sex differences were found in the analgesic effects of asimadoline when tested with a mechanical stimulus, but PNU50488H appeared to be more potent in female than in male rats. When a thermal stimulus was used, PNU50488H and asimadoline produced antinociceptive effects in female rats, but in male rats asimadoline had no analgesic effect.
Boyer et al. (1998); to determine whether the greater antinociception in male rats following i.c.v. administration of morphine is mediated, at least in part, by a difference in the RVM of male and female rats.	Sprague Dawley rats; thermal TW test	Morphine; microinjection into RVM	No	No	Male rats showed greater antinociception than female rats at all doses and times following morphine administration.
Cicero et al. (1996); to establish whether there are gender-related differences in the antinociceptive activity of morphine in male and female rats and to evaluate whether sex steroid hormones may be involved. To determine the ED_{50} values of morphine and measure morphine levels in the serum of male and female rats.	Sprague Dawley rats; thermal HP test, TF test; chemical AC test	Morphine, s.c.	No	Yes	Male rats displayed enhanced sensitivity to morphine as evidenced by higher peak antinociceptive effects, greater magnitude of antinociceptive effects, and an ED_{50} dose of 50% less in male compared to female rats regardless of noxious stimulus used. GTX produced no differences in the antinociceptive effects of morphine in male and female rats. No sex differences were found in serum concentrations of morphine.
Cicero et al. (1997); to measure peak blood and brain levels of morphine and the elimination half-life of the drug at doses that produce maximal differences in morphine-induced antinociception in male and female rats. To determine whether sex differences observed with morphine are also seen with another μ agonist, alfentanil.	Sprague Dawley rats; thermal HP test	Morphine, s.c.; alfentanil, s.c.	No	No	Male rats were more sensitive to the antinociceptive effects of morphine, with the ED_{50} of morphine being ~50% less in males than females. Male rats were more sensitive to the antinociceptive effects of alfentanil. No sex differences were observed in the peak levels of morphine in the blood or brain, in the elimination half-life of morphine in the blood, or in the disappearance of morphine from the brain.

(continued)

Table I. Continued

Reference; Purpose of Study	Species; Test	Opioid Agonist; Route	EC Effects Rated?	GTX Effects Rated?	Results
Islam et al. (1993); to evaluate changes in morphine antinociception in rats as functions of age (6, 12, 18, and 24 months), gender, and gonadal status (intact, GTX) across a dose range (1, 2.5, 5, and 10 mg/kg) and time course (30–120 min) on the TF test.	Sprague Dawley rats; thermal TF test	Morphine, s.c.	No	Yes	In sham-operated males, the ED_{50} for morphine decreased with age. but in sham-operated females, it increased with age. OVX eliminated the age-related increase in ED_{50} in female rats.
Kavaliers and Choleris (1997); to evaluate sex differences in the antinociceptive effects of the κ-specific opioid agonist U69,593. To determine the involvement of the NMDA receptor in the analgesic responses of male and female mice to U69,593.	CD-1 and CF-1 strain equivalent mice; thermal HP test	U69,593, i.p.; NPC 12626 (a competitive NMDA-receptor antagonist), i.p.	No	No	No sex differences were found in the analgesic effects of U69,593. NPC 12626 attenuated the antinociceptive effects of U69,593 in male, but not female mice.
Kepler et al. (1989); to evaluate the dose-response and time-response of central morphine analgesia in sham-operated male, castrated male, OVX female, and sham-operated female rats during estrus, proestrus, and met-/diestrus on the spinally mediated TF and supraspinally mediated jump tests.	Sprague Dawley rats; thermal TF test; electric shock jump test	Morphine, i.c.v.	Yes	Yes	Male rats displayed sign. greater peak and total morphine analgesia than female rats on both tests. GTX produced small but sign. decreases in morphine analgesia in both male and female rats. While female rats in proestrus and estrus displayed sign. greater analgesia than OVX rats or rats in a combined met-/diestrous phase at some doses, the ED_{50} did not sign. alter as a function of EC phase or OVX.
Kepler et al. (1991); to evaluate whether gender or adult GTX alters the analgesic responses following i.c.v. administration of either the μ-selective agonist DAMGO or the δ-selective agonist DSLET as measured by the TF and jump tests.	Sprague Dawley rats; thermal TF test; electric shock jump test	DAMGO, i.c.v.; DSLET, i.c.v.	No; females tested only during estrus	Yes	Sham-operated males demonstrated sign. greater analgesia with DAMGO but not DSLET on the TF test than did sham-operated females. Sex differences were not observed for DAMGO or DSLET analgesia on the jump test. GTX failed to consistently affect DAMGO or DSLET analgesia.

Abbreviations: AC = abdominal constriction; CNS = central nervous system; EC = estrous cycle; GTX = gonadectomy; HP = hot-plate; i.c.v. = intracerebroventricular; i.p. = intraperitoneally; i.t. = intrathecal; OVX = ovariectomy; PW = paw-withdrawal; RVM = rostroventral medulla; s.c. = subcutaneously; sign. = significant(ly); TF = tail-flick; TW = tail-withdrawal.

in the female rat. Findings from these studies suggest that female rats' sensitivity to morphine varies during the phases of the estrous cycle. However, the data are not definitive as to which cycle phases are associated with the greatest antinociceptive effects.

INFLUENCE OF GONADECTOMY ON THE ANTINOCICEPTIVE EFFECTS OF OPIOID AGONISTS

Six studies evaluated the effects of gonadectomy or ovariectomy on antinociceptive responses (Banerjee et al. 1983; Kepler et al. 1989, 1991; Islam et al. 1993; Ali et al. 1995; Cicero et al. 1996). In male rats, the data are contradictory on the influence of gonadectomy on responsiveness to opioid analgesics. Kepler et al. (1989) found that the antinociceptive effects of morphine are *decreased,* while Ali et al. (1995) found that they are *enhanced* following gonadectomy in male rats. Two studies reported no differences in antinociceptive responses of gonadectomized male rats to morphine (Cicero et al. 1996), DAMGO, or DSLET (Kepler et al. 1991).

The data on the influence of ovariectomy on responsiveness to opioids are also conflicting. Findings from three studies (Banerjee et al. 1983; Kepler et al. 1989; Islam et al. 1993) suggest that the antinociceptive effects of morphine are *decreased* in ovariectomized rats. In contrast, Ali et al. (1995) suggest that ovariectomy *increases* the antinociceptive effects of morphine in rats, and two studies found no differences in antinociceptive responses of female rats to morphine (Cicero et al. 1996), or to DAMGO or DSLET (Kepler et al. 1991) following ovariectomy. These contradictory findings are not readily explainable and will require additional investigation.

Half of the studies administered the opioid agonist through the subcutaneous route. Only two studies (Kepler et al. 1989, 1991) administered opioid agonists through the i.c.v. route, and only one study (Dawson-Basoa and Gintzler 1996) used the intrathecal (i.t.) route. Only five studies evaluated gender differences in the analgesic effects of *selective* opioid agonists (Kepler et al. 1991; Dawson-Basoa and Gintzler 1996; Bartok and Craft 1997; Kavaliers and Choleris 1997; Binder et al. 2000).

SEX DIFFERENCES IN THE ANTINOCICEPTIVE EFFECTS OF CHOLINERGIC AGENTS

Cholinergic agents such as neostigmine produce analgesia following i.t. administration in human volunteers (Hood et al. 1995; 1996; Eisenach et al. 1997; Hood et al. 1997) and in patients with chronic pain (Klamt et al. 1996) or acute postoperative pain (Lauretti et al. 1996; Krukowski et al. 1997; Pan et al. 1998). A recent retrospective review of the studies cited above demonstrated that women exhibited twice as much sensitivity to the analgesic effects of neostigmine compared to men (summary reported in Chiari et al. 1999). This retrospective review led to a series of experiments that looked for sex differences in the antinociceptive effects of cholinergic agents in normal rats (Chiari et al. 1999) and in rats following spinal nerve ligation or intraplantar injection of capsaicin (Lavand'homme and Eisenach 1999).

In the experiments involving normal rats (Chiari et al. 1999), male and female rats with indwelling i.t. catheters received injections of neostigmine (a cholinergic agonist), bethanechol (a muscarinic agonist), or RJR-2403 (a neuronal nicotinic agonist), either alone or with atropine (a muscarinic antagonist), mecamylamine (a nicotinic antagonist), or phentolamine (an α-adrenergic antagonist). Antinociceptive effects were evaluated using a noxious heat stimulus to the rat's hindpaw. Neostigmine produced dose-dependent antinociceptive effects with five times greater potency in female compared to male rats. Neostigmine-induced antinociception was reversed in male rats by atropine but was not affected by mecamylamine. However, in female rats, neostigmine-induced antinociception was partially reversed by either atropine or mecamylamine and was completely reversed after an i.t. injection of both antagonists. In addition, the neural nicotinic agonist, RJR-2403, was more potent in females than in males. However, no sex differences in antinociceptive effects were observed with the muscarinic agonist, bethanechol. Phentolamine partially reversed the antinociceptive effects of RJR-2403 in female rats. These findings demonstrate a large sex difference in the antinociceptive effects of i.t. neostigmine that is primarily the result of a nicotinic component in the pain-modulatory mechanism of females. The findings with phentolamine suggest that part of this nicotinic component may rely on the release of spinal norepinephrine.

The purpose of a second set of experiments (Lavand'homme and Eisenach 1999) was to determine whether there were sex differences in the antinociceptive effects of cholinergic agents in two models of allodynia and to test their pharmacological mechanisms. In these experiments, male and female rats with indwelling i.t. catheters received injections of neostigmine, bethanechol, or RJR-2403, either alone or with atropine, mecamylamine, phentolamine, or saline control. The effects of these agents were determined on mechanical allodynia produced by either intraplantar injection of capsaicin or by ligation of spinal nerves. Neostigmine and RJR-2403, but not bethanechol, were more potent in female as compared to male rats in decreasing allodynia after nerve injury, and antagonist studies were also consistent with a nicotinic component in females. Phentolamine did not reverse the effect of neostigmine. In contrast, for capsaicin-induced allodynia, neostigmine plus mecamylamine, but not neostigmine alone or RJR-2403, was more potent in female than in male rats. These data demonstrate a sex difference in the effects of i.t. administration of neostigmine after nerve-injury-induced allodynia similar to that observed in normal rats that received acute noxious thermal stimulation. However, findings from this study suggest that this sex difference is not universal to all pain models because it was not present after intradermal injection of capsaicin. In addition, the interaction among spinal noradrenergic mechanisms in female rats was not consistent in all pain models.

Findings from these two studies (Chiari et al. 1999; Lavand'homme and Eisenach 1999) support the need to explore sex differences in antinociceptive responses. More detailed investigations are warranted to evaluate the influence of hormonal status on antinociceptive responses and to determine whether sex differences exist in various models of acute and chronic pain.

HUMAN STUDIES OF SEX-RELATED DIFFERENCES IN ANALGESIC RESPONSES

Little is known about sex-related differences in the pharmacokinetics and pharmacodynamics of analgesics in humans. In a recent review (Miaskowski and Levine 1999) we summarized data from the human studies on sex-related differences in responses to opioid analgesics. This chapter presents a summary of that review as well as additional findings that were published subsequent to its completion.

SEX-RELATED DIFFERENCES IN ANALGESIC RESPONSES TO NSAIDS

Nonsteroidal anti-inflammatory drugs (NSAIDs) are widely used to manage acute and chronic pain problems. Only one study (Walker and Carmody 1998) has evaluated for gender differences in the pharmacokinetics and pharmacodynamics of an NSAID (ibuprofen). The investigators induced pain in young, healthy participants through electrical stimulation of the earlobe. This procedure allowed for the measurement of pain detection thresholds and maximal pain tolerance. Only male participants exhibited a statistically significant analgesic response to ibuprofen. The sex-related difference in analgesic response could not be attributed to any pharmacokinetic differences (i.e., C_{max}, area under the curve measurement, half-life, clearance, or volume of distribution). The authors concluded that this reduced effectiveness of ibuprofen in women compared to men has potential clinical significance, especially as a factor in the reported response variability of NSAIDs (Walker 1995). Additional studies are warranted to evaluate sex-related differences in analgesic responses to acetaminophen, aspirin, and other NSAIDs.

SEX-RELATED DIFFERENCES IN THE CONSUMPTION OF OPIOID ANALGESICS

Table II provides summary data from 14 papers that reported on the results of 18 studies that evaluated sex-related differences in analgesic consumption during the postoperative period. The primary aim of most of the studies listed in Table II was to evaluate the pharmacokinetic and/or pharmacodynamic properties of one or more opioid analgesics that were administered in the immediate postoperative period. All of these studies used patient-controlled analgesia (PCA) devices to administer the analgesic. Only two of these studies (Gourlay et al. 1988; Burns et al. 1989) stated that one of their specific aims was to evaluate for sex differences in the postoperative use of opioid analgesics. Most of these PCA studies did not evaluate analgesic responses directly (i.e., a decrease in pain) but rather used the consumption of the analgesic medication as the outcome measure. Most of the studies used μ-opioid analgesics. The untested, yet underlying assumption in these studies was that patients titrated their analgesic medication to the minimum effective plasma concentration (i.e., a concentration that would produce an optimal balance between adequate analgesia and an acceptable level of side effects).

In these 18 studies, a total of 2055 patients (1014 males, 1041 females) were evaluated. In approximately 56% (10/18) of the studies, males (n = 959) consumed more opioid analgesics in the immediate postoperative period than did females (n = 953). More specifically, males consumed more diamorphine (five studies; 28 males, 21 females), fentanyl (one study; 13 males, 17 females), and morphine (four studies; 918 males, 915 females) than did females. In these studies, males used considerably more opioids than did females (i.e., on average 2.4 times more opioids, range 1.1–5.5 times more). These findings are compatible with the suggestion that a sexual dimorphism exists in the *use* of opioid analgesics for the management of acute postoperative pain. In all of the studies that demonstrated a sex-related difference in analgesic consumption, except one (Sidebotham et al. 1997), either there were no differences in body weight between the males and the females, or weight was evaluated as part of the statistical analysis and was found *not* to be related to sex differences in analgesic consumption.

In eight of the studies (55 males, 88 females), no sex differences were found in the consumption of pethidine (two studies; 15 males, 21 females), nalbuphine (two studies; 20 males, 36 females), morphine (three studies; 13 males; 23 females), or ketobemidone (one study; 7 males, 8 females). It is unclear at the present time why these studies did not find sex differences in analgesic consumption. Many of these studies enrolled relatively small numbers of patients, and several of them probably lacked sufficient statistical power to detect sex-related differences. Another possible methodological reason for the negative findings in two of the studies (Bennett et al. 1982; Bahar et al. 1985) was the inequality in the number of men and women enrolled in the study.

One of the major limitations of most of these PCA studies is that the analgesic effects of the opioid were not measured in the participants. Only analgesic consumption (using a PCA device), which may be effected by factors other than pain intensity or pain relief (Bond 1971; Dalrymple et al. 1972, 1973; Parbrook et al. 1973a,b; Dalrymple and Parbrook 1976; Boyle and Parbrook 1977; Peck 1986; Egan and Ready 1994; Taylor et al. 1996; Badner et al. 1997; Tsui et al. 1997), was used as the variable to evaluate for sex differences. In fact, only three studies (Bennett et al. 1982; Lehmann and Tenbuhs 1986; Burns et al. 1989) confirmed that there were no differences in pain intensity scores between men and women who were receiving analgesic medication through a PCA device (two of these studies found no sex differences in analgesic consumption, and one found increased analgesic consumption in males).

We can only speculate on the possible explanations for the conflicting findings on sex-related differences in postoperative analgesic consumption. One possible explanation is that men and women tolerated different levels of postoperative pain and titrated their dose of analgesic accordingly. An alternative explanation, noted in two of the studies (Gourlay et al. 1988; Tsui et al. 1996), is that sex differences in analgesic consumption might be related to various psychological factors or personality traits that affect men's and women's perceptions of pain and their use of PCA devices. These factors might include anxiety, fears of addiction, previous experience with pain, expectations regarding postoperative pain and pain relief, and patient education regarding postoperative pain management (Bond 1971; Dalrymple et al. 1972, 1973; Parbrook et al. 1973a,b; Dalrymple and Parbrook 1976; Boyle and Parbrook 1977; Peck 1986; Egan and Ready 1994; Taylor et al. 1996; Badner et al. 1997; Tsui et al. 1997). Another explanation for the sex differences in analgesic consumption might be differential side effects in men and women, if patients titrated their analgesic dose depending on a tolerable level of side effects (Petros et al. 1992; Tsui et al. 1997, 1988; Liu et al. 1998).

SEX-RELATED DIFFERENCES IN ANALGESIC RESPONSES TO KAPPA-LIKE OPIOIDS

The opioid analgesics available for clinical use can be divided into two major classes based on the predominant opioid receptor subtype at which they are thought to act to produce analgesia, namely μ or κ. Almost all of the

Table II

Summary of the patient controlled analgesic studies of sex-related differences in the analgesic effects of opioid agonists

Reference	Opioid Agonist	Sample Size; Mean Age (years) ± SD	Gender Differences in Analgesic Consumption	Gender Differences in Pharmacokinetics
McQuay et al. 1980; study 1	Immediate postop. period = i.m. buprenorphine; PCA = diamorphine	M = 6, F = 4; age = 62.7 ± 2.9	Males made significantly more demands than females (6.5 vs. 2.0 μg/min, respectively; 3.3 times as much). No differences in weight between males and females.	No difference in plasma levels of buprenorphine
McQuay et al. 1980; study 2	Immediate postop. period = i.v. buprenorphine; PCA = diamorphine	M = 6, F = 4; age = 62.7 ± 2.0	Males made significantly more demands than females (8.6 vs. 4.8 μg/min, respectively; 1.8 times as much). No differences in weight between males and females.	No difference in plasma levels of buprenorphine
Bullingham et al. 1981	Immediate postop. period = sublingual buprenorphine; PCA = diamorphine	M = 6, F = 4; age = 59.8 ± 3.7	Males made significantly more demands than females (8.3 vs. 1.5 μg/min, respectively; 5.5 times as much). No differences in weight between males and females.	No difference in plasma levels of buprenorphine
Watson et al. 1982; study 1	Immediate postop. period = 0.3 mg buprenorphine; PCA = diamorphine	M = 5, F = 4; age = 66.2 ± 2.9	Males made significantly more demands than females (18.8 vs. 8.6 μg/min, respectively; 2.2 times as much). No differences in weight between males and females.	Not evaluated
Watson et al. 1982; study 2	Immediate postop. period = 0.6 mg buprenorphine; PCA = diamorphine	M = 5, F = 5; age = 59.9 ± 3.8	Males made significantly more demands than females (13.0 vs. 4.3 μg/min, respectively; 3.0 times as much). No differences in weight between males and females.	Not evaluated
Bennett et al. 1982	PCA = morphine	M = 2, F = 8; age = 41.4 ± 9.8	No gender differences; body weight was not related to analgesic consumption.	Not evaluated
Tamsen et al. 1982a	PCA = pethidine	M = 11, F = 9; age = 33 ± 11	No gender differences; body weight was not related to analgesic consumption.	No differences in plasma concentration or MEC of pethidine
Tamsen et al. 1982b	PCA = ketobemidone	M = 7, F = 8; age = 31 ± 9	No gender differences; body weight was not related to analgesic consumption.	No differences in distribution volume, total plasma clearance, half-life, plasma concentration, or MEC of ketobemidone

Dahlström et al. 1982	PCA = morphine	M = 4, F = 6; age = 38 ± 15	No gender differences; body weight was not related to analgesic demands.	No differences in distribution volume, total plasma clearance, half-life, plasma concentration, or MEC of morphine
Bahar et al. 1985; study 1	PCA = nalbuphine	M = 1, F = 15; age = 46 ± 3	No gender differences; no differences in weight between males and females.	Not evaluated
Bahar et al. 1985; study 2	PCA = morphine	M = 7, F = 9; age = 43 ± 3	No gender differences; no differences in weight between males and females.	Not evaluated
Bahar et al. 1985; study 3	PCA = pethidine	M = 4, F = 12; age = 43 ± 3	No gender differences; no differences in weight between males and females.	Not evaluated
Lehmann et al. 1986	PCA = nalbuphine	M = 19, F = 21; age = 46.6 ± 14.5	No gender differences; no differences in weight between males and females.	Not evaluated
Gourlay et al. 1988	PCA = fentanyl	M = 13, F = 17; age = 47.0 ± 13.9	Males required significantly more fentanyl than females; body weight was not predictive of analgesic requirements.	No difference in MEC of fentanyl
Burns et al. 1989	PCA = morphine	M = 46, F = 54; age = 46.3 ± 14.9	Males consumed significantly more morphine than females (71.4 mg vs. 48.8 mg, respectively; 1.5 times as much); body weight did not correlate with analgesic consumption.	Not evaluated
De Kock et al. 1991	PCA = morphine	M = 111, F = 89; age = 52.7 ± 15.6	Males consumed significantly more morphine than females (95 mg vs. 63 mg in patients <40 years of age respectively; 1.4 times as much); body weight did not correlate with morphine requirements.	Not evaluated
Tsui et al. 1996	PCA = morphine	M = 603, F = 630; age = 52.6 ± 16.5	Males consumed significantly more morphine than females: 1st to 16th hour, 27.3 vs. 24.1 $\mu g \cdot kg^{-1} \cdot h^{-1}$, respectively (1.1 times as much); 17th to 41st hour, 20.3 vs. 15.0 $\mu g \cdot kg^{-1} \cdot h^{-1}$ (1.4 times as much); 42nd to 66th hour, 19.8 vs. 14.3 $\mu g \cdot kg^{-1} \cdot h^{-1}$ (1.4 times as much); dose of PCA was ordered by body weight.	Not evaluated
Sidebotham et al. 1997	PCA = morphine	M = 158, F = 142; age = 49.4 ± 20.5	Males consumed significantly more morphine than females (141.7 mg vs. 102.7 mg respectively; 1.4 times as much); body weight was not evaluated.	Not evaluated

Abbreviations: F = female; i.m. = intramuscular; i.v. = intravenous; M = male; MEC = minimum effective concentration; PCA = patient-controlled analgesia. Adapted with permission from Miaskowski and Levine (1999).

human studies discussed above used μ opioids (morphine, diamorphine, meperidine, and ketobemidone). In 1995, our laboratory began a systematic evaluation of opioid agonists that are thought to produce analgesia by an action at the κ-opioid receptor (e.g., pentazocine, nalbuphine, butorphanol; Reisine and Pasternak 1996).

All of our studies were conducted using the same postoperative pain paradigm. All patients underwent standardized surgery by the same oral surgeon for the removal of third molar teeth. The surgical procedure always included the removal of at least one bony impacted mandibular third molar. This procedure is associated with moderate to severe postoperative pain.

Prior to surgery, patients received intravenous (i.v.) diazepam and a local anesthetic (mepivacaine without vasoconstrictor to obtain a nerve block of short duration). After surgery, each patient was randomly assigned, in an open, double-blinded fashion, to receive a test drug through an i.v. line. The drug was administered at least 80 minutes after the onset of the local anesthetic and was only given if the patient had a pain rating that was greater than 2.5 cm on a 10-cm visual analogue scale (VAS). Baseline pain intensity was defined as the VAS pain rating just prior to administration of the test drug. The duration of most of the experiments was 5 hours. Following administration of the study drug, pain ratings were taken every 20 minutes for a total of 2.5 hours. The magnitude of the analgesic response for each patient was defined as the difference between the pain rating at each time point following test drug administration and baseline VAS pain rating.

The first study (Gordon et al. 1995) evaluated the effects of preoperative administration of baclofen on the analgesia produced by postoperative administration of morphine (predominantly a μ-opioid agonist) or pentazocine (predominantly a κ-opioid agonist). Baclofen is a $GABA_B$ agonist that is commonly used to treat spasticity associated with multiple sclerosis or spinal cord injury. Studies in animals have shown that baclofen, administered intrathecally (Wilson and Yaksh 1978; Yaksh and Reddy 1981; Zieglgansberger 1988) or supraspinally (Levy and Proudfit 1979), produces antinociceptive effects.

The results showed that the analgesic efficacy of morphine was enhanced by the preoperative administration of baclofen. However, no sex differences were found in the analgesic responses to either morphine alone or morphine given in combination with baclofen. In contrast, in the pentazocine experiments, regardless of drug group (i.e., pentazocine alone or pentazocine with pretreatment with baclofen), women (n = 22) reported consistently better analgesic effects than men (n = 12). These data suggest that the administration of a drug that relieves pain by an action at the κ-opioid receptor produces better analgesia in women compared to men (Gordon et al. 1995).

To confirm our initial findings, we investigated gender differences in the analgesic effects of i.v. pentazocine (Gear et al. 1996a). Again, the analgesic efficacy of pentazocine was greater in women (n = 10) than in men (n = 8). With this confirmation of the gender difference in the analgesic effects of pentazocine, we continued to investigate the hypothesis that sex differences in responses to analgesic medications are a characteristic of κ-opioid analgesics. To determine whether sex differences were associated with κ-like opioids, the analgesic effects of two additional drugs in this class (nalbuphine and butorphanol) were compared in men and women who underwent surgery for removal of third molar teeth (Gear et al. 1996b). Consistent with the findings with pentazocine, 10 mg of i.v. nalbuphine prolonged the duration of analgesia in women (n = 12) significantly more than it did in men (n = 16). As shown in Fig. 1A, both men and women experienced analgesia for the first 60 minutes following the administration of nalbuphine, although the women experienced a greater analgesic effect. The analgesic effects of nalbuphine begin to decline after 60 minutes in men, whereas women experienced analgesia for the entire duration of the experiment. At the conclusion of the experiment, men reported a significant amount of pain, while women continued to report analgesic effects from nalbuphine. Similar analgesic effects were observed with 2 mg butorphanol administered to male (n = 12) and female (n = 8) patients experiencing postoperative dental pain (Fig. 1B).

The next study was conducted to determine whether, within the range of doses usually given in clinical practice, the observed sex differences in analgesia produced by κ-opioid agonists are due to the presence of a rightward shift in the dose-response relationship of men compared to women (Gear et al. 1999). Specifically, we tested the hypothesis that men, given a sufficiently large dose of nalbuphine, would experience analgesia equivalent to that observed in women. Since there were no previous studies of analgesic efficacy with κ opioids, we compared the analgesic effects produced by nalbuphine with those produced by placebo within each sex. In addition, we evaluated sex differences in placebo responses. Different groups of male and female patients who were experiencing moderate to severe postoperative pain were given either a placebo (0.9% saline) or one of three doses (5, 10, or 20 mg) of nalbuphine.

As illustrated in Fig. 2, although responses to placebo were similar in men and women, women experienced a significantly greater analgesic response than men for all doses of nalbuphine. Unexpectedly, men who received the 5-mg dose of nalbuphine experienced significantly *greater* pain than those who received placebo. Only the 20-mg dose of nalbuphine in men produced significant analgesia compared to placebo (Fig. 3). While no

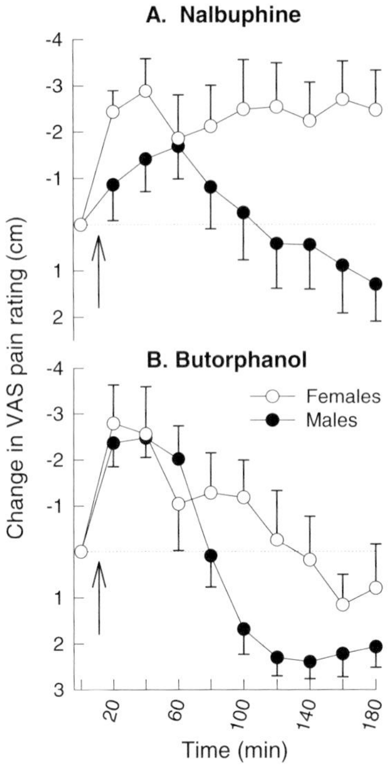

Fig. 1. The change in postoperative pain level following administration of (a) nalbuphine or (b) butorphanol. Change in pain rating (ordinate), recorded on a 10-cm visual analogue scale (VAS), represents changes from baseline level at various times. Arrows indicate time of administration of nalbuphine or butorphanol. Data are plotted as means ± SEM. (Reprinted with permission from Gear et al. 1996b.)

antianalgesic effect was observed in women, only the 10-mg dose of nalbuphine produced significant analgesia compared to placebo.

Taken together, the results of these studies support the hypothesis that among patients experiencing postoperative pain, women obtain better analgesia than men using opioid analgesics of the κ-opioid class (i.e., pentazocine, butorphanol, and nalbuphine). One might argue that sex differences in weight or pharmacokinetics might account for the sex differences in analgesic responses observed. However, several lines of evidence contradict these alternative hypotheses. First in the studies with pentazocine (Gear et al. 1996a) and butorphanol (Gear et al. 1996b), no differences in weight were found between the male and female participants. In the other study with pentazocine (Gordon et al. 1995) and in the study with nalbuphine (Gear et al. 1996b), differences in weight between men and women were accounted for by using weight as a covariate in the statistical analyses. In addition, in a recent study of the dose-response relationship of nalbuphine (Gear et al. 1999), we were unable to overcome the sex differences in analgesic responses by increasing the dose of nalbuphine.

While sex differences in pharmacokinetics might explain the sex differences in analgesic responses observed with this class of opioid agonist, previous studies have shown no sex differences in the pharmacokinetics of

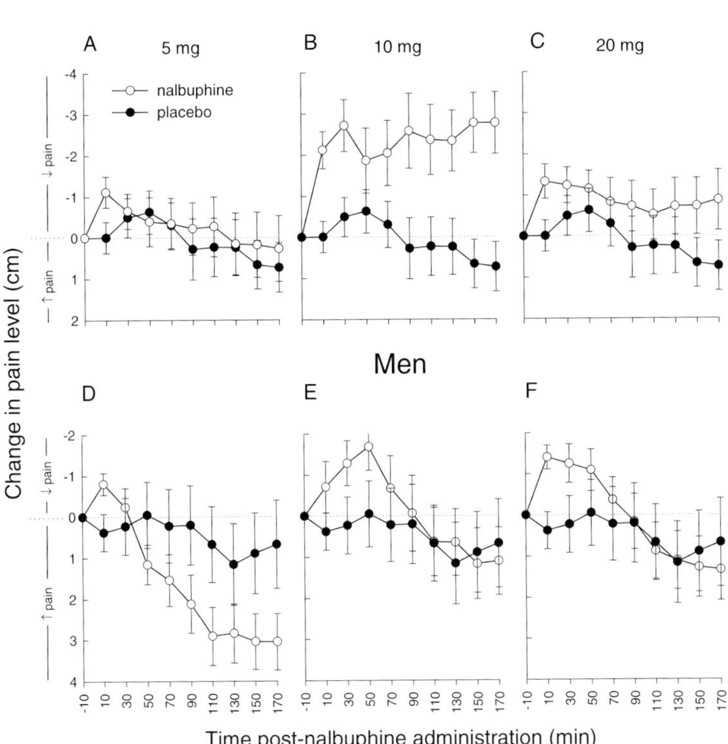

Fig. 2. The effect on postoperative pain of various doses of nalbuphine compared to placebo in women (panels A–C) and men (panels D–F), plotted as a change in postoperative pain level over the 3 hours following administration. Change in pain level (ordinate), recorded on a 10-cm VAS, represents changes from baseline level at various times. Decreased pain scores (i.e., analgesia) are above the baseline. (Reprinted with permission from Gear et al. 1999.)

butorphanol (Shyu et al. 1994) and nalbuphine (Wilson et al. 1986; Jaillon et al. 1989). In a study population consisting almost exclusively of females (Berkowitz et al. 1969), pentazocine had a half-life of 126 minutes. In a different study that included only male participants (Ehrnebo et al. 1977), the half-life of pentazocine was 203 minutes. Although the plasma half-life of pentazocine may be longer in males, we observed that the analgesia produced by pentazocine is of shorter duration in males than in females. Therefore, the sex differences in analgesic responses that we observed with butorphanol, nalbuphine, and pentazocine (Gordon et al. 1995; Gear et al. 1996a,b, 1999) are not explained by pharmacokinetic differences between men and women. In addition, our studies explain the failure of other studies to find an analgesic effect with the more selective κ-opioid agonist enandoline,

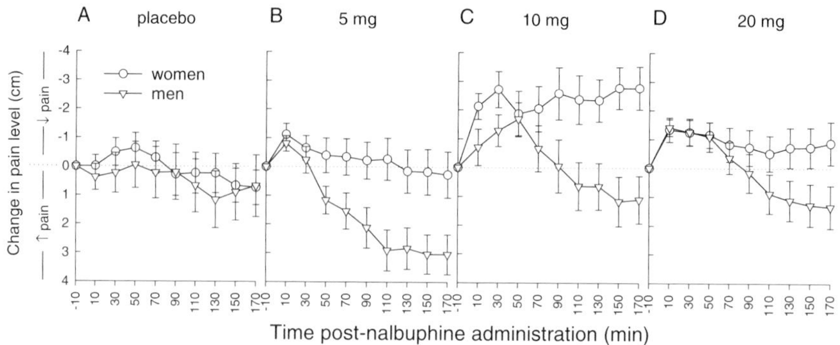

Fig. 3. The effect of placebo or various doses of nalbuphine on postoperative pain in women and men plotted as a change in postoperative pain level over the 3 hours following administration (see Fig. 2 legend for details). (Reprinted with permission from Gear et al. 1999.)

given the fact that in two such studies the entire study sample consisted of men (Pande et al. 1996a,b).

DISCREPANCIES BETWEEN ANIMAL AND HUMAN STUDIES OF SEX-RELATED DIFFERENCES IN ANALGESIC RESPONSES

Findings from the limited number of animal studies suggest that males exhibit significantly greater antinociceptive effects than females when given the predominantly μ-opioid agonist morphine subcutaneously. However, findings from the PCA studies in humans suggest the opposite. In addition, the exact role that sex steroid hormones play in modulating these sex-related differences in antinociception remains to be elucidated in both animals and humans.

Recent animal studies that used selective κ-opioid agonists (Bartok and Craft 1997; Binder et al. 2000) found that these drugs elicited significantly greater antinociceptive effects in female than in male rats. These findings are consistent with data in humans.

Additional research in both animals and humans is warranted to determine the extent to which sex differences in pharmacokinetics and pharmacodynamics of nonopioid and opioid analgesics are mediated by sex steroid hormones. Systematic investigations are needed to determine whether sex differences persist with repeated dosing of analgesic medications in models of both acute and chronic pain. Investigators must consider sex as a significant variable that may affect the outcome of analgesic trials in both animals and humans.

REFERENCES

Ali BH, Sharif, SI, Elkadi A. Sex differences and the effect of gonadectomy on morphine-induced antinociception and dependence in rats and mice. *Clin Exp Pharmacol Physiol* 1995; 22:342–344.

Badner NH, Komar WE, Craen RA. Patient attitudes regarding PCA and associated costs. *Can J Anesth* 1997; 44:255–258.

Bahar M, Rosen M, Vickers MD. Self-administered nalbuphine, morphine and pethidine. *Anaesthesia* 1985; 40:529–532.

Banerjee P, Chatterjee TK, Ghosh JJ. Ovarian steroids and modulation of morphine-induced analgesia and catalepsy in female rats. *Eur J Pharmacol* 1983; 96:291–294.

Bartok RE, Craft RM. Sex differences in opioid antinociception. *J Pharmacol Exp Ther* 1997; 282:769–778.

Bennett R, Batenhorst R, Graves DA, et al. Variation in postoperative analgesic requirements in the morbidly obese following gastric bypass surgery. *Pharmacotherapy* 1982; 2:50–53.

Berkowitz BA, Asling JH, Shnider SM, Way EL. Relationship of pentazocine plasma levels to pharmacologic activity in man. *Clin Pharmacol Ther* 1969; 10:320–328.

Beierle I, Meibohm B, Derendorf H. Gender differences in pharmacokinetics and pharmacodynamics. *Int J Clin Pharmacol Ther* 1999; 37(11):529–547.

Binder W, Carmody J, Walker J. Effects of gender on anti-inflammatory and analgesic actions of two κ-opioids. *J Pharmacol Exp Ther* 2000; 292:303–309.

Bond MR. The relationship of pain to the Eysenck Personality Inventory, Cornell Medical Index, and Whitely Index of hypochondriasis. *Br J Psychiatry* 1971; 119:671–678.

Boyer JS, Morgan MM, Craft RM. Microinjection of morphine into the rostral ventromedial medulla produces greater antinociception in male compared to female rats. *Brain Res* 1998; 796:315–318.

Boyle P, Parbrook GD. The interrelation of personality and postoperative factors. *Br J Anaesth* 1977; 49:259–264.

Bullingham RES, McQuay HJ, Dwyer D, Allen MC, Moore RA. Sublingual buprenorphine used postoperatively: clinical observations and preliminary pharmacokinetic analysis. *Br J Clin Pharmacol* 1981; 12:117–122.

Burns JW, Hodsman NBA, McLintock TTC, et al. The influence of patient characteristics on the requirements for postoperative analgesia: a reassessment using patient-controlled analgesia. *Anesthesia* 1989; 44:2–6.

Chiari A, Tobin JR, Pan H-L, Hood DD, Eisenach JC. Sex differences in cholinergic analgesia: a supplemental nicotinic mechanism in normal females. *Anesthesiology* 1999; 91;1447–1454.

Cicero TJ, Nock B, Meyer ER. Gender-related differences in the antinociceptive properties of morphine. *J Pharmacol Exp Ther* 1996; 279:767–773.

Cicero TJ, Nock B, Meyer ER. Sex-related differences in morphine antinociceptive activity: relationship to serum and brain morphine concentrations. *J Pharmacol Exp Ther* 1997; 282:939–994.

Dahlström B, Tamsen A, Paalzow L, Hartvig P. Patient-controlled analgesic therapy, Part IV: pharmacokinetics and analgesic plasma concentrations of morphine. *Clin Pharmacokinet* 1982; 7:266–279.

Dalrymple DG, Parbrook GD. Personality assessment and postoperative analgesia. A study in male patients undergoing elective gastric surgery. *Br J Anaesth* 1976; 48:593–597.

Dalrymple DG, Parbrook GD, Steel DF. The effect of personality in postoperative pain and vital capacity impairment. *Br J Anaesth* 1972; 44:902.

Dalrymple DG, Parbrook GD, Steel DF. Factors predisposing to postoperative pain and pulmonary complications: a study of female patients undergoing elective cholecystectomy. *Br J Anaesth* 1973; 45:589–598.

Dawson-Basoa ME, Gintzler AR. Estrogen and progesterone activate spinal kappa-opiate receptor analgesic mechanisms. *Pain* 1996; 64:607–615.

De Kock M, Scholtes JL. Postoperative PCA in abdominal surgery. Analysis of 200 consecutive patients. *Acta Anaesthesiol Belg* 1991; 42:85–91.

Egan KJ, Ready LB. Patient satisfaction with intravenous PCA or epidural morphine. *Can J Anaesth* 1994; 41:6–11.

Ehrnebo M, Boreus LO, Lonroth U. Bioavailability and first-pass metabolism of oral pentazocine in man. *Clin Pharmacol Ther* 1977; 22:888–892.

Eisenach JC, Hood DD, Curry R. Phase I human safety assessment of intrathecal neostigmine containing methyl- and propyl-parabens. *Anesth Analg* 1997; 85;842–846.

Gear RW, Gordon NC, Heller PH, et al. Gender difference in analgesic response to the kappa-opioid pentazocine. *Neurosci Lett* 1996a; 205:207–209.

Gear RW, Miaskowski C, Gordon NC, et al. Kappa-opioids produce significantly greater analgesia in women than in men. *Nat Med* 1996b; 2:1248–1250.

Gear RW, Miaskowski C, Gordon, et al. The kappa-opioid nalbuphine produces gender and dose dependent analgesia and antianalgesia in patients with postoperative pain. *Pain* 1999; 83(2):339–345.

Gordon NC, Gear RW, Heller PH, et al. Enhancement of morphine analgesia by the GABA-B agonist baclofen. *Neuroscience* 1995; 69:345–349.

Gourlay GK, Kowalski SR, Plummer JL, Cousins MJ, Armstrong PJ. Fentanyl blood concentration—analgesic response relationship in the treatment of postoperative pain. *Anesth Analg* 1988; 67:329–337.

Hood DD, Eisenach JC, Tuttle R. Phase I safety assessment of intrathecal neostigmine in humans. *Anesthesiology* 1995; 82:331–343.

Hood DD, Mallak KA, Eisenach JC, Tong CY. Interaction between intrathecal neostigmine and epidural clonidine in human volunteers. *Anesthesiology* 1996; 85:315–325.

Hood DD, Mallak KA, James RC, Tuttle R, Eisenach JC. Enhancement of analgesia from systemic opioid in humans by cholinesterase inhibition. *J Pharmacol Exp Th*er 1997; 282:86–92.

Islam A, Cooper M, Bodnar R. Interactions among aging, gender, and gonadectomy effects upon morphine antinociception in rats. *Physiol Behav* 1993; 54:45–53.

Jaillon P, Gardin ME, Lecocq B, et al. Pharmacokinetics of nalbuphine in infants, young health volunteers, and elderly patients. *Clin Pharmacol Ther* 1989; 46:226–233.

Kavaliers M, Choleris E. Sex differences in N-methyl-D-aspartate involvement in κ-opioid and non-opioid predator-induced analgesia in mice. *Brain Res* 1997; 768:30–36.

Kando JC, Yonkers KA, Cole JO. Gender as a risk factor for adverse events to medications. *Drugs* 1995; 50:1–6.

Kepler KL, Kest B, Kiefel JM, Cooper ML, Bodnar RJ. Roles of gender, gonadectomy and estrous phase in the analgesic effects of intracerebroventricular morphine in rats. *Pharmacol Biochem Behav* 1989; 34:119–127.

Kepler KL, Standifer KM, Paul D, et al. Gender effects and central opioid analgesia. *Pain* 1991; 45:87–94.

Klamt JC, Dos Reis MP, Neto JB, Prado WA. Analgesic effect of subarachnoid neostigmine in two patients with cancer pain. *Pain* 1996; 66:389–391.

Krukowski JA, Hood DD, Eisenach JC, Mallak KA, Parker RL. Intrathecal neostigmine for post-cesarean section analgesia: dose response. *Anesth Analg* 1997; 84:1269–1275.

Lauretti GR, Dos Reis MP, Prado WA, Klamt JC. Dose-response study of intrathecal morphine versus intrathecal neostigmine, their combination, or placebo for postoperative analgesia in patients undergoing anterior and posterior vaginoplasty. *Anesth Analg* 1996; 82:1182–1187.

Lavand'homme PM, Eisenach JC. Sex differences in cholinergic analgesia. II. Differing mechanisms in two models of allodynia. *Anesthesiology* 1999; 91:1455–1461.

Lehmann KA, Tenbuhs B. Patient-controlled analgesia with nalbuphine, a new narcotic agonist-antagonist, for the treatment of postoperative pain. *Eur J Clin Pharmacol* 1986; 31:267–276.

Levy RA, Proudfit HK. Analgesia produced by microinjection of baclofen and morphine at brain stem sites. *Eur J Pharmacol* 1979; 57:43–55.

Liu SS, Allen HW, Olsson GI. Patient-controlled epidural analgesia with bupivacaine and fentanyl on hospital wards: prospective experience in 1,030 surgical patients. *Anesthesiology* 1998; 88:688–695.

McQuay HJ, Bullingham RES, Paterson GMC, Moore RA. Clinical effects of buprenorphine during and after operation. *Br J Anaesth* 1980; 52:1013–1019.

Merkatz RB, Temple R, Subel S, Feiden K, Kessler DA. Women in clinical trials of new drugs. A change in Food and Drug Administration policy. The Working Group of Women in Clinical Trials. *N Engl J Med* 1993; 329:292–296.

Miaskowski C, Levine JD. Does opioid analgesia show a gender preference for females? *Pain Forum* 1999; 8(1):34–44.

Pan PM, Huang CT, Wei TT, Mok MS. Enhancement of analgesic effect of intrathecal neostigmine and clonidine on bupivacaine spinal anesthesia. *Reg Anesth Pain Med* 1998; 23:49–56.

Pande AC, Pyke RE, Greiner M, et al. Analgesic efficacy of the kappa-receptor agonist, enadoline, in dental surgery pain. *Clin Neuropharmacol* 1996a; 19:92–97.

Pande AC, Pyke RE, Greiner M, et al. Analgesic efficacy of enadoline versus placebo or morphine in postsurgical pain. *Clin Neuropharmacol* 1996b; 19:451–456.

Parbrook GD, Dalrymple DG, Steel DF. Personality assessment and postoperative pain and complications. *J Psychosom Res* 1973a; 17:277–285.

Parbrook GD, Steel DF, Dalrymple DG. Factors predisposing to postoperative pain and pulmonary complications. A study of male patients undergoing elective gastric surgery. *Br J Anaesth* 1973b; 45:21–33.

Peck CL. Psychological factors in acute pain management. In: Cousins MJ, Phillips GD (Eds). *Acute Pain Management*. New York: Churchill Livingstone, 1986, pp 251–274.

Petros JG, Rimm EB, Robillard RJ. Factors influencing urinary tract retention after elective cholecystectomy. *Surg Gynecol Obstet* 1992; 174:497–500.

Reisine T, Pasternak G. Opioid analgesics and antagonists. In: Hardman JG, Limbird LE (Eds). *Goodman and Gilman's The Pharmacologic Basis of Therapeutics*. New York: McGraw-Hill, 1996, pp 521–555.

Shyu WC, Morgenthien EA, Pittman KA, Barbhaiya RH. The effects of age and sex on the systemic availability and pharmacokinetics of transnasal butorphanol. *Eur J Clin Pharmacol* 1994; 47:57–60.

Sidebotham D, Dijkhuizen MRJ, Schug SA. The safety and utilization of patient controlled analgesia. *J Pain Symptom Manage* 1997; 14:202–209.

Tamsen A, Bondesson U, Dahlström B, Hartvig P. Patient-controlled analgesic therapy, Part III: Pharmacokinetics and analgesic plasma concentrations of ketobemidone. *Clin Pharmacokinet* 1982a; 7:151–165.

Tamsen A, Hartvig P, Fagerlund C, Dahlström B. Patient-controlled analgesic therapy, Part I: Pharmacokinetics of pethidine in the pre- and postoperative periods. *Clin Pharmacokinet* 1982b; 7:149–163.

Taylor NM, Hall GM, Salmon P. Patients' experiences of patient-controlled analgesia. *Anaesthesia* 1996; 51:525–528.

Tsui SL, Tong WN, Irwin M, et al. The efficacy, applicability and side effects of postoperative intravenous patient-controlled morphine analgesia: an audit of 1233 Chinese patients. *Anaesth Intens Care* 1996; 24:658–664.

Tsui SL, Irwin MG, Wong CM, et al. An audit of the safety of an acute pain service. *Anaesthesia* 1997; 52:1042–1047.

Walker JS. NSAIDs: an update on their analgesic effects. *Clin Exp Physiol Pharmacol* 1995; 22:855–860.

Walker JS, Carmody JJ. Experimental pain in healthy human subjects: gender differences in nociception and in response to ibuprofen. *Anesth Analg* 1998; 86:1257–1262.

Watson PJQ, McQuay HJ, Bullingham RES, Allen MC, Moore RA. Single-dose comparison of buprenorphine 0.3 and 0.6 mg I.V. given after operation: clinical effects and plasma concentrations. *Br J Anaesth* 1982; 54:37–43.

Wilson PR, Yaksh TL. Baclofen is antinociceptive in the spinal intrathecal space of animals. *Eur J Pharmacol* 1978; 51:323–330.

Wilson SJ, Errick JK, Balkon J. Pharmacokinetics of nalbuphine during parturition. *Am J Obstet Gynecol* 1986; 155:340–344.

Yaksh TL, Reddy SV. Studies in the primate on the analgetic effects associated with intrathecal actions of opiates, alpha-adrenergic agonists and baclofen. *Anesthesiology* 1981; 54:451–467.

Zieglgansberger W. Dorsal horn neuropharmacology: baclofen and morphine. *Ann NY Acad Sci* 1988; 31:150–156.

Correspondence to: Christine Miaskowski, RN, PhD, FAAN, Department of Physiological Nursing, University of California, San Francisco, CA 94143-0610, USA. Fax: 415-476-8899; email: chris.miaskowski@nursing.ucsf.edu.

Part III

Sex-Related Factors in Clinical Pain Conditions

Sex, Gender, and Pain, Progress in Pain Research and Management, Vol. 17, edited by R.B. Fillingim, IASP Press, Seattle, © 2000.

12

Epidemiologic Perspectives on Sex Differences in Pain

Linda LeResche

Department of Oral Medicine, University of Washington, Seattle, Washington, USA

EPIDEMIOLOGY

What percentage of adults in the United States have experienced chronic pain in the past year? What are the rates at which men and women in their twenties develop back pain? Do migraine episodes last longer in women or in men? Does hormone replacement therapy increase a woman's risk of developing musculoskeletal pain? Are women or men more likely to become disabled from pain? These are the kinds of questions that epidemiologic research can answer. Epidemiology is defined as "the study of the distribution, determinants and natural history of disease in populations" (Lilienfeld and Lilienfeld 1980). Epidemiologists have traditionally focused their research on well-defined diseases such as cancer and heart disease. However, epidemiologic methods are being increasingly employed to study pain and other symptomatic conditions (Gordis 1988), and a wealth of information is being accumulated on the epidemiology of pain. This chapter provides a broad overview of issues related to gender and pain from an epidemiologic perspective. Readers interested in more information on the epidemiology of specific pain conditions are referred to the recently published International Association for the Study of Pain (IASP) task force book entitled *Epidemiology of Pain* (Crombie et al. 1999), which presents systematic reviews of the available epidemiologic data on a range of chronic pain conditions.

In studying the distribution and determinants of diseases and disorders, it is standard practice for epidemiologists to calculate rates of diseases or symptoms by age and gender, and to investigate gender as a risk factor for developing the conditions of interest. Thus, it is possible to glean a great deal of information about gender and pain in populations from existing epidemiologic studies, even if these studies were originally designed to investigate other questions (e.g., the relationship of pain to social class). An understanding of the patterns of pain in the population by gender and age can provide important clues about factors that may contribute to the etiology and persistence of pain. For example, a pain condition that shows a female predominance throughout the lifespan (i.e., in childhood and old age as well as during the reproductive years) is more likely to be related to structural differences between the sexes or to gender roles than to the influence of hormonal factors that vary over time. Later in this chapter, I will review patterns of pain by age and gender, and suggest some hypotheses about factors that may be influencing these patterns.

As we have discussed previously (Dworkin et al. 1992), three perspectives distinguish the epidemiologic approach to understanding pain—the population perspective, the developmental perspective, and the ecological perspective. Because not everyone who develops a pain problem seeks treatment, the study of patients in treatment settings can provide only a limited picture of the distribution and determinants of pain. The population perspective suggests that to understand the full spectrum of pain problems, these conditions must be studied in the general populations, not only in persons seeking treatment. The population perspective is especially important for understanding gender differences in pain, because women are more likely than men to seek health care for many conditions, including many pain problems (Unruh 1996). In addition, there may be gender-specific preferences in the type of practitioner visited and the kinds of treatment sought. Thus, studies in a specific treatment setting could lead to a false impression of the degree to which a given pain problem affects each gender. For example, in secondary and tertiary care centers where temporomandibular disorder (TMD) pain is treated, the ratio of female patients to male patients ranges from about 5:1 to 9:1 (Bush et al. 1993), whereas in the community the female to male prevalence ratio is only about 2:1 (LeResche 1997).

The developmental perspective suggests that studying pain across the life cycle is essential, because factors that influence the risk of having a specific pain condition may vary with age. To ask whether there are gender differences in the prevalence of a given pain condition may be too simplistic, since, at least for some pain conditions, gender-specific prevalence may vary significantly with age (e.g., the probability of experiencing migraine headache may be similar for boys and girls at age 12, whereas a 30-year-old woman is much more likely than a 30-year-old man to have this kind of pain).

Finally, epidemiologists view the development and maintenance of any disorder in an ecological perspective—that is, disease agents, characteristics of the host, and characteristics of the environment are all considered important in whether and how a condition manifests itself in a given person. This perspective is similar to the biopsychosocial perspective on pain (Engel 1960), which suggests that biological, psychological, and social factors interact in pain experience. As described elsewhere in this volume, men and women differ, at least to some extent, in the biological and psychological substrates underlying pain. In addition, girls and boys undergo different socialization processes, and men and women are exposed to different risk factors for pain due to their differing occupational and social roles. When gender differences in pain are identified, the ecological perspective is heuristic for interpreting these differences and providing hypotheses for further study (e.g., concerning specific host and environmental factors for each gender that might be associated with pain).

EPIDEMIOLOGIC MEASURES

The basic measures epidemiologists use to describe the distribution, determinants and natural history of disease in populations include prevalence, incidence, duration, and risk. These measures are discussed below.

Prevalence is defined as the proportion of persons in the population with a disease or condition at a particular time. To calculate a prevalence rate, we must know both the number of persons with the condition (the numerator of the prevalence rate) and the total population at risk of having the condition (the denominator). If the enumeration is done at a single point in time (or approximates this kind of measure), the prevalence rate is called a *point prevalence* rate. Other commonly reported kinds of prevalence rates include *period prevalence* (e.g., number of cases in the population over a 3- or 6-month period) or *lifetime prevalence* (number of persons who experience the condition at some time over the course of their life). Period prevalence is probably the most appropriate type of prevalence measure for chronic pain conditions, since it is better able to capture significant pain problems that may be frequent or persistent, but may not be present at the exact time of the survey.

Incidence is defined as the rate of onset of the condition over a defined time period (usually 1 year). To calculate an incidence rate, we must know the number of new cases appearing in a population over the time period (the numerator of the incidence rate) as well as the number of persons at risk of developing the condition (the denominator). It is important to remember that persons at risk include all those capable of developing the condition (e.g., females in the case of uterine cancer) who do not already have the condition, or who have no history of the condition.

Duration is simply the length of time the condition lasts. For episodic or recurrent conditions, like many pain conditions, the total duration can be computed by summing the durations of individual episodes. Prevalence, incidence, and duration are related such that:

$$\text{Prevalence} = \text{Incidence} \times \text{Mean Duration.}$$

For chronic or recurrent conditions (Von Korff and Parker 1980; Von Korff 1992):

$$\text{Lifetime Prevalence} = \text{Incidence} \times \text{Mean Episode Duration} \times \text{Mean No. Episodes.}$$

Risk is defined as the likelihood that persons who do not have a specific condition (but who have particular attributes, or are exposed to certain "risk factors") will develop the condition. Male or female sex (an attribute) can be thought of as a risk factor for developing specific kinds of pain. Some might even consider female gender as a risk factor for developing *any* kind of pain problem. However, in attempting to identify causes of pain that can be modified, as well as to develop our understanding of pain mechanisms, it may be more productive to think of sex or gender as a marker for a range of more specific risk factors (e.g., hormonal factors and occupational risks) that could have a more direct effect on pain.

In the remainder of this chapter, I will examine the available evidence related to gender as a risk factor for specific pain problems, review population-based epidemiologic data concerning age- and gender-specific prevalence rates for common chronic pain conditions, and discuss possible reasons for observed gender differences in pain from the developmental and ecological perspectives.

IS FEMALE GENDER A RISK FACTOR FOR PAIN?

Many recent reviews of gender and pain (Fillingim and Maixner 1995; Unruh 1996; Berkley 1997) have noted that the prevalence of most pain conditions appears to be higher in women than in men. If this is the case, two questions arise: (1) What is the magnitude of the observed differences; and (2) Do they indicate a higher risk for developing pain related specifically to female sex (a biological host characteristic), or to some other risk factor (e.g., occupational exposures, lower rates of exercise) that might be related to female gender? Data from epidemiologic studies can shed light on the first question—the magnitude of sex differences in prevalence for the most common pain conditions. To answer the second question—whether being female is, per se, a risk factor for pain—we must use measures such as odds ratios that assess the influence of female sex as a risk factor for pain, controlled for other potential risk factors. Unfortunately, few epidemiologic studies have analyzed data in this way. Thus, while we can systematically review the magnitude of the prevalence differences of specific pain conditions in the two sexes, it is not possible at this time to assess the degree to which these differences are attributable to female sex, or the degree to which they are attributable to different rates of exposure to other risk factors in men and women.

Table I summarizes data from epidemiologic studies of the general population for a range of common pain conditions. The prevalence rate for the pain condition in females compared to the prevalence rate in males in the same population is shown as a ratio. A number greater than 1 indicates a higher rate in women than in men (e.g., a ratio of 1.2 indicates that the rate is 20% higher in women than in men). As Table I shows, the median prevalence

Table I
Gender prevalence ratios for various pain conditions: studies of the adult general population

Pain Site/Condition	No. Studies	F:M Prevalence Ratio		References
		Range	Median	
Headache (general)	15	1.1–3.1	1.3	Scher et al. 1999, Table II
Migraine	14	1.6–4.0	2.5	Scher et al. 1999, Table I
Temporomandibular (TMD) pain	10	1.2–2.6	1.5	Drangsholt and LeResche 1999, Table III
Burning mouth pain	2	1.3–2.5	1.9	Lipton et al. 1993; Tammiala-Salonen et al. 1993
Neck pain	5	1.0–3.3	1.4	Ariëns et al. 1999, Table I
Shoulder pain	5	1.0–2.2	1.3	van der Windt and Croft 1999, Table II
Back pain	4	0.9–1.3	1.2	Von Korff et al. 1988; Walsh et al. 1992; Croft and Rigby 1994; Wright et al. 1995
Knee pain	4	1.0–1.9	1.6	McCarney and Croft 1999, Table I
Abdominal pain	4	1.2–1.3	1.25	Von Korff et al. 1988; Agréus et al. 1994; Kay et al. 1994; Adelman et al. 1995
Fibromyalgia	4	2.0–6.8 (+ all cases female in 1 study)	4.3	Jacobsson et al. 1989; Mäkelä and Heliövaara 1991; Prescott et al. 1993; Wolfe et al. 1995

ratios indicate a female predominance for all the pain conditions examined. However, it is also important to note that some studies of neck, shoulder, back, and knee pain indicated equal prevalence among the two sexes, or even, in one case, a higher rate in males than in females (i.e., a ratio of 0.9 for one study of back pain). Prevalence ratios on the order of 2.0 or greater, which were found in some studies of all the pain conditions except back pain and abdominal pain, may indicate substantial differences in risk that warrant further focused investigation.

POSSIBLE SOURCES OF GENDER DIFFERENCES IN PAIN

What is it about being female that might lead to increased rates of pain onset, a greater number of pain episodes, or longer pain duration, and consequently, higher pain prevalence? Because pain is a multidimensional experience, if we see gender differences in the prevalence of chronic pain, differences could be occurring at several levels. Perhaps there are anatomical or physiological differences between men and women in the nociceptive systems that transmit or modulate pain signals (Gear et al. 1996; Berkley 1997). Women may be more perceptually sensitive than men and thus more readily able to detect physiological signals (Fillingim and Maixner 1995). Men and women may also differ in their cognitive and emotional experiences of pain, and in their approaches to coping with pain, i.e., pain appraisal (Unruh 1996), such that women are more likely to assess a pain sensation as important and worthy of attention. The genders may differ in their pain behaviors, including pain report. The issue of willingness to report pain and how the differential socialization of males and females can influence pain report is especially important for epidemiologic studies, given that self-report is a primary source of data for the pain epidemiologist (LeResche 1995). Finally, the social and occupational roles of men and women differ, and those roles may present different risks for developing pain. Risk for maintaining a pain condition, once it has developed, may also be related to different roles for the two genders within the context of the family, the workplace, the welfare system, and the health care delivery system (e.g., Crook 1993). Most likely, differences operate simultaneously at a number of levels to influence the prevalence rates of pain in the two genders shown in Table I.

However, because Table I presents only overall prevalence ratios for women and men, it may provide a picture of gender and pain that is too simplistic. From a developmental perspective, it is clear that biological, psychological, and social factors may vary for both men and women at different points in the life cycle. Biological changes for both sexes include growth, puberty, and senescence. In addition, females undergo specific hormonally related changes including menarche, menopause, and possibly pregnancy and childbearing. Social role changes that can occur across the life cycle include marriage, divorce, parenthood, education, employment, retirement, and widowhood. These changes in social role are frequently accompanied by psychological changes. All these biological, psychological, and social changes may be experienced differently by the two genders, and consequently may contribute to differences in the pain experience and pain behavior of males and females. For example, both boys and girls undergo puberty, but in females puberty marks the beginning of monthly menstrual cycles that provide women with a set of physiological signals from their bodies that are not experienced by men. As Berkley (1997) has suggested, these sometimes painful physiological signals could have a sensitizing effect on pain perception or result in behavioral and social role responses (e.g., taking medication, staying in bed) that can generalize to other types of pain. Because of the dramatic changes over the life cycle that have the potential to interact with gender to influence pain, it seems important to take a closer look at the epidemiology of pain conditions not only by gender, but also by age.

PATTERNS OF PAIN PREVALENCE BY AGE AND GENDER

Because little information is available concerning rates of pain onset (incidence) or the duration of pain episodes by age and gender, this review of epidemiologic data on pain must focus on the *prevalence* of pain by age and gender. In thinking about the prevalence data to be presented here, it is important to remember that for chronic and recurrent pain conditions, prevalence is a product of the incidence or onset rate, the number of episode recurrences, and the average episode duration. Thus, if we see a higher prevalence rate of a specific pain condition in one sex, that difference may be due to a higher onset rate, a higher probability of recurrence, a longer episode duration, or some combination of these components.

In keeping with the epidemiologic perspectives mentioned earlier, studies were selected for review in this section only if they were truly population-based. Investigations of particular occupational groups or clinic attendees are not included. A more comprehensive review encompassing clinical studies as well as population-based research has been provided by Unruh (1996). The data presented here are also limited to adults. Although similar analysis of the age- and sex-specific prevalence of pain conditions in children could provide important insights into gender differences across the entire lifespan, such a review is beyond the scope of this chapter. See McGrath (1999) for a systematic review of the epidemiology of pain conditions in children and adolescents.

The goal of this section is to try to discern the *patterns* of pain prevalence for men and women across the adult life cycle. Because different authors have studied different populations, have used different case definitions and different sampling approaches, and have created age groupings for their study populations somewhat differently, the absolute prevalence rates found across studies are likely to differ. However, if several population-based studies, despite their methodological differences, find a consistent *pattern* of prevalence for a specific pain condition by gender and age, the prevalence pattern may provide clues about factors that increase the risk of developing that pain problem.

CHRONIC PAIN

People who are interested in gender and pain frequently want to know the overall prevalence of chronic pain in men and women. I know of no studies that have specifically set out to answer this question. Most studies of chronic pain have focused on particular pain complaints. However, a few population-based surveys have assessed more than one chronic pain condition. One such study was conducted among 1016 enrollees of a health maintenance organization (HMO) in Seattle (Von Korff et al. 1988). Using similar measures for all pain problems, the investigators inquired into the presence of back pain, headache, abdominal pain, chest pain, and temporomandibular pain. Respondents were asked to report pains occurring in the last 6 months that had lasted at least a day and were not fleeting or minor. Fig. 1 shows the percentage of persons in each age/sex group who reported experiencing at least one of the five pain conditions investigated. The prevalence of pain was higher in women than in men at all ages. However, the discrepancy between men and women diminished with age.

Persons with multiple pain conditions have more significant levels of psychological disturbance than persons with a single chronic pain condition (e.g., Dworkin et al. 1990). Fig. 2 shows the percentage of persons in each age/sex group in the Seattle survey who had three or more of the five pain conditions assessed. Although the prevalence of three or more pain conditions did not exceed 13% for any group, the prevalence of three or more pain problems was significantly higher in women than in men in all age groups except those 65 years of age and older. Taken together, the data in Figs. 1 and 2 appear to indicate that, at least up until age 65, women are

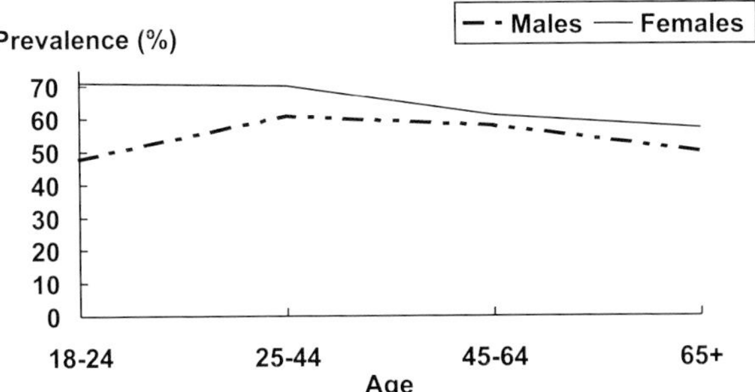

Fig. 1. Age- and sex-specific prevalence of one or more of the five pain conditions studied (back pain, headache, chest pain, abdominal pain, and temporomandibular pain). Data are from a sample of 1016 adult enrollees of a Seattle health maintenance organization (HMO) (Von Korff et al. 1988).

more likely to experience pain than men, and in particular, that women are more likely to experience multiple pains. Of course, several factors could affect these data, including a differential willingness of the two genders to report pain. I will discuss these factors at the conclusion of this chapter.

SPECIFIC PAIN CONDITIONS

Back pain. Back pain is one of the most common pain conditions in the general population, affecting 58–84% of all adults at some point in their lifetime (Dionne 1999). However, the pattern of back pain prevalence by age and gender is not consistent from study to study. For example, in the HMO sample described above (Von Korff et al. 1988), back pain prevalence was substantially higher among women than among men at younger ages,

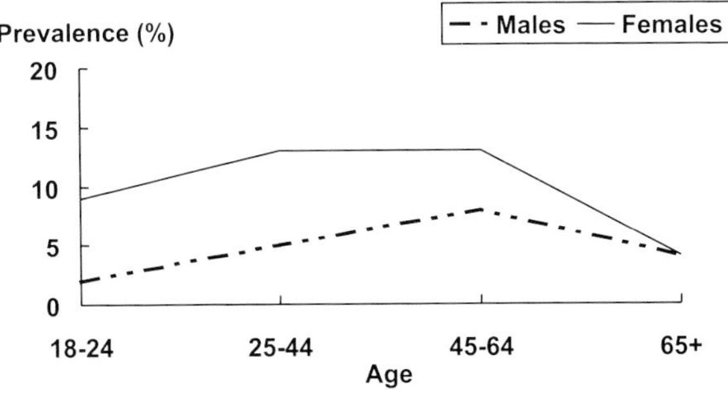

Fig. 2. Age- and sex-specific prevalence of the presence of three or more of the five pain conditions studied (see Fig. 1 for details) (Von Korff et al. 1988).

but prevalence increased steadily with age in men. For persons aged 45–64, the prevalence rate for men exceeded that of women, whereas rates for both sexes were similar after age 65.

In contrast, a study of 2667 persons aged 20–60 from small towns and rural areas in Great Britain (Walsh et al. 1992) found back pain prevalence rates to be higher in young men in their twenties than in women of comparable age (35% vs. 27%). Rates increased only very slightly for men with age, but fluctuated with age for women.

Two other studies in Great Britain were consistent in finding higher back pain prevalence rates in women than in men at all ages. Both studies also found that prevalence discrepancies between the sexes were greatest among those over 65 years of age. One of these studies inquired into "problems with a bad back" in a household sample of about 9000 people throughout Great Britain, and found increasing prevalence rates with age for both sexes up to age 64 (Croft and Rigby 1994). The other study (Wright et al. 1995) surveyed over 34,000 persons in the northwest of England, asking about the presence of "sciatica, lumbago or recurring backache" in the past year. In men, prevalence rates rose from ages 18–39 to ages 40–64 and dropped slightly over age 65. For women, rates also increased from ages 18–39 to ages 40–64, but held steady thereafter.

A few epidemiologic studies of back pain have focused exclusively on the elderly (Lavsky-Shulan et al. 1985; Bergström et al. 1986; Woo et al. 1994). These studies have consistently found higher rates of back pain among women than among men; however, the reported age-specific prevalence patterns differed from study to study. One study (Lavsky-Shulan et al. 1985) showed a decline in prevalence with age, the second (Woo et al. 1994) showed a rising prevalence of back pain with age for men, but not for women, and the third (Bergström et al. 1986) showed a rise, then a decline in prevalence with age in women aged 70–79. Thus, it appears that the data for back pain—the most prevalent and one of the most disabling pain conditions—present no clear, consistent pattern across the studies reviewed. Urban-rural differences as well as socioeconomic, occupational, and cohort differences may be so powerful for back pain that specific influences of age and gender on prevalence are difficult to discern (Walsh et al. 1992; Croft and Rigby 1994).

Joint pain. As might be expected, joint pain shows an increase in prevalence across the adult lifespan in both men and women. The age- and gender-specific prevalence patterns for joint pain differ somewhat, depending on the joint involved. However, one large epidemiologic study in the north of England (Lawrence et al. 1966) found, for both knee pain and finger joint pain, that prevalence rates were similar in young men and young women, but that at older ages, the curves for women and men diverged, with higher prevalence in women than in men.

Abdominal pain. Three population-based studies of gastrointestinal abdominal pain (Agréus et al. 1994; Kay et al. 1994; Adelman et al. 1995) consistently found the prevalence of abdominal pain to decline steadily with age after about age 40. This pattern of declining prevalence was consistent for both sexes. All studies also found rates of abdominal pain to be somewhat higher in women than in men at all ages. These patterns were consistent whether the subjects were residents of an urban county (Copenhagen County, Denmark; Kay et al. 1994), persons living in rural areas and small towns in Sweden (Agréus et al. 1994), or members of an HMO in Howard County, Maryland, near Washington, D.C. (Adelman et al. 1995). In one study that assessed pain in different regions of the abdomen, the same age- and sex-specific prevalence pattern (i.e., higher rates in women, declining with age in both sexes) was found whether pain was located in the upper, mid-, or lower abdomen (Agréus et al. 1994). All these studies focused on gastrointestinal pain and excluded menstrual pain. It is, however, possible that some abdominal pain in women is referred pain of gynecological origin (Giamberardino et al. 1997; see Chapter 8, this volume). Whatever the reason for the observed pattern, the available data on the prevalence of abdominal pain by age and sex appear highly consistent, and show a higher prevalence for women than for men across the adult lifespan, with prevalence rates declining with age for both sexes.

Headache and migraine. Another very common complaint that occurs at somewhat higher rates in women than in men, and appears to decline in prevalence with age, is headache. Scores of studies have investigated the epidemiology of headache; a meta-analysis of these studies is presented in Chapter 13 of the IASP task force book on pain epidemiology (Scher et al. 1999). Fig. 3 of that chapter presents a computed age- by sex-specific prevalence curve, based on 29 epidemiologic studies of headache conducted in North America. The shape of the curve suggests an almost unchanging prevalence rate across the adult life cycle for men, with about 60% of males experiencing headache at any given age. The curve for women is relatively flat, with prevalence rates of approximately 75–80%, until about age 45, when rates begin to decline. By about age 60, prevalence rates for men and women appear similar. It is important to note that the studies summarized in this meta-analysis used a number of different definitions of headache; the meta-analysis showed that, particularly for men, case definition explained a great deal of the variability in prevalence rates. Depending on the case definition used, prevalence curves for specific types of nonmigraine headaches (e.g., tension-type headache; Rasmussen et al. 1991) could show a somewhat different pattern than that described for headache in general by Scher and colleagues.

Many epidemiologic studies have focused specifically on migraine headache, and most of these have used fairly similar case definitions. These studies, conducted in a variety of cultures, have consistently replicated the finding of a clear bell-shaped curve for age-specific prevalence in both sexes, with rates rising over the reproductive years and declining after age 40. Rates for women are substantially higher than for men at all adult ages (see Stewart et al. 1994 and Scher et al. 1999 for reviews.)

Temporomandibular disorder pain. Another set of pain conditions that follows the same age-by sex-specific prevalence pattern as migraine is temporomandibular disorder pain, i.e., pain in the muscles of mastication or the temporomandibular joint. Data from three studies conducted in North America (Locker and Slade 1988; Von Korff et al. 1988; Goulet et al. 1995) indicate a peak prevalence for both sexes at 40–50 years of age (age groupings in the studies vary), and a steep decline thereafter. Again, prevalence is higher in women than in men across the entire adult lifespan.

Chronic widespread pain and fibromyalgia. Although chronic widespread pain and fibromyalgia are less prevalent than most of the pain conditions reviewed above, their epidemiology is of interest because of the observation that the vast majority of patients presenting for treatment of fibromyalgia are women (see Chapter 14). Chronic widespread pain is defined by the standardized criteria of the American College of Rheumatology (ACR) (Wolfe et al. 1990) as pain of longer than 3 months' duration in two contralateral quadrants of the body. Two population-based studies have examined the prevalence of chronic widespread pain based on these criteria. The first (Croft et al. 1993) surveyed a sample of persons enrolled in two general practices in Cheshire, England, in an area that included both a suburb of Manchester and a rural town. Prevalence data were based on 1340 survey respondents. For men, rates of chronic widespread pain rose until about age 65, dropped in those 65–74 years of age, and then rose again in the very elderly. For women, the shape of the curve was similar, although the first prevalence peak appeared at a younger age for women than for men. For all the ages surveyed, except ages 55–64, prevalence rates were substantially higher for women than for men.

The second study was a community survey of 3006 persons from randomly selected households in Wichita, Kansas (Wolfe et al. 1995). In this study, prevalence rates were consistently higher for women than for men, and rose across the adult lifespan through age 69, but dropped off in the very elderly. Thus, the two studies were similar in finding higher rates in women than in men. Both studies also found low rates in young adulthood and steeply rising prevalence in middle age, especially for women. However, the pattern found for the elderly differs in the two studies, perhaps because of relatively small sample sizes in the oldest age groups.

In addition to studying chronic widespread pain, Wolfe et al. (1995) conducted examinations on a sample of respondents to assess how many of them met ACR examination criteria for fibromyalgia (i.e., pain on palpation in at least 11 of 18 designated body sites, as well as chronic widespread pain). The age- and sex-specific prevalence pattern for fibromyalgia was very similar to that found for chronic widespread pain in the same study. However, the absolute prevalence rates were lower for fibromyalgia, and the gender difference was more dramatic for fibromyalgia than for chronic widespread pain.

SUMMARY AND CONCLUSIONS

The data presented in this chapter suggest that the relationship between gender and the occurrence of pain is far from simple. Although women are more likely than men to experience one or more chronic pain conditions, and in particular, to experience multiple pain problems, prevalence patterns differ from condition to condition, and gender-specific prevalence for most conditions varies across the life cycle. Although women are more likely than men to report pain at most body sites, this is not the case for every pain condition at every stage of life. For back pain, gender differences in prevalence are small, and the available data are not consistent with regard to prevalence by gender and age. Definitive information on chest pain is also lacking, not because of inconsistent results, but because few epidemiologic studies have focused specifically on chest pain (as opposed to heart disease).

For other pain conditions, however, the age- and sex-specific prevalence patterns are more clear. Joint pain, chronic widespread pain, and fibromyalgia all appear to *increase* in prevalence with age in both genders at least up until approximately age 65, and all show higher prevalence in women than in men. A recent review by van der Windt and Croft (1999) indicates that shoulder pain also shows this pattern. The pattern of increasing pain prevalence with age could result from an increased susceptibility to pain as body structures age, or from progressive, degenerative conditions (which are known to be relevant in at least some cases), or possibly from the accrual of cases in the population with age. To ascertain the relative importance of these factors would require studies of pain incidence, in addition to pain prevalence. Since at least some data suggest a possible decline in joint pain and fibromyalgia among the very elderly (Bergström et al. 1986; Wolfe et al. 1995), research is needed on whether persons with these conditions recover over time, or are at increased risk for disability or even mortality, which removes them from community populations as they age.

While abdominal pain also consistently shows somewhat higher prevalence in women than in men, prevalence *decreases* with age for this condition. The prevalence of headache (other than migraine) also appears to decrease somewhat with age, at least in women. It is intriguing to consider what biological, psychological, or social changes associated with aging might actually be *protective* against the onset or continuation of these conditions. Likely candidates for investigation might be life stress, diet, or work-related factors.

Finally, migraine headache and painful temporomandibular disorders are substantially more common in women than in men, and prevalence follows a bell-shaped curve, with peak prevalence in the reproductive years. This prevalence pattern suggests a possible relationship to factors that are present from young adulthood into middle age, but are less common in the elderly. Hormonal factors have long been postulated as risk factors for migraine (e.g., Somerville 1972; Stewart et al. 1991; see Chapter 13 of this volume). Recently, research has suggested that hormonal factors may also play a role in temporomandibular pain (LeResche et al. 1997; Dao et al. 1998; see Chapter 15 of this volume). Interestingly, both the excellent incidence data available for migraine and the more limited data available for temporomandibular pain suggest that both these pain problems are uncommon in children and that incidence rates rise sharply beginning at puberty. This trend strengthens the possibility that hormonal factors may play some role in the onset or maintenance of these pain conditions. Of course, it is likely that psychological as well as biological factors associated with life cycle changes also influence the onset and maintenance of these pain conditions (LeResche 1997). In any case, the prevalence pattern of these pain problems raises a number of hypotheses regarding possible risk factors that could be further investigated not only with epidemiologic methods, but also through basic and clinical research.

While the age- and sex-specific prevalence patterns suggest a number of specific hypotheses related to particular pain conditions, the fact that most common pain conditions show at least somewhat higher prevalence in women than in men also indicates that some generic gender factor or factors may pertain. These factors could include a greater perceptual sensitivity to stimuli in women such that signals that might not be noticed by men are detected by women, a cognitive difference between the sexes such that the threshold for labeling stimuli as painful is lower for women than for men, or a difference in the upbringing of men and women, which makes it more acceptable for women than for men to report the experience of pain. There is some empirical support for each of these hypothesized factors (Unruh 1996; Berkley 1997). However, further research is needed to identify the degree to which biological, psychological, and social factors contribute to the observed prevalence differences. Because nearly all the epidemiologic research on pain has been conducted in Western Europe and North America, studies using similar methods in cultures where the roles of men and women differ from those already studied could help clarify this issue.

In conclusion, a review of the epidemiologic literature indicates that definite gender and age differences exist in the prevalence of many chronic pain conditions. Very little information is available to clarify whether these prevalence differences are due to different incidence rates, different probabilities of recurrence, different duration of pain episodes, or some combination of these factors. However, I hope that this systematic examination of the existing epidemiologic data may help to generate hypotheses in our search for a better understanding of chronic pain in both sexes.

ACKNOWLEDGMENTS

During the preparation of this chapter the author was supported in part by Grants No. DE12470 and DE08773 from the National Institute of Dental and Craniofacial Research and the National Institutes of Health Office of Research on Women's Health.

REFERENCES

Adelman AM, Revicki DA, Magaziner J, Hebel R. Abdominal pain in an HMO. *Fam Med* 1995; 27:321–325.

Agréus L, Svardsudd K, Nyren O, Tibblin G. The epidemiology of abdominal symptoms: prevalence and demographic characteristics in a Swedish adult population. *Scand J Gastroenterol* 1994; 29:102–109.

Ariëns GAM, Borghouts JAJ, Koes BW. Neck pain. In: Crombie IK, Croft PR, Linton SJ, LeResche L, Von Korff M (Eds). *Epidemiology of Pain.* Seattle: IASP Press, 1999, pp 235–255.

Bergström G, Bjelle A, Sundh V, Svanborg A. Joint disorders at ages 70, 75 and 79 years—a cross-sectional comparison. *Br J Rheumatol* 1986; 25:333–341.

Berkley KJ. Sex differences in pain. *Behav Brain Sci* 1997; 20:371–380.

Bush FM, Harkins SW, Harrington WG, Price DD. Analysis of gender effects on pain perception and symptom presentation in temporomandibular pain. *Pain* 1993; 53:73–80.

Croft PR, Rigby AS. Socioeconomic influences on back problems in the community in Britain. *J Epidemiol Community Health* 1994; 48:166–170.

Croft P, Rigby AS, Boswell R, Schollum J, Silman A. The prevalence of chronic widespread pain in the general population. *J Rheumatol* 1993; 20:710–713.

Crombie IK, Croft PR, Linton SJ, LeResche L, Von Korff M (Eds). *Epidemiology of Pain.* Seattle: IASP Press, 1999.

Crook J. Comparative experiences of men and women who have sustained a work related musculoskeletal injury. *Abstracts: 7th World Congress on Pain.* Seattle: IASP Press, 1993, pp 293–294.

Dao TTT, Knight K, Ton-That V. Modulation of myofascial pain by the reproductive hormones: a preliminary report. *J Prosthet Dent* 1998; 79:663–670.

Dionne, CE. Low back pain. In: Crombie IK, Croft PR, Linton SJ, LeResche L, Von Korff M (Eds). *Epidemiology of Pain.* Seattle: IASP Press, 1999, pp 283–297.

Drangsholt M, LeResche L. Temporomandibular disorder pain. In: Crombie IK, Croft PR, Linton SJ, LeResche L, Von Korff M (Eds). *Epidemiology of Pain.* Seattle: IASP Press, 1999, pp 203–233.

Dworkin SF, Von Korff MR, LeResche L. Multiple pains and psychiatric disturbance: an epidemiologic investigation. *Arch Gen Psychiatry* 1990; 47:239–244.

Dworkin SF, Von Korff M, LeResche L. Epidemiologic studies of chronic pain: a dynamic-ecologic perspective. *Ann Behav Med* 1992; 14:3–11.

Engel G. A unified concept of health and disease. *Perspect Biol Med* 1960; 3:459–485.

Fillingim RB, Maixner W. Gender differences in the responses to noxious stimuli. *Pain Forum* 1995; 4:209–221.

Gear RW, Miaskowski C, Gordon NC, et al. Kappa-opioids produce significantly greater analgesia in women than in men. *Nat Med* 1996; 2:1248–1250.

Giamberardino MA, Berkley KJ, Iezzi S, de Bigontina P, Vecchiet L. Pain threshold variations in somatic wall tissues as a function of menstrual cycle, segmental site and tissue depth in non-dysmenorrheic women, dysmenorrheic women and men. *Pain* 1997; 71:187–197.

Gordis L. Challenges to epidemiology in the next decade. *Am J Epidemiol* 1988; 128:1–9.

Goulet J-P, Lavigne GJ, Lund J P. Jaw pain prevalence among French-speaking Canadians in Quebec and related symptoms of temporomandibular disorders. *J Dent Res* 1995; 74:1738–1744.

Jacobsson L, Lindegarde F, Manthorpe R. The commonest rheumatic complaints of over six weeks' duration in a twelve month period in a defined Swedish population. *Scan J Rheumatol* 1989; 18:353–360.

Kay L, Jorgensen T, Jensen KH. Epidemiology of abdominal symptoms in a random population: prevalence, incidence, and natural history. *Eur J Epidemiol* 1994; 10:559–566.

Lavsky-Shulan M, Wallace RB, Kohout FJ, et al. Prevalence and functional correlates of low back pain in the elderly. *J Am Geriatr Soc* 1985; 33:23–28.

Lawrence JS, Bremner JM, Bier F. Osteo-arthrosis: prevalence in the population and relationship between symptom and x-ray changes. *Ann Rheum Dis* 1966; 25:1–23.

LeResche L. Gender differences in pain: epidemiologic perspectives. *Pain Forum* 1995; 4:228–230.

LeResche L. Epidemiology of temporomandibular disorders: implications for the investigation of etiologic factors. *Crit Rev Oral Biol Med* 1997; 8:291–305.

LeResche L, Saunders K, Von Korff M, Barlow W, Dworkin SF. Use of exogenous hormones and risk of temporomandibular disorder pain. *Pain* 1997; 69:153–160.

Lilienfeld AM, Lilienfeld DE. *Foundations of Epidemiology,* 2nd ed. New York: Oxford University Press, 1980.

Lipton JA, Ship JA, Larach-Robinson D. Estimated prevalence and distribution of reported orofacial pain in the United States. *J Am Dent Assoc* 1993; 124:115–121.

Locker D, Slade G. Prevalence of symptoms associated with temporomandibular disorders in a Canadian population. *Community Dent Oral Epidemiol* 1988; 16:310–313.

Mäkelä M, Heliövaara M. Prevalence of primary fibromyalgia in the Finnish population. *BMJ* 1991; 303:216–219.

McCarney R, Croft PR. Knee pain. In: Crombie IK, Croft PR, Linton SJ, LeResche L, Von Korff M (Eds). *Epidemiology of Pain.* Seattle: IASP Press, 1999, pp 299–313.

McGrath PA. Chronic pain in children. In: Crombie IK, Croft PR, Linton SJ, LeResche L, Von Korff M (Eds). *Epidemiology of Pain*. Seattle: IASP Press, 1999, pp 81–101.

Morris JN. *Uses of Epidemiology*, 3rd ed. Edinburgh: Churchill Livingstone, 1975.

Prescott E, Kjoller M, Jacobson S, et al. Fibromyalgia in the adult Danish population. I: Prevalence study. *Scand J Rheumatol* 1993; 22:233–237.

Rasmussen BK, Jensen R, Schroll M, Olesen J. Epidemiology of headache in a general population—a prevalence study. *J Clin Epidemiol* 1991; 44:1147–1157.

Scher AI, Stewart WF, Lipton RB. Epidemiology of migraine and headache: a meta-analytic approach. In: Crombie IK, Croft PR, Linton SJ, LeResche L, Von Korff M (Eds). *Epidemiology of Pain*. Seattle: IASP Press, 1999, pp 159–170.

Somerville BW. The influence of progesterone and estradiol upon migraine. *Headache* 1972; 12:93–102.

Stewart WF, Linet MS, Celentano DD, Van Natta M, Ziegler D. Age- and sex-specific incidence rates of migraine with and without visual aura. *Am J Epidemiol* 1991; 134:1111–1120.

Stewart WF, Shechter A, Rasmussen BK. Migraine prevalence: a review of population-based studies. *Neurology* 1994; 44(Suppl 4):S17–S23.

Tammiala-Salonen T, Hiidenkari T, Parvinen T. Burning mouth in a Finnish adult population. *Community Dent Oral Epidemiol* 1993; 21:67–71.

Unruh AM. Gender variations in clinical pain experience. *Pain* 1996; 65:123–167.

Van der Windt DAWM, Croft PR. In: Crombie IK, Croft PR, Linton SJ, LeResche L, Von Korff M (Eds). *Epidemiology of Pain*. Seattle: IASP Press, 1999, pp 257–281.

Von Korff M. Epidemiologic and survey methods: chronic pain assessment. In: Turk DC, Melzack R (Eds). *Handbook of Pain Assessment*. New York: Guilford Press, 1992, pp 391–408.

Von Korff M, Parker RD. The dynamics of the prevalence of chronic episodic disease. *J Chron Dis* 1980; 33:79–85.

Von Korff M, Dworkin SF, LeResche L, Kruger A. An epidemiologic comparison of pain complaints. *Pain* 1988; 32:173–183.

Walsh K, Cruddas M, Coggon D. Low back pain in eight areas of Britain. *J Epidemiol Community Health* 1992; 46:227–230.

Wolfe F, Smythe HA, Yunus MB, et al. The American College of Rheumatology 1990 criteria for the classification of fibromyalgia. *Arthritis Rheum* 1990; 33:160–172.

Wolfe F, Ross K, Anderson J, Russell IJ, Herbert L. The prevalence and characteristics of fibromyalgia in the general population. *Arthritis Rheum* 1995; 38:19–28.

Woo J, Ho SC, Lau J, Leung PC. Musculoskeletal complaints and associated consequences in elderly Chinese aged 70 years and over. *J Rheumatol* 1994; 21:1927–1931.

Wright D, Barrow S, Fisher AD, Horsley SD, Jayson MIV. Influence of physical, psychological and behavioural factors on consultations for back pain. *Br J Rheumatol* 1995; 34:156–161.

Correspondence to: Linda LeResche, ScD, Department of Oral Medicine, Box 356370, University of Washington, Seattle, WA 98195, USA. Tel: 206-616-6049; Fax: 206-685-8412; email: leresche@u.washington.edu.

Sex, Gender, and Pain, Progress in Pain Research and Management, Vol. 17, edited by R.B. Fillingim, IASP Press, Seattle, © 2000.

13

Sex Differences in Recurrent Headache Disorders: Overview and Significance

Kenneth A. Holroyd and Gay L. Lipchik

Department of Psychology, Ohio University, Athens, Ohio, USA

This chapter reviews information on sex differences in recurrent headache disorders, including prevalence, impact, psychological correlates, psychophysiology, and response to treatment. We examine the influence on recurrent headache disorders of female reproductive hormones, which are thought to be inextricably linked to sex differences in headache prevalence. Finally, we discuss which observed sex differences represent only minor demographic variance, and which may provide important insights into recurrent headache disorders and their treatment.

EPIDEMIOLOGY

There are clear sex differences in headache prevalence, with women being more likely than men to experience most recurrent headache disorders (see Table I). On average, women are two to three times as likely as men to suffer migraines (18% of females, 6% of males) or to experience disabling (daily or near-daily) tension headaches (5% of females, 2% of males). Although no gender differences are seen in children prior to puberty, with migraine occurring in approximately 4% of boys and girls (Waters and O'Connor 1971; Goldstein and Chen 1982), after puberty there is a striking increase of migraine in women. Migraine prevalence peaks between the ages of 40 and 45, when migraine is 3.3 times more common in women than in men (Stewart et al. 1992). The female prevalence decreases after menopause, although it still remains more than double that of males, suggesting that gender differences in reproductive hormones do not fully account for gender differences in migraine prevalence (Stewart et al. 1992).

Table I
Overview of epidemiology of headache disorders

Migraine

Migraine affects 15–25% of women and 4–8% of men (O'Brien et al. 1994; Stewart et al. 1994; Rasmussen 1995)

In women, prevalence peaks between the ages of 40 and 45 (Stewart et al. 1992)

In men, prevalence peaks between the ages of 30 and 40 (Lipton and Stewart 1993)

51.1% of women with migraine, compared to 38.1% of men, miss an estimated 6 work days per year due to migraine (Stewart et al. 1996)

Women are more likely than men to experience aura, scalp tenderness, nausea, and vomiting (Celentano et al. 1990)

Women report migraines of longer duration and greater intensity than men (Celentano et al. 1990)

Women are more likely than men to consult a physician for their migraines (Lipton et al. 1998)

Women are more likely than men to be prescribed medication for their headaches; women receive about 40% more prescriptions for their migraines than men (Krobot et al. 1999)

Episodic Tension-Type Headache

Female to male prevalence ratio is 5:4 for episodic tension-type headache (Rasmussen et al. 1991)

Headache prevalence peaks between the ages of 30 and 39 in both genders (Schwartz et al. 1998)

Chronic Tension-Type Headache

Female to male prevalence is 2:1 for chronic tension-type headache (Rasmussen et al. 1991; Schwartz et al. 1998)

In women, prevalence of chronic tension-type increases around age 45, peaking between ages 50 and 59 (Schwartz et al. 1998)

In men, there is no relation between age and prevalence of chronic tension-type headache (Schwartz et al. 1998)

Cluster Headache

Male to female prevalence ratio is about 5:1 (Diamond and Dalessio 1986)

The only primary headache disorder that is more prevalent in men than in women is cluster headache, which occurs with less frequency than migraine or tension-type headache. Cluster headaches occur with a male to female ratio of about 5:1 (Diamond and Dalessio 1986). In a conservative estimate, cluster headaches are experienced by 400,000 men and 80,000 women in the United States, with a prevalence rate of about 0.4% for men and 0.08% for women (Kudrow 1987). The onset of cluster headache can occur at any age, although this problem is most frequent in individuals between 20 and 40 years of age.

SOCIAL IMPACT OF HEADACHE DISORDERS

Sex differences in the impact of headaches on work attendance and productivity are substantial. Women with migraine experience greater disability with their headaches than do men with migraine. For example, it is estimated that 51.1% of women with migraine, compared to 38.1% of men with migraine, miss at least six work days per year because of migraines (Stewart et al. 1996). Each year, employed women with migraine in the United States incur an estimated 18.8 million days of restricted activity because of migraines, compared to 2.7 million days for employed men with migraine (Stang et al. 1994).

Although approximately 19% of migraine sufferers miss work, a larger percentage of migraine sufferers discontinue normal activities (50%) or cancel family (31%) or social activities (30%) (Pryse-Philips et al. 1992). The disruption in family, social, and recreational activities also differentially effects women, who assume a larger share of these responsibilities. Women are more than twice as likely as men to report that their headaches interfere with their family relationships (Kryst and Scherl 1994) and social life as well as their leisure activities (Lacroix and Barbaree 1990).

CONSULTING BEHAVIOR

Females with either tension-type headaches or migraines are more likely than their male counterparts to seek treatment for their headaches (Celentano et al. 1990, 1992; Rasmussen et al. 1992; Lipton et al. 1998). This sex difference in consulting behavior is, of course, not limited to headaches (e.g., Wilensky and Cafferata 1983). However, any relationship between sex and consulting behavior must be interpreted in the context of other demographic and headache variables that also influence consulting behavior.

Among American Migraine Study respondents (*N* = 2479) who reported at least one migraine per year, 68% of women, but only 57% of men had consulted a physician specifically for headaches (Lipton et al. 1998). The determinants of treatment seeking also differed somewhat for men and women. Among women, severity of pain, attack frequency, attack duration, disability, and number of associated symptoms of migraine (e.g., nausea, vomiting, photophobia, phonophobia, and visual or sensory symptoms), were all independent predictors of consultation. However, for men these relationships were not evident, although there was a trend for higher levels of consultation with more severe pain. The authors suggested that the severity and the nature of headache symptoms are likely to determine whether a woman will seek headache treatment; in contrast, men appear less inclined than women to seek treatment, irrespective of the severity of pain or the migraine symptoms they experience.

Females also are more likely than males to receive a headache diagnosis when they do seek treatment (Linet et al. 1989; Rasmussen et al. 1992; Stewart and Lipton 1993; Lipton et al. 1998; Krobot et al. 1999). For example, in the American Migraine Study, 66% of women but only 58% of men reported receiving a diagnosis of migraine (Lipton et al. 1998). A similar sex difference in diagnosis has been reported where linked medical records were accessed to rule out the possibility that the physician failed to communicate the diagnosis to the patient, or that the patients forgot their diagnosis (Stang et al. 1996). However, a study that compared primary care physicians' diagnoses with algorithm-based headache diagnoses based on information from medical records makes it clear that factors other than the sex of the patient, such as comorbid tension headaches or depression, or frequency of headache days, can affect the diagnosis (Stang et al. 1994).

More limited evidence suggests that females are more likely than males to receive prescription medication for their headaches when they do consult a physician. A comprehensive study of drug therapy in primary practice using German health insurance records provides information not only about sex differences in medication use, but also about the appropriateness of the medications prescribed (Krobot et al. 1999). The investigators examined the prescription records of 21,209 individuals who had received a migraine diagnosis. Women received about 40% more prescriptions than men (2.1 vs. 1.5 prescriptions per year; this number refers to prescription density, a variable that takes into account the length of time the patient was in the care of a physician). Women received more prescriptions than men for all migraine medication categories (antiemetic, abortive, and prophylactic) except the analgesic/NSAID category. The type of drugs that were prescribed for headaches did not differ for men and women; however, 73% of prescriptions were for drugs that are not recommended in current practice guidelines as a primary migraine therapy, and 55% of these prescriptions were for analgesics combined with other substances (ergot, barbiturate, etc.). These data suggest that more medicine does not necessarily mean more effective treatment.

CLASSIFICATION AND DIAGNOSIS

The Headache Classification Committee of the International Headache Society (IHS; Olesen 1988) has recently updated diagnostic criteria for all headache disorders. The vast majority (probably over 95%) of patients who seek medical assistance have benign, idiopathic headaches such as migraine and tension-type headache. The diagnostic criteria for migraine, tension-type headache, cluster headache, and headaches associated with substance abuse or withdrawal are presented in Tables II and III. (For detailed descriptions of diagnostic criteria, see Diamond and Dalessio 1992; Rapoport and Sheftell 1996; Holroyd et al. 1998; Olesen 2000.)

HEADACHE PRECIPITANTS

Headache precipitants identified by headache sufferers are listed in Table IV. Headache precipitants are not universal, do not necessarily precipitate an attack on every exposure, and are not necessarily specific to a particular type of headache. Headache triggers may include a variety of psychosocial, hormonal, dietary, and environmental factors (Radnitz 1990; Blau 1993; Rasmussen 1993; Robbins 1994; Rains et al. 1996). Recent general population studies identify stress, sleep difficulties, and hormonal factors as the most frequently identified triggers (Rasmussen 1993). Significant headache improvement may result from teaching patients to avoid, modify, or cope more effectively with headache precipitants.

Psychological stress. The most frequently identified headache trigger identified by both female and male headache sufferers is stress (Nikiforow and Hokkanen 1978; Rasmussen 1993; Robbins 1994; Rains et al. 1996). Recurrent headache sufferers do not report a greater number of major life stressors than matched controls, although they do report more minor daily life stressors than controls (Holm et al. 1986; De Benedittis and Lorenzetti 1992).

Hormonal factors. Reproductive hormones are associated with headache disorders, and this topic is covered below in the section "Origins of Sex Differences: Reproductive Hormones?"

Sleep patterns. The relationship between headache and sleep remains unclear; however, a large proportion of headache sufferers identify insufficient or unrefreshing sleep as a headache precipitant (Rasmussen 1993). Women are more likely than men to identify delayed sleep onset and restless sleep as precipitants (Rasmussen 1993). Prolonged or unusually deep sleep may precipitate headaches in some individuals (Sahota and Dexter 1990). Patients who identify sleep difficulties as headache precipitants should be instructed in sleep hygiene and should be advised to maintain regular sleep schedules. For some, headaches may arise as a consequence of a sleep disorder, such as sleep apnea, that merits evaluation by a sleep specialist (Paiva et al. 1995).

Table II
Diagnostic criteria for migraine, tension-type headache, and cluster headache

1. Migraine

1.1 Migraine without aura

A. At least five attacks fulfilling B–D

B. Headache attacks lasting 4–72 hours (untreated or unsuccessfully treated)

C. Headache has at least two of the following characteristics:
1) Unilateral location; 2) Pulsating quality; 3) Moderate or severe intensity (inhibits or prohibits daily activity); 4) Aggravated by walking stairs or similar routine physical activity

D. During headache at least one of the following:
1) Nausea and/or vomiting or 2) Photophobia and phonophobia

1.2 Migraine with aura

A. At least two attacks fulfilling B

B. At least three of the following characteristics:
1) One or more fully reversible aura symptoms indicating focal cerebral cortical and/or brain-stem dysfunction; 2) At least one aura symptom develops gradually over more than 4 minutes, or 2 or more symptoms occur in succession; 3) No aura symptom lasts more than 60 minutes. If more than one aura symptom is present, accepted duration is proportionately increased; 4) Headache follows aura with an interval of less than 60 minutes (it may also begin before or simultaneously with the aura)

2. Tension-Type Headache

2.1 Episodic tension-type headache

A. At least 10 previous headache episodes fulfilling B–D
Number of days with such headache <180 days/year (<15 days/month)

B. Headache lasting from 30 minutes to 7 days

C. At least two of the following:
1) Pressing/tightening (nonpulsating) quality; 2) Mild or moderate intensity (may inhibit, but does not prohibit daily activity); 3) Bilateral location; 4) Is not aggravated by walking stairs or similar routine physical activity

D. Both of the following:
1) No nausea or vomiting (anorexia may occur) and 2) Photophobia and phonophobia are absent, or one but not the other is present

2.2 Chronic tension-type headache

A. Average headache frequency >15 days/month, 180 days/year for 6 months fulfilling B–C

B. At least two of the following:
1) Pressing/tightening; 2) Mild or moderate severity (may inhibit, but does not prohibit daily activity; 3) Bilateral location; 4) Is not aggravated by walking stairs or similar routine physical activity

C. Both of the following:
1) No vomiting; 2) No more than one of the following: nausea, photophobia, or phonophobia

3. Cluster Headache

A. At least five previous headache episodes fulfilling B–D

B. Severe unilateral, supraorbital and/or temporal pain lasting 15–180 minutes untreated

C. Headache is associated with at least one of the following signs that must be present on the pain side:
1) Conjunctival injection; 2) Lacrimation; 3) Nasal congestion; 4) Rhinorrhea;
5) Forehead and facial sweating; 6) Miosis; 7) Ptosis; 8) Euelid edema

D. Frequency of attacks: from 1 every other day to 8 per day

Source: Headache Classification Committee of the International Headache Society (Olesen 1988).

Table III
Two proposed diagnostic criteria for headaches aggravated by chronic medication use

IHS Criteria[a]	2nd International Workshop Criteria[b]
Headache Characteristics	
1. More than 14 headache days/month	1. More than 20 headache days/month
2. Headache is diffuse, pulsating, and distinguished from migraine by absent attack pattern and/or absent associated symptoms (for ergotamine-induced headache)	2. Daily headache duration exceeds10 hours
Relationship to Medication Use	
1. Ergotamine a. Onset is preceded by daily ergotamine intake (oral = 2 mg, rectal = 1 mg)	1. Intake of analgesics or abortive medication on more than 20 days per month
2. Analgesics a. At least 50 g aspirin or equivalent/month b. At least 100 tablets/month of analgesics combined with barbiturates or other non-narcotic compounds c. Narcotic analgesic use	2. Regular intake of analgesics and/or ergotamine in combination with barbiturates, codeine, caffeine, antihistamines, or tranquilizers
3. Headache disappears within 1 month after withdrawal of substance	3. Increase in the severity and frequency of headaches after discontinuation of drug intake

Source: [a]Headache Classification Committee of the International Headache Society (Olesen 1988); [b]Diener and Wilkonson (1988).

Dietary factors. Almost 30% of headache sufferers report that dietary factors sometimes trigger their headaches (e.g., Robbins 1994). However, most of the data on dietary factors come from surveys and clinical reports. Few double-blind studies of dietary triggers have been conducted, and clinical opinions differ regarding the benefits to be expected from dietary alterations (Medina and Diamond 1978; Blau and Thavapalan 1988). Nonetheless, a diet that eliminates possible dietary precipitants can serve as a valuable assessment device (Rapoport and Sheftell 1996).

Environmental factors. Various environmental factors, such as exposure to chemicals or vapors, glare, or fluorescent lights (see Table IV), have been identified as headache precipitants (e.g., Blau and Thavapalan 1988; Rasmussen 1993). Women are more likely than men to identify weather changes, perfume, and cigarette smoke as migraine precipitants (Robbins 1994). The type of headache triggered by an environmental precipitant also may differ between women and men. For example, exposure to chemicals or vapors is more likely to trigger migraine in women, but more likely to trigger tension-type headache in men (Rasmussen 1993). Patients should be

Table IV
Precipitating factors for headache identified by patients

- Stress
  - During stress
  - After stress (i.e., "let-down headache")
- Lack of food
  - Fasting
  - Insufficient food
  - Delayed or missed meals
- Specific foods
  - Alcoholic beverages
  - Chocolate
  - Aged cheese
  - Aged meats
  - Monosodium glutamate (used in Chinese restaurants, many processed foods, seasonings)
  - Aspartame (sugar substitute found in diet foods)
  - Caffeine (coffee, tea, cola)
  - Nuts
- Physical exertion
- Fatigue
- Sleep
  - Excessive sleep
  - Unrefreshing sleep
  - Insufficient sleep
  - Sleep problems*
  - Delayed onset
  - Restless sleep
  - Snoring*
- Hormones (women only)
  - Menstrual period (before, during, after)
  - Postmenopausal changes
  - Oral contraceptives
  - Hormone supplements
  - Pregnancy
- Environment
  - Exposure to chemicals or chemical vapors
  - Weather changes*
  - Heat
  - Cold
  - Fluorescent light
  - Bright light, glare
  - Noise
  - Perfume*
  - Cigarette smoke*

Source: Adapted from Blau and Thavapalan (1988), Radnitz (1990), Rasmussen (1993), Robbins (1994).
* More frequently reported by women than men.

instructed to avoid or restrict their exposure to various environmental factors identified as headache triggers (Table IV). This can often be accomplished with little lifestyle disruption.

PSYCHOPHYSIOLOGY

Recent research on psychophysiological mechanisms has largely focused on tension-type headaches and has emphasized central as well as peripheral mechanisms (Olesen 1991; Schoenen and Wang 1997; Jensen 1999; G.L. Lipchik et al., unpublished manuscript). The psychophysiological abnormality most consistently observed in tension headache has been elevated pericranial muscle tenderness in response to manual palpitation (e.g., Jensen et al. 1993; Lipchik et al. 1996, 1997, unpublished manuscript; Jensen et al. 1998). This pericranial allodynia has been observed in both episodic and chronic tension headache, even when subjects are assessed when headache-free. Other psychophysiological findings, such as a reduced peripheral pain threshold or elevated electromyographic (EMG) activity in pericranial muscles, have been observed inconsistently in tension headache (Andrasik et al. 1982; Schoenen et al. 1991; Jensen et al. 1993). Bendtsen and colleagues (1996) have postulated that the elevation in pericranial muscle tenderness observed in frequent tension headache reflects an abnormality in central pain transmission, specifically a neuroplasticity in second-order neurons in the dorsal horn and trigeminal nucleus that causes low threshold mechanoreceptors to be wired into pain transmission circuits in this brain region.

Sex differences have been observed in all of the above psychophysiological measures, as shown by the results from a Danish population study in which 1000 randomly selected subjects received a detailed psychophysiological evaluation (Jensen et al. 1992). Females exhibited higher levels of tenderness than males in all 14 pericranial muscles examined; over half of females, but less than a quarter of males, obtained total tenderness scores that reflected some degree of tenderness. Pain thresholds to algometer pressure applied at the temporalis muscle were about 20% lower in females than in males. These results are of particular interest because they were obtained in a randomly selected population sample; these findings thus were not subject to the selection biases that can occur in clinical samples. Similar sex differences in tenderness and pain thresholds of pericranial muscles have been observed in other studies (Rieder et al. 1983; Fischer 1987), although there have been negative findings as well.

In both population samples and clinical samples of tension-type headache sufferers, women exhibit higher levels of pericranial muscle tenderness than men, and both male and female headache sufferers exhibit higher levels of tenderness than their respective healthy controls (Jensen et al. 1993; G.L. Lipchik et al., unpublished manuscript). For example, Fig. 1 displays the proportion of male and female chronic tension-type headache sufferers exhibiting tenderness to 500 g force applied by finger palpation to each of 10 pericranial muscles. Although males and females did not differ in headache activity, females exhibited substantially higher levels of overall tenderness than males ($P < 0.0001$), with this sex difference observed across all 10 muscles ($P \leq 0.01$).

Sex differences in pericranial muscle tenderness may reflect important sex differences in pain mechanisms; however, they may also reflect the greater readiness of females to display pain behaviors (Miaskowski 1999). Signal detection methodology (Lloyd and Appel 1976) may help investigators disentangle these two explanations. To the extent that sex differences in tenderness reflect physiological differences in pain mechanisms, an understanding of these physiological differences may shed light on pain mechanisms in a variety of disorders that have chronic muscular pain as a prominent feature. Sex differences in pericranial muscle tenderness thus deserve further study.

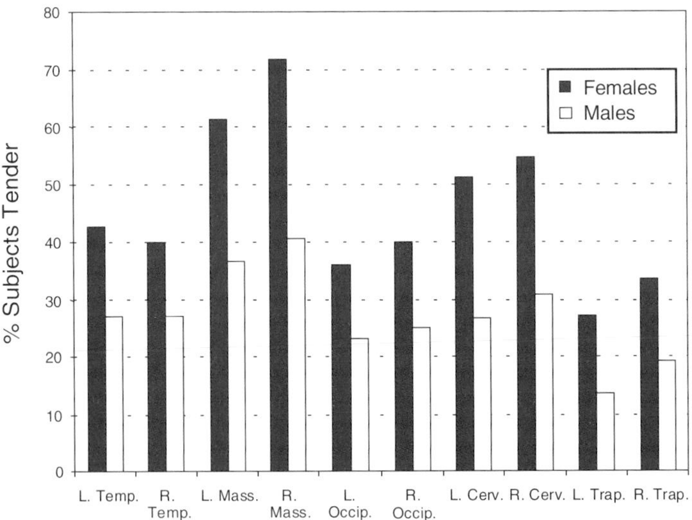

Fig. 1. Pericranial muscle tenderness in male and female chronic tension-type headache sufferers in response to palpation (500 g force; $P < 0.01$ for all muscles). L. = left; R. = right; Temp. = temporalis; Mass. = masseter; Occip. = occipitalis; Cerv. = cervical; Trap. = trapezius.

PSYCHOPATHOLOGY

Recurrent migraine and chronic tension-type headaches substantially increase the risk for both anxiety and mood disorders for both males and females (e.g., Brandt et al. 1990; Breslau and Davis 1992; Merikangas et al. 1993; Breslau et al. 1994b; Merikangas 1994; Holroyd et al. 2000). The epidemiological data are clearest for migraine, where longitudinal studies have examined relationships between migraine and psychopathology. For example, Breslau and colleagues (1994a) followed a random sample of young adults 21–30 years of age for 3.5 years. Women were significantly more likely than men to receive lifetime diagnoses of both migraine (24% vs. 9%) and major depression (24% vs. 13%) by age 30, with the relative female risk increasing for migraine in the late teens and for major depression after about age 20. Longitudinal data also indicate that women are more than four times as likely as men to develop migraine and more than twice as likely to develop major depression, confirming that female sex remains a significant risk factor for both disorders over time. Particularly noteworthy is the finding that migraine dramatically increased the risk of depression, tripling the probability that an individual would develop major depression. As a result, by age 33 the majority (53%) of migraine sufferers, but fewer than 1 in 6 individuals without migraine had received a lifetime diagnosis of major depression. This figure is particularly dramatic given that it must underestimate the eventual comorbidity between migraine and depression in this relatively young sample.

The nature of the relationship between recurrent headache disorders and anxiety/mood disorders remains unclear, though it is unlikely to be the case that the strain of living with recurrent headaches simply increases the risk of anxiety and mood disorders. In fact, the relationship appears bidirectional, because major depression also increases the likelihood of subsequently developing migraine (Breslau et al. 1994a); perhaps there is a common genetic vulnerability for both disorders. Glover (1993) has reviewed features common to the biology of migraine and depression, and Silberstein (1995) and others have hypothesized that a dysfunction in the serotonergic system increases the risk for both disorders. However, preliminary examination of the co-transmission pattern of anxiety/mood disorders and migraine has failed to reveal evidence of a shared genetic predisposition for migraine and major affective disorders (Breslau et al. 1994b). Any investigations into a common vulnerability will have to take into account the large sex differences in the prevalence of both disorders.

ORIGINS OF SEX DIFFERENCES: REPRODUCTIVE HORMONES?

The significantly higher prevalence of headache disorders in women, and the increased incidence of migraine at menarche and menstruation, have focused attention on the possible role of female reproductive hormones, especially cyclic changes of estradiol and progestin, in the pathogenesis of migraine (e.g., Silberstein and Merriam 1993; MacGregor 1997). Evidence suggests that the abrupt fall of estrogens that occurs before menstruation gives rise to migraine in susceptible women (Somerville 1972, 1975a,b). Similarly, the alterations in estrogens that occur with oral contraceptive use, menopause, and following pregnancy are believed to be related to migraine in some women (Bousser et al. 1993; Silberstein 1993). Fluctuations in estrogens are hypothesized to influence migraine through modifications of serotonin metabolism (Martignoni et al. 1987), through changes involving catecholaminergic systems that lead to cerebral vasoconstriction followed by vasodilation (Welch et al. 1984; Martignoni et al. 1987), and through cyclic failure of endogenous opioid systems (Facchinetti et al. 1989). Fluctuations in estrogen levels also induce changes in prostaglandins that sensitize nociceptors, promote the development of neurogenic inflammation, and possibly influence descending pain-modulatory systems (Silberstein and Merriam 1993). Nonetheless, the exact mechanisms whereby estrogen triggers migraine are unknown. Insufficient data are available to draw conclusions about the relationship of reproductive hormones to tension-type headache. Well-controlled and methodologically sound investigations of reproductive hormones might significantly enhance our understanding of the pathogenesis of headache disorders in both women and men.

MENSTRUAL MIGRAINE

Migraine episodes occur at the time of menses in about 60–70% of women who experience migraines (Nattero 1982; Silberstein 1998), and exclusively in about 7–14% (Epstein et al. 1975; MacGregor 1997). Menstrual migraine begins at menarche in about one-third of female migraineurs (Nattero 1982). Migraine with onset at menarche is most likely to show menstrual periodicity (Granella et al. 1993). Most menstrually related migraine attacks are characterized by severe and intense pain lasting 2–3 days, which is likely to be accompanied by prominent nausea and vomiting. Attacks without aura are most common (Bousser et al. 1993; MacGregor 1997).

Although the term "menstrual migraine" is used frequently, definitions vary widely. Migraine attacks occurring *only* at the time of menstruation (occurring on day 1 of menstruation ± 2 days), and at no other time, are considered true menstrual migraine by several researchers (Bousser et al. 1993; MacGregor 1997). This definition is supported by diary records kept by women over three cycles that revealed a marked increase in migraine around the first day of menstruation (MacGregor et al. 1990). Attacks occurring both at menstruation and at other times of the month may be best categorized as "menstrually triggered migraine" (Silberstein 1998) or "menstrually related migraine." Some investigators assert that the differentiation between menstrually triggered migraine and true menstrual migraine is necessary because women with true menstrual migraine are most likely to have an exclusive hormonal trigger for their headaches, which is an important factor in identifying mechanisms and effective management (MacGregor 1997).

PREMENSTRUAL HEADACHE

In distinction from true menstrual migraine, as defined above, a significant percentage of women report they are more likely to experience migraine premenstrually, often along with other premenstrual symptoms such as negative affect, inability to concentrate, and water retention (MacGregor 1997; Silberstein 1998). Moreover, several studies have found an increase in nonmigraine headaches premenstrually, particularly in women who fulfill criteria for premenstrual syndrome (PMS) (Keenan and Lindamer 1992). However, it is difficult to establish a relationship between PMS and headaches, as the existence of PMS remains a topic of debate among researchers.

ORAL CONTRACEPTIVES

Oral contraceptives (OC) have been variously reported to increase the incidence or severity of migraine, to alleviate headaches, and to result in no change in headache activity. This conflicting evidence may be due, at least in part, to methodological problems in studies investigating the impact of OC on headaches. Double-blind, placebo-controlled studies have revealed no change in headache frequency or severity in women taking OC (Silberstein and Merriam 1991). Moreover, studies reporting an increase in frequency or severity of headaches in women taking OC were conducted primarily in the 1960s and 1970s and examined OC with a higher estrogen content than is typical today. OC may thus be less of a factor in precipitating or aggravating headaches than was previously thought. Nonetheless, OC containing low levels of estrogen can precipitate migraine attacks in some women, with attacks occurring most frequently during the drug-free interval of the cycle.

PREGNANCY

Approximately 55–80% of women with migraine report improvement or disappearance of migraine during pregnancy (for review, see Bousser et al. 1993; Silberstein 1997). The improvement is typically most pronounced following the first trimester, and is more likely to occur in migraine without aura than in migraine with aura. Improvement is most likely to occur if headaches had been regularly associated with menstruation. Most women with tension-type headaches report little change in headache activity during pregnancy (Rasmussen 1992).

For a small minority of pregnant women, migraine does not improve, or worsens, especially in the case of migraine with aura (Bousser et al. 1993). Migraine may also appear for the first time during pregnancy; most reported cases involve migraine with aura, probably because patients with these dramatic neurological symptoms are more likely to seek treatment (Uknis and Silberstein 1991; Granella et al. 1993).

During the first postpartum week, approximately 35–45% of women experience headaches. Women with a prior history of migraine, especially if it was menstrually related, are more likely to develop postpartum migraine (Stein 1981; Stein et al. 1984).

Rising or sustained high levels of estrogen may be responsible for the improvement in headaches during pregnancy, and their fall at the time of delivery may trigger postpartum migraine (see Chapter 6 for a discussion of pregnancy-induced analgesia). This mechanism, however, cannot account for the worsening or new onset of migraine that sometimes occurs during pregnancy. Rather, the key to migraine genesis may be the intrinsic estrogen receptor sensitivity of the hypothalamic neurons; in most women, rising or sustained estrogen levels decrease migraine episodes, but in some women these changes might induce migraine (Silberstein and Merriam 1991).

MENOPAUSE

Although migraine prevalence decreases with advancing age, at menopause migraine frequency and severity can either decrease, remain unchanged, or worsen, with some women reporting a continuation of the monthly periodicity of their headaches (Hering and Rose 1992). The type of menopause may play a significant role. Women going through physiological menopause experience a more favorable course with their migraines than do women whose menopause is surgically induced by hysterectomy or ovariectomy (Granella et al. 1993; Neri et al. 1993). Worsening of migraine is most likely to occur in women whose menopause is surgically induced.

Women whose migraines prior to menopause were closely linked to their menstrual periods are more likely to experience postmenopausal improvement in their headaches. The premenstrual fall in estrogen levels that triggered their headaches is now replaced by a low, but stable level of estrogen (Welch et al. 1984). However, women whose migraines were not triggered by falling estrogen levels may not experience a decrease in their migraines after menopause.

The effect of postmenopausal hormone replacement therapy (HRT) on migraine is also variable. Some studies report an exacerbation of migraine, while others suggest no change, and others suggest an amelioration of migraine following HRT consisting of estrogen administered alone or in combination with testosterone (Silberstein and Merriam 1993). Controlled studies of the impact of menopause and of HRT on headache disorders are needed.

TREATMENT

BEHAVIORAL INTERVENTIONS

Behavioral interventions may permit nonpharmacological management of headache problems or at least the use of less aggressive drug therapy, and may facilitate the management of difficult-to-treat headache problems such as drug-induced headache or near-daily migraine-like headaches (sometimes termed "transformed migraine"). Three types of behavioral interventions are frequently used in the management of recurrent migraine and tension-type headaches: relaxation training, EMG and thermal (hand-warming) biofeedback training, and stress-management or cognitive-behavioral therapy. Detailed descriptions of these behavioral treatment procedures and clinical details concerning their use have been published elsewhere (Blanchard and Andrasik 1985; Martin 1993; Penzien and Holroyd 1994; Holroyd et al. 1998).

SEX DIFFERENCES IN EFFICACY OF BEHAVIORAL INTERVENTIONS

Because of the higher prevalence of tension and migraine headaches in women than in men, and the greater propensity of women to seek treatment, about three-quarters of participants in clinical trials have been women (Holroyd and Penzien 1986, 1990; Bogaards and ter Kuile 1994). The small number of male participants in many trials probably has limited the ability of investigators to detect sex differences in treatment response. However, even in larger studies where such analyses would be possible, information about sex differences in treatment response typically has not been reported.

Where meta-analytic reviews of the behavioral treatment literature have examined the relationship between the sex composition of the patient sample and treatment outcome, no dramatic sex differences in treatment response have been detected (Holroyd and Penzien 1986, 1990; Bogaards and ter Kuile 1994), although such secondary analyses provide a relatively insensitive way of addressing this question. It can be seen in Table V that mean reductions in both tension-type headaches and migraines reported with the most commonly used relaxation and biofeedback therapies have been moderate, though substantially larger than have been observed with placebo. Meta-analyses have failed to detect reliable differences in the effectiveness of these various behavioral interventions, let alone sex differences in response to individual interventions.

Individual studies that have examined gender differences in response to behavioral treatments have mostly found little evidence of sex differences in treatment response, although they typically had insufficient statistical power to detect moderate or small sex differences in treatment response (e.g., Ford et al. 1983; Blanchard and Andrasik 1985; Blanchard et al. 1985; Holroyd et al. 1988). However, there have been some exceptions. Diamond and colleagues (1979) reported sex differences in treatment response in a retrospective evaluation (N = 556) of a behavioral treatment package that combined several biofeedback (thermal and EMG) and relaxation training procedures. Most patients had received migraine or combined migraine and

Table V
Mean percentage improvement by type of treatment and headache diagnosis

	BF	Relax	BF and Relax	CBT	Placebo	HM Control
Tension-Type Headache						
Mean improvement (%)	48	36	59	53	16	1
No. of treatment groups	28	37	9	15	21	16
Improvement range (%)	–18 to 96	4 to 99	37 to 89	27 to 76	–70 to 74	–33 to 26
Migraine						
Mean improvement (%)	37	32	33	49	9	5
No. of treatment groups	5	10	10	7	4	12
Improvement range (%)	13 to 86	3 to 78	21 to 87	29 to 76	–37 to –7	–20 to 19

Note: BF = biofeedback training (EMG biofeedback training for tension-type headache, thermal biofeedback training for migraine); relax = relaxation training; CBT = cognitive-behavioral therapy; placebo = placebo and control conditions; HM control = headache-monitoring control.
Source: Data for tension-type headaches are from Borgards and ter Kuile (1994). Data on migraine treatments are based on all studies included in an evidence report sponsored by the Agency for Health Care Policy and Research (Duke University 1999).

tension-type headache diagnoses. At a short-term evaluation completed by 407 patients, 77% of women but only 61% of men ($P < 0.005$) reported that behavioral treatment had been helpful, and females also were more likely than males to report long-term benefit.

Overall, the literature provides little evidence of significant sex differences in response to behavioral treatment, although few trials have conducted statistical tests with adequate power to detect small to moderate sex differences in treatment response. Patient characteristics such as comorbid psychopathology, overuse of analgesic or ergotamine-containing medications, or continuous or near-continuous pain are probably more strongly associated than gender with treatment outcome.

IMPLICATIONS OF THE REPRODUCTIVE CYCLE FOR BEHAVIORAL MANAGEMENT OF HEADACHES

The fact that headaches are often influenced by hormonal changes associated with the female reproductive cycle has important implications for treatment. Clinicians often assume that headaches associated with hormonal changes, or aggravated by hormonal preparations, are less responsive than other headaches to either behavioral therapy or pharmacological treatment.

Menstrual-related migraine. The few studies that have evaluated the effectiveness of behavioral treatments for menstrual migraine have yielded conflicting results. As shown in Table VI, two studies (Szekely et al. 1986; Gauthier et al. 1991) have reported reasonable reductions in menstrual migraine with relaxation/biofeedback therapies, while one study (study 2 by Kim and Blanchard 1992) reported only marginal reductions in menstrual migraines. In addition, one study (study 1 by Kim and Blanchard 1992) reported reasonable improvement, whereas another (Solbach et al. 1984) reported almost no improvement in overall headache activity in women identified as experiencing both menstrual and nonmenstrual migraines. These studies differed in their definition of menstrual migraine; as a result, headaches that were considered menstrually related in one study were not considered menstrually related in another study. The inability to unambiguously identify menstrually related migraine has limited investigators' ability to address the effectiveness of behavior therapy for this type of headache.

Nevertheless, one of the strongest of the available studies provides reasonable evidence that menstrually related migraines need not be refractory to behavioral therapy. Gauthier and colleagues (1991) compared improvements in headaches associated with menstruation (occurring within 3 days of the beginning of menstruation) and in headaches occurring at other times in women who received either thermal or cephalic vasomotor biofeedback

Table VI
Response of menstrual migraines to behavioral treatment

Reference (No. Subjects)	Definition of MM	Results	Comments
Gauthier et al. 1991 ($N = 39$)	–3 to +3 days from start of menstruation	MM = NMM; 49% of patients had >50% reduction in MM	Not clear if subjects on oral contraceptives were excluded
Kim and Blanchard 1992, Study 1 ($N = 98$)	Self-identification	MM = NMM; 42% of patients had >50% reduction in MM	MM and NMM not distinguished in diary recordings
Kim and Blanchard 1992, Study 2 ($N = 15$)	Self-identification and verification by diary	MM = NMH; 27% of patients had >50% reduction in MM	Reductions in neither MM nor NMN significant
Szekeley et al. 1986 ($N = 8$)	–7 to +7 days from start of menstruation	MM = NMM; 50% of patients had >50% reduction in MM	Cluster and tension headache included; improvements not significant
Solbach et al. 1984 ($N = 136$)	–3 to +3 days from start of menstruation	Direct comparison not reported*; ~13% reduction in headaches in MM patients†	MM and NMM not distinguished in diary recordings

Abbreviations: MM = menstrual migraine; NMM = nonmenstrual migraine.
* Indirect comparison suggested MM < NMM.
† Reduction in frequency from pretreatment to final 12-week block.

training. Similar improvements were observed in menstrual and nonmenstrual headaches, with about half of the women showing clinically significant (greater than 50%) improvement in each type of headache. Improvements in menstrual and nonmenstrual headaches were equally likely to be maintained at a 6-month follow-up.

Pregnancy. Behavioral interventions are attractive for managing headaches during pregnancy because, unlike drugs, they would not be expected to pose risks to the developing baby. Moreover, such interventions may reduce the nausea and vomiting associated with pregnancy. On the other hand, health care professionals are often skeptical about the efficacy of these therapies, because headaches during pregnancy are influenced by dramatic hormonal changes that are unlikely to be altered by behavioral treatment. During the second or third trimester, some women experience a remission of their migraines without treatment, which makes it difficult to evaluate the effectiveness of headache therapies during pregnancy. Uncontrolled studies (Hicking et al. 1990) thus provide only preliminary evidence of the effectiveness of behavioral therapy.

One study (Marcus et al. 1995) suggests that behavioral therapy may be a promising treatment during pregnancy. In this study, 31 pregnant women were randomized to either a 2-month (eight-session) treatment that included relaxation, thermal biofeedback training to increase finger temperature, and physical therapy exercises, or to a pseudotherapy control treatment that included much of the same educational material along with thermal biofeedback training to *decrease* finger temperature. For most women the treatment program was initiated during the second trimester (18th week of pregnancy on average) and thus was completed before delivery. Women who received the active treatment showed substantially larger mean reductions in headache activity (81% vs. 33% reduction) and were more likely to show clinically significant improvements (73% vs. 29% of women) following treatment as compared to women in the control condition. Moreover, improvements were maintained throughout the perinatal period and at 3- and 6-month follow-up evaluations (Scharff et al. 1996). These initial findings should encourage greater experimentation with behavioral intervention to manage headaches during pregnancy.

Menopause. Little attention has been paid to the evaluation of therapies in postmenopausal women, possibly because headaches often improve at menopause. Clinical trials that have been large enough to include a reasonable sample of postmenopausal women have failed to report results specifically for this subgroup of women. Data from available clinical trials should thus be only cautiously generalized to postmenopausal women.

Clinical observations suggest that the efficacy of both drug and behavioral therapies is reduced when headaches are aggravated by HRT. When a patient taking HRT does not respond to standard behavior or drug therapy for headache problems, a reduction in estrogen dose may improve therapeutic response (Kudrow 1975). The lack of controlled therapeutic trials in postmenopausal women, and particularly in women on HRT, leave the clinician with few guidelines for modifying treatment for these women. Studies are needed to evaluate the effectiveness of behavioral therapy and preventive drug therapy for headache in women taking HRT.

DRUG THERAPY

There is little evidence to suggest any striking sex differences in response to drug therapies for headaches, although analyses of sex differences in response to drug therapies are typically not reported in clinical trials (good overviews of drug trials include Goadsby 1997; Silberstein et al. 1998; Olesen 2000). A meta-analysis of 47 clinical trials (including over 1200 patients) that was conducted to evaluate the most widely used preventive therapy for migraine (propranolol HCl) found no evidence of sex differences in treatment response (Holroyd et al. 1991). In contrast, trial outcome varied with other characteristics of patient samples (e.g., mean chronicity of headache disorder) and with clinical trial methodology (e.g., type of outcome measure used). Individual clinical trials of propranolol HCl typically either have not reported data on sex differences in treatment response, or have found no significant sex differences in treatment response.

Menstrual migraine. Double-blind, placebo-controlled clinical trials are scarce for the numerous proposed drug treatments for menstrual migraine. Moreover, as discussed above, the lack of a universally accepted definition of menstrual migraine makes comparisons across available studies difficult. In clinical practice, menstrual migraine is typically treated by the perimenstrual use of the same prophylactic medications (antidepressants, β-blockers, calcium channel blockers, and ergotamine derivatives) used to treat nonmenstrual migraine (Silberstein 1998).

Some evidence suggests that nonsteroidal anti-inflammatory drugs (NSAIDs), administered prophylactically, are quite effective in treating menstrual migraine (Solbach et al. 1984; Nattero et al. 1991; Giacovazzo et al. 1993). NSAIDs used prophylactically need to be taken in adequate doses for several days prior to the onset of menses as well as throughout the vulnerable time. If the first type of NSAID is not effective, other classes of NSAIDs should be tried (Silberstein 1998).

Ergot derivatives (including ergotamine tartrate, ergonovine, and dihydroergotamine) can be used effectively as abortive or prophylactic migraine treatments (D'Alessandro et al. 1983; Gallagher 1989; Silberstein et al. 1990). However, the use of ergots has largely been replaced by the 5-HT1 (serotonin) agonists (sumatriptan, rizatriptan, zolmitriptan, etc.). Recent placebo-controlled studies have found various triptans to be an effective and well-tolerated treatment for migraine attacks occurring just before or during menses (Facchinetti et al. 1995; Loder and Silberstein 1999; Salonen and Saiers 1999), but many of the study participants did not have exclusively menstrual migraine.

If estrogen withdrawal is the trigger for menstrual migraine, then estrogen replacement prior to menstruation should be an effective preventative. Several estrogen preparations have been investigated with varying results. The best results have been obtained with percutaneous estradiol gel, which was found to be highly effective in two double-blind, placebo-controlled studies in women with true menstrual migraine (de Lignieres et al. 1986; Dennerstein et al. 1988). It is important to produce a stable level of estrogen when using estrogen replacement in order to prevent exacerbation of symptoms; in this regard, percutaneous estrogens produce higher, more stable levels than do other estrogen replacements.

Other successful hormonal manipulations include synthetic androgens, antiestrogens, dopamine agonists, and luteinizing-hormone-releasing hormone analogues (for review, see Bousser and Massiou 1993; Silberstein 1998). However, the evidence consists mostly of open-label studies or anecdotal case reports.

In conclusion, diverse treatment options are available for menstrual migraine. Additional double-blind, placebo-controlled investigations using a universally accepted definition of menstrual migraine are necessary to establish the efficacy of various drug therapies.

Oral contraceptives. Treatment of migraine in women taking OC does not differ from the usual treatment of migraine. Women receiving OC with a high estrogen content may benefit from trying a pill with a lower estrogen content. For women in whom migraine is confined to the pill-free (or placebo) week, extended regimens using the active pill continuously for up to 3 or 4 months can be considered.

Women with migraine receiving OC should receive a closer follow-up than those not receiving OC because the risk for ischemic stroke is elevated in women who have migraine compared to the general population (Tzourio et al. 1993). Women who experience a change in their usual pattern of headache, such as severe headache of sudden onset, daily headache, neurological symptoms, or significant increase in frequency or severity of headache while taking OC should discontinue OC use and should receive a neurological evaluation to rule out subarachnoid hemorrhage or arterial or venous thrombosis (Bousser and Massiou 1993).

Pregnancy. Treatment of headache during pregnancy and the postpartum period (if breast-feeding) is challenging because few data are available about the risks of prophylactic or abortive medications used for migraine and tension-type headache during pregnancy, delivery, and breast-feeding. If medication is necessary, drugs with a short elimination half-life and inert metabolites (ibuprofen, flurbiprofen, diclofenac, and mefenamic acid) may be employed (Bousser and Massiou 1993). Ergotamine tartrate and parenteral dihydroergotamine are contraindicated during pregnancy. Behavioral treatments, as described above, should be considered.

Menopause. Treatment of menopausal and postmenopausal headaches does not differ from typical headache treatment, although few investigations of the treatment of menopausal headaches have been conducted. Similarly, few published studies have assessed the effects of HRT on migraine, although it has been suggested that women with migraine and menopausal symptoms resulting from erratic estrogen secretions may benefit from HRT that stabilizes the estrogen fluctuations. However, HRT for the treatment of menopause may aggravate migraine or interfere with the effectiveness of prophylactic migraine medications and behavioral interventions. A reduction in estrogen dose may improve therapeutic response in this situation; however, almost any change in estrogen regimen may be helpful in some instances, including changing the type of estrogen (e.g., from an organic conjugated estrogen to a pure synthetic estrogen, or vice versa), switching from interrupted to continuous administration or from oral to parenteral dosing, or adding androgens (Silberstein 1993). Surgical menopause (hysterectomy or ovariectomy) is not recommended for the treatment for migraine at any age (Silberstein 1993) as it fails to result in an improvement in migraine and has can result in worse headaches (Granella et al. 1993).

CONCLUSIONS

Sex differences in the prevalence of recurrent headache disorders are so dramatic as to have been evident for decades. Similarly, the fact that some headache disorders such as migraine are influenced by female reproductive hormones has been evident for some time. Nonetheless, research on the pathophysiology and treatment of recurrent headache disorders—with the exception of research that has focused specifically on the influence of reproductive hormones on migraine—has paid relatively little attention to possible sex differences in psychophysiological mechanisms or treatment response. This omission may have reflected the belief that pathophysiological mechanisms and effective treatments are the same for men and women, although in females, reproductive hormones can aggravate common headache mechanisms. Our review found no evidence that convincingly challenges this belief, but was limited by the infrequency with which sex differences are examined in the literature. We suspect that this belief has thus been self-fulfilling in that it has discouraged the detailed examination of sex differences in either psychophysiological mechanisms or treatment responses.

In spite of dramatic and well-documented sex differences in the prevalence of recurrent headache disorders, relatively minor sex differences have been reported in symptom presentation. It must be kept in mind, however, that the absence of sex differences in defining diagnostic criteria would tend to minimize the differences that could be observed. Relatively dramatic sex differences in the impact of headaches and in health care utilization are reasonably well documented, however. By all measures, the impact of recurrent headache disorders is greater for females than males, and females are more likely than males to seek and to receive treatment for recurrent headache disorders. Some evidence also suggests that headache disorders are more likely to be accurately diagnosed in females than in males, possibly because a female patient is typical and thus the most recognizable presentation. It is unclear, however, whether accurate diagnosis leads to more appropriate treatment, because headache disorders are often not appropriately managed in many settings.

Sex differences in psychophysiological mechanisms of headache have received surprisingly little attention. In the case of tension-type headache, recent research suggests that a sensitization or other alteration in pain transmission circuits may underlie the persistent muscle tenderness that characterizes tension-type headache pain. It is unclear whether the relatively large sex differences in muscle tenderness that are observed in tension-type headache reflect sex differences in the vulnerability of underlying psychophysiological mechanisms or whether they indicate sex differences in the behavioral display of pain behaviors. However, to the extent that this research clarifies the origin of sex differences in psychophysiological mechanisms underlying persistent pain in tension-type headache, it may also shed light on the source of sex differences in other forms of musculoskeletal pain disorders. Little information is available about sex differences in neuronal or neurovascular mechanisms that have been hypothesized to underlie migraine. Greater attention has been directed to the influence of female reproductive hormones in migraine. Sex differences in migraine prevalence appear to be partially explained by the aggravating effects of female reproductive hormones. We therefore reviewed the role of reproductive hormones in migraine, highlighting the ways hormonal factors can influence migraine management. Treatments that stabilize reproductive hormone levels, for example estrogen supplementation for menstrual migraine and the elimination of the pill-free week for women taking OC, appear to reduce these hormonally related migraine episodes. However, few data are available regarding the effects of menopause or HRT on headache, despite the relevance of such data for the clinical management of headache disorders in large numbers of women. The reproductive cycle is complex, and the exact mechanisms underlying migraine episodes triggered by various hormonal events remain unclear. Further studies using strict criteria and controls are needed.

In the few instances where sex differences in response to treatment have been reported, females have tended to show a slightly better response to therapy than males. For the most part, however, no data on sex differences in treatment response are reported in clinical trials of either behavioral or drug therapies. As a result, it is widely assumed that sex differences in treatment response need not be a major consideration in treatment planning, except where headaches are thought to be influenced by female reproductive hormones. However, study samples have been overwhelmingly female, raising the possibility that available outcome data are more accurate for females than for males. We therefore recommend that data on sex differences in treatment response be reported in all future clinical trials with adequate sample size.

ACKNOWLEDGMENT

Support for preparation of this chapter was provided in part by NS32374 from the National Institute of Neurological Disorders and Stroke.

REFERENCES

Andrasik F, Blanchard EB, Arena JG, Saunders NL. Barron KD. Psychophysiology of recurrent headache: methodological issues and new empirical findings. *Behav Ther* 1982; 13:407–429.

Bendtsen L, Jensen R, Olesen J. Qualitatively altered nociception in chronic myofascial pain. *Pain* 1996; 65:259–264.

Blanchard EB, Andrasik F. *Management of Chronic Headaches: a Psychological Approach.* Elmsford, NY: Pergamon Press, 1985.

Blanchard EB, Andrasik F, Evans DD, et al. Behavioral treatment of 250 chronic headache patients: a clinical replication series. *Behav Ther* 1985; 16:308–327.

Blau JN. Diagnosing migraine: are the criteria valid or invalid? *Cephalalgia* 1993; 13:21–24.

Blau JN, Thavapalan M. Preventing migraine: a study of precipitating factors. *Headache* 1988; 28:481–483.

Bogaards MC, ter Kuile MM. Treatment of recurrent tension headache: a meta-analytic review. *Clin J Pain* 1994; 10:174–190.

Bousser MG, Massiou H. Migraine in the reproductive cycle. In: Olesen J, Tfelt-Hansen P, Welch KMA (Eds). *The Headaches.* New York: Raven Press, 1993, pp 413–419.

Bousser MG, Ratinahirana H, Darbois X. Migraine and pregnancy: a prospective study of 703 women after delivery. *Neurology* 1993; 40:437.

Brandt J, Celentano D, Stewart W, Linet M, Folstein MF. Personality and emotional disorder in a community sample of migraine headache sufferers. *Am J Psychiatry* 1990; 147:303–308.

Breslau N, Davis GC. Migraine, major depression and panic disorder: a prospective epidemiologic study of young adults. *Cephalalgia* 1992; 12:85–90.

Breslau N, Davis GC, Schultz LR, Peterson EL. Migraine and major depression: a longitudinal study. *Headache* 1994a; 34:387–393.

Breslau N, Merikangas K, Bowden CL. Comorbidity of migraine and major affective disorders. *Neurology* 1994b; 44 (Suppl 7):S17–S22.

Campbell JK, Penzien DB, Wall EM. Evidence-based guidelines for migraine headache: behavioral and physical treatments. Available via the Internet: http://www.aan.com under Practice Guidelines. Accessed May 2000.

Celentano DD, Linet MS, Stewart WF. Gender differences in the experience of headache. *Soc Sci Med* 1990; 30:1289–1295.

Celentano DD, Stewart WF, Lipton RB, Reed ML. Medication use and disability among migraineurs: a national probability sample survey. *Headache* 1992; 32:223–228.

D'Alessandro R, Gamberini G, Lozito A, Sacquengna T. Menstrual migraine: intermittent prophylaxis with a time-release pharmacologic formulation of dihydroergotamine. *Cephalalgia* 1983; 15 (Suppl 1):156–158.

De Benedittis G, Lorenzetti A. Minor stressful life events (daily hassles) in chronic primary headache: relationship with MMPI personality patterns. *Headache* 1992; 32:330–332.

de Lignieres B, Vincens M, Mauvais-Jarvis P, et al. Prevention of menstrual migraine by percutaneous oestradiol. *BMJ* 1986; 293:1540.

Dennerstein L, Morse C, Burrows G, et al. Menstrual migraine: a double blind trial of percutaneous estradiol. *Gynecol Endocrinol* 1988; 2:113–120.

Diamond S, Dalessio DJ. *The Practicing Physician's Approach to Headache.* Baltimore: Williams & Wilkins, 1986, pp 66–75.

Diamond S, Dalessio DJ. *The Practicing Physician's Approach to Headache.* Baltimore: Williams & Wilkins, 1992.

Diamond S, Mediana J, Diamond-Falk J, DeVeno T. The value of biofeedback in the treatment of chronic headache: a five-year retrospective study. *Headache* 1979; 19:90–96.

Duke University. *Behavioral and Physical Treatments for Migraine Headache,* Technical Review 2.2, AHCPR Document No. PB99-127946, Agency for Health Care Policy and Research, February 1999. Available via the Internet: http://www.ahrq.gov/. Accessed May 2000.

Epstein MT, Hockaday JM, Hockaday TDR. Migraine and reproductive hormones throughout the menstrual cycle. *Lancet* 1975; 543–548.

Facchinetti F, Martignoni E, Nappi G, et al. Premenstrual failure of α-adrenergic stimulation on hypothalamus-pituitary responses in menstrual migraine. *Psychosom Med* 1989; 51:550–558.

Facchinetti F, Bonellie G, Kangasniemi P, Pascual J, Shuaib A. The efficacy and safety of subcutaneous sumatriptan in the acute treatment of menstrual migraine. *Obstet Gynecol* 1995; 86:911–918.

Fischer AA. Pressure algometry over normal muscles. Standard values, validity and reproducibility of pressure threshold. *Pain* 1987; 30:115–126.

Ford MR, Strobel CF, Strong P, Szarek BL. Quieting response training: Predictors of long-term outcome. *Biofeed Self Regul* 1983; 8:393–408.

Gallagher RM. Menstrual migraine and intermittent ergonovine therapy. *Headache* 1989; 29:366–377.

Gauthier JG, Fournier A, Roberge C. The differential effects of biofeedback in the treatment of menstrual and non-menstrual migraine. *Headache* 1991; 31:82–90.

Giacovazzo M, Gallo MF, Guidi V, Rico R, Scaricabarozzi I. Nimesulide in the treatment of menstrual headache. *Drugs* 1993; 46(1):140–141.

Glover V, Jarman J, Sandler M. Migraine and depression: biological aspects. *J Psychiatr Res* 1993; 27:918–924.

Goadsby PJ, Silberstein SD (Eds). *Headache,* Bluebooks in Practical Neurology, Vol. 17. Boston: Butterworth-Heinemann, 1997.

Goldstein M, Chen TC. The epidemiology of disabling headache. In: Critchley M, Friedman AR, Goring S, Sicuteri F (Eds). *Advances in Neurology*, Vol. 33. New York: Raven Press, 1982, pp 377–390.

Granella F, Sances G, Zanferrari C, et al. Migraine without aura and reproductive life events: a clinical epidemiological study in 1300 women. *Headache* 1993; 33:385–389.

Hering R, Rose FC. Menstrual migraine, headache. *Q Current Treat Res* 1992; 3:27–31.

Holm JE, Holroyd K, Hursey KG, Penzien D. The role of stress in recurrent tension headaches. *Headache* 1986; 26:160–167.

Holroyd KA, Penzien DB. Client variables in the behavioral treatment of recurrent tension headache: a meta-analytic review. *J Behav Med* 1986; 9:515–536.

Holroyd KA, Penzien DB. Pharmacological vs. nonpharmacological prophylaxis of recurrent migraine headache: a meta-analytic review of clinical trails. *Pain* 1990; 42:1–13.

Holroyd KA, Holm JE, Hursey KG, et al. Treatment of recurrent vascular headache: a comparison of a home-based behavioral treatment vs. abortive pharmacological treatment. *J Consult Clin Psychol* 1988; 56:218–223.

Holroyd KA, Penzien DD, Cordingley G. Propranolol in the management of recurrent migraine: a meta-analytic review. *Headache* 1991; 31:333–340.

Holroyd KA, Lipchik GL, Penzien DB. Psychological management of recurrent headache disorders: empirical basis for clinical practice. In: Dobson KS, Craig KD (Eds). *Best Practice: Developing and Promoting Empirically Supported Interventions.* Newbury Park, CA: Sage, 1998.

Holroyd K, Stensland M, Lipchik G, et al. Psychosocial correlates and impact of chronic tension-type headaches. *Headache* 2000; 40:3–16.

Jensen R. Pathophysiological mechanisms of tension-type headache: a review of epidemiological and experimental studies. *Cephalalgia* 1999; 19:602–621.

Jensen R, Rasmussen BK, Pedersen B, Lous I, Olesen J. Cephalic muscle tenderness and pressure pain threshold in a general population. *Pain* 1992; 48:197–203.

Jensen R, Rasmussen BK, Pedersen B, Olesen J. Muscle tenderness and pressure pain thresholds in headache: a population study. *Pain* 1993; 52:193–199.

Jensen R, Bendtsen, L Olesen J. Muscular factors are of importance in tension-type headache. *Headache* 1998; 38:10–17.

Keenan PA, Lindamer LA. Non-migraine headache across the menstrual cycle in women with and without premenstrual syndrome. *Cephalalgia* 1992; 12:356–359.

Kim M, Blanchard EB. Two studies of the non-pharmacological treatment of menstrually-related migraine headaches. *Headache* 1992; 32:197–202.

Krobot KJ, Steinberg HW, Pfaffenrath V. Migraine prescription density and recommendations: results of the PCAOM study. *Cephalalgia* 1999; 19:511–519.

Kryst S, Scherl E. A population-based survey of the social and personal impact of headache. *Headache* 1994; 34:344–350.

Kudrow L. The relationship of headache frequency to hormone use in migraine. *Headache* 1975; 15:36–40.

Kudrow L. Cluster headaches. In: Blau JN (Ed). *Migraine: Clinical, Therapeutic, Conceptual and Research Aspects.* London: Chapman & Hall, 1987, pp 113–133.

Lacroix R, Barbaree HE. The impact of recurrent headache on behavior lifestyle and health. *Behav Res Ther* 1990; 28:235–242.

Linet MS, Stewart WF, Celentano DD, Ziegler D, Sprecher M. An epidemiologic study of headache among adolescents and young adults. *JAMA* 1989; 261:2211–2216.

Lipchik GL, Holroyd KA, France CR, et al. Central and peripheral mechanisms in chronic tension-type headache. *Pain* 1996; 64:467–475.

Lipchik GL, Holroyd KH, Talbot F, Greer M. Pericranial muscle tenderness and exteroceptive suppression of temporalis muscle activity: a blind study of chronic tension-type headache. *Headache* 1997; 37:368–376.

Lipton RB, Stewart WF. Migraine in the United States: a review of epidemiology and health care use. *Neurology* 1993; 48 (Suppl 3):S6–S10.

Lipton RB, Stewart WS, Simon D. Medical consultation for migraine: results from the American Migraine Study. *Headache* 1998; 38:87–96.

Lloyd MA, Appel N. Signal detection theory and the psychophysics of pain: an introduction and review. *Anesthesiology* 1976; 44:147–150.

Loder E. Silberstein S. Efficacy of zolmitriptan in the acute treatment of menstrual migraine. *Headache* 1999; 39:366.

MacGregor EA. Menstruation, sex hormones, and migraine. In: Mathew NT (Ed). *Neurologic Clinics: Headache,* Vol. 15. Philadelphia: W.B. Saunders, 1997, pp 125–141.

MacGregor EA, Chia H, Vohrah RC, Wilkinson M. Migraine and menstruation: a pilot study. *Cephalalgia* 1990; 10:305–310.

Marcus DA, Scharff L, Turk DC. Nonpharmacological management of headache during pregnancy. *Psychosom Med* 1995; 57:527–535.

Martignoni E, Sance SG, Nappi G. Significance of hormonal changes in migraine and cluster headache. *Gynecol Endocrinol* 1987; 1:295–319.

Martin PK. *Psychological Management of Chronic Headaches: a Functional Perspective.* New York: Guilford Press, 1993.

Medina JL, Diamond S. The role of diet in migraine. *Headache* 1978; 5:1020–1026.

Merikangas KR. Psychopathology and headache syndromes in the community. *Headache* 1994; 34:S17–S26.

Merikangas KR, Merikangas JR, Angst J. Headache syndromes and psychiatric disorders: association and family transmission. *J Psychiatr Res* 1993; 27:197–210.

Miaskowski C. The role of sex and gender in pain perception and responses to treatment. In: Gatchel RJ, Turk DC (Eds). *Psychosocial Factors In Pain: Critical Perspectives.* New York: Guilford Press, 1999, pp 401–411.

Nattero G. Menstrual headache. In: Critchley M (Ed). *Advances in Neurology,* Vol. 33. New York: Raven Press, 1982, pp 215–226.

Nattero G, Allais G, De Lorenzo C. Biological and clinical effects of naproxen sodium in patients with menstrual migraine. *Cephalalgia* 1991; 11(Suppl 11):201–202.

Neri I, Granella F, Nappi RE, et al. Features of headache at the menopause: a clinical-epidemiological study. *Maturitas* 1993; 17:31–37.

Nikiforow R, Hokkanen E. An epidemiological study of headache in an urban and rural population in Northern Finland. *Headache* 1978; 18:137–145.

O'Brien B, Goeree R, Streiner D. Prevalence of migraine headache in Canada: A population-based survey. *Int J Epidemiol* 1994; 25:1020–1026.

Olesen JC. Classification and diagnostic criteria for headache disorders, cranial neuralgias, and facial pain: Headache Classification Committee of the International Headache Society. *Cephalalgia* 1988; 8 (Suppl 7).

Olesen J. Clinical and pathophysiological observations in migraine and tension-type headache explained by integration of vascular, supraspinal and myofacial inputs. *Pain* 1991; 46:125–132.

Olesen J. Classification of headache. In: Olesen J, Michael K, Welch A, Tfelt-Hansen P (Eds). *The Headaches.* New York: Raven Press, 2000, pp 9–16.

Paiva T, Batista A, Martins P, Martins A. The relationship between headaches and sleep disturbances. *Headache* 1995; 35:590–596.

Penzien DB, Holroyd KA. Psychosocial interventions in the management of recurrent headache disorders. 2: Description of treatment techniques. *Behav Med* 1994; 20:64–73.

Pryse-Philips W, Findlay H, Tugwell P, et al. A Canadian population survey on the clinical, epidemiologic and societal impact of migraine and tension-type headache. *Can J Neurol Sci* 1992; 19:333–339.

Radnitz CL. Food-triggered migraine: a critical review. *Ann Behav Med* 1990; 12:51–65.

Rains JC, Penzien DB, Hursey KG. Precipitants of episodic migraine: behavioral, environmental, hormonal, and dietary factors. *Headache* 1996; 36:247–275.

Rapoport AM, Sheftell FD. *Headache Disorders: A Management Guide for Practitioners.* Philadelphia: Saunders, 1996.

Rasmussen BK. Migraine and tension-type headache in a general population: psychosocial factors. *Int J Epidemiol* 1992; 21:1138–1143.

Rasmussen BK. Migraine and tension-type headache in a general population: precipitating factors, female hormones, sleep pattern and relation to lifestyle. *Pain* 1993; 53:65–72.

Rasmussen BK. Epidemiology of headache. *Cephalalgia* 1995; 14:45–68.

Rasmussen BK, Jensen R, Schroll M, Olesen J. Epidemiology of headache in a general population—a prevalence study. *J Clin Epidemiol* 1991; 44:1147–1157.

Rasmussen BK, Jensen R, Olesen J. Impact of headache on sickness absence and utilization of medical services: a Danish population study. *J Epidemiol Community Health* 1992; 46:443–446.

Rieder CE, Martinoff JT, Wilcox SA. The prevalence of mandibular dysfunction. I. Sex and age distribution of related signs and symptoms. *J Prosth Dent* 1983; 50:81–88.

Robbins L. Precipitating factors in migraine: a retrospective review of 494 patients. *Headache* 1994; 34:214–216.

Sahota PK, Dexter JD. Sleep and headache syndromes: a clinical review. *Headache* 1990; 35:80–84.
Salonen R, Saiers J. Sumatriptan is effective in the treatment of menstrual migraine: a review of prospective studies and retrospective analyses. *Cephalalgia* 1999; 19:16–19.
Scharff L, Marcus DA, Turk DC. Maintenance of effects in the nonmedical treatment of headaches during pregnancy. *Headache* 1996; 36:285–290.
Schoenen J, Wang W. Tension type headache. In: Goadsby PJ, Silberstein SD (Eds). *Headache*, Bluebooks in Practical Neurology, Vol. 17. Boston: Butterworth-Heinemann, 1997, pp 177–200.
Schoenen J, Bottin D, Hardy F, Gerard P. Cephalic and extracephalic pressure pain thresholds in chronic tension-type headache. *Pain* 1991; 47:145–149.
Schwartz BS, Stewart WF, Simon D, Lipton RB. A population-based study of the epidemiology of tension-type headache. *JAMA* 1998; 279:381–383.
Silberstein SD. Headaches and women: treatment of the pregnant and lactating migraineur. *Headache* 1993; 33:533–540.
Silberstein SD. Migraine and pregnancy. In: Mathew NT (Ed). *Neurologic Clinics: Advances in Headache,* Vol. 15. Philadelphia: W.B. Saunders, 1997, pp 209–231.
Silberstein SD. Menstrual migraine. *Semin Headache Manage* 1998; 3:4–9.
Silberstein SD, Merriam GR. Estrogens, progestins, and headache. *Neurology* 1991; 22:239–244.
Silberstein SD, Merriam GR. Sex hormones and headache. *J Pain Symptom Manage* 1993; 8:98–114.
Silberstein SD, Lipton RB, Breslau N. Migraine: association with personality characteristics and psychopathology. *Cephalalgia* 1995; 15:358–369.
Silberstein SD, Shulman EA. McFadden-Hopkins M. Repetitive intravenous DHE in the treatment of refractory headache. *Headache* 1990; 30:334–339.
Silberstein SD, Lipton RB, Goadsby PJ. *Headache in Clinical Practice.* Oxford: Isis Medical Media, 1998.
Solbach P, Sargent J, Coyne L. Menstrual migraine headache: results of a controlled, experimental outcome study of non-drug treatments. *Headache* 1984; 24:75–78.
Somerville BW. The role of estradiol withdrawal in the etiology of menstrual migraine. *Neurology* 1972; 22:355–365.
Somerville BW. Estrogen-withdrawal migraine: I. Duration of exposure required and attempted prophylaxis by premenstrual estrogen administration. *Neurology* 1975a; 22:239–244.
Somerville BW. Estrogen-withdrawal migraine: II. Attempted prophylaxis by continuous estradiol administration. *Neurology* 1975b; 25:245–250.
Stang PE, Osterhaus JT, Celentano DD. Migraine: patterns of healthcare use. *Neurology* 1994; 44 (Suppl 44):S47–S55.
Stang P, Sternfeld B, Sidney S. Migraine headache in a prepaid health plan: ascertainment, demographics, physiological, and behavioral factors. *Headache* 1996; 36:69–76.
Stein GS. Headaches in the first post partum week and their relationship to migraine. *Headache* 1981; 21:201–205.
Stein G, Morton J, Marsh A, et al. Headaches after childbirth. *Acta Neurol Scand* 1984; 69:74–79.
Stewart WF, Lipton RB. Migraine headache: epidemiology and health care utilization. *Cephalalgia* 1993; 13:41–46.
Stewart WF, Lipton RB, Celentano DD, Reed ML. Prevalence of migraine headache in the United States: relationship to age, income, race and other sociodemographic factors. *JAMA* 1992; 267:64–69.
Stewart WF, Shechter A, Rasmussen BK. Migraine prevalence: a review of population-based studies. *Neurology* 1994; 44:S17–S23.
Stewart WF, Lipton RB, Simon D. Work-related disability: results from the American Migraine Study. *Cephalalgia* 1996; 16:231–238.

Szekely B, Botwin D, Eidelman BH, et al. Nonpharmacological treatment of menstrual headache: relaxation-biofeedback behavior therapy and person-centered insight therapy. *Headache* 1986; 26:86–92.
Tzourio C, Iglesias S, Hubert JB, et al. Migraine and risk of ischemic stroke: a case-control study. *BMJ* 1993; 308:289–292.
Uknis A, Silberstein SD. Review article: migraine and pregnancy. *Headache* 1991; 31:372–374.
Waters WE, O'Connor PJ. Epidemiology of headache and migraine in women. *J Neurol Neurosurg Psychiatry* 1971; 34:148–153.
Welch KMA, Darnley D, Simkins RT. The role of estrogen in migraine: a review. *Cephalalgia* 1984; 4:227–236.
Wilensky GR, Cafferata GL. Women and the use of health services. *Am Econ Rev* 1983; 73:128–133.

Correspondence to: Kenneth A. Holroyd, PhD, Department of Psychology, Ohio University, Room 225, Porter Hall, Athens, OH 45701, USA. Tel: 740-593-1085; email: holroyd@oak.cats.ohiou.edu.

Sex, Gender, and Pain, Progress in Pain Research and Management, Vol. 17, edited by R.B. Fillingim, IASP Press, Seattle, © 2000.

14

Sex-Related Influences in Fibromyalgia

Laurence A. Bradley and Graciela S. Alarcón

Division of Clinical Immunology and Rheumatology, University of Alabama at Birmingham, Birmingham, Alabama, USA

DEFINITION, DIAGNOSIS, AND CLINICAL FEATURES

PRIMARY CLINICAL MANIFESTATIONS

Fibromyalgia is a chronic musculoskeletal disorder that is characterized by widespread pain, exquisite tenderness at multiple anatomical sites, and other clinical manifestations such as fatigue and sleep disturbance (Yunus 1994). It is a disorder that primarily affects women. Indeed, both clinical and population-based studies indicate that between 75% and 95% of persons who suffer from fibromyalgia are women (Wolfe et al. 1995).

The symptom complex associated with fibromyalgia has been recognized for decades. However, it was not until 1990 that reliable classification criteria for this syndrome were developed and published by the Multicenter Committee of the American College of Rheumatology (ACR) (Wolfe et al. 1990). These criteria are (1) widespread pain that persists for at least 3 months; and (2) tenderness in at least 11 of 18 specific anatomical sites. The ACR defined widespread pain as (a) pain in the right and left sides of the body, (b) pain above and below the waist, and (c) axial skeletal pain (i.e., pain of the cervical spine, anterior chest, thoracic spine, or low back).

The ACR Multicenter Committee defined tenderness as the verbal report of pain in response to pressure that is applied with a force of approximately 4 kg with either the thumb (in the clinical setting) or a calibrated dolorimeter (in the research setting). The 18 anatomical sites or "tender points" used for classification were identified empirically. That is, of 30 anatomic sites evaluated in the ACR classification study, the 18 tender points were those that best distinguished patients with fibromyalgia from patients with various other chronic pain syndromes and rheumatic disorders, specifically, low back pain, rheumatoid arthritis (RA), and systemic lupus erythematosus. These tender points are found bilaterally at the following sites: (a) occiput, at the insertion of the suboccipital muscles; (b) lower cervical area, at the anterior aspect of the intertransverse spaces between C5–C7; (c) trapezius, at the midpoint of the upper border; (d) supraspinatus, at the origin of the muscle, above the spine of the scapula near the medial border; (e) second rib, at the second costochondral junction; (f) gluteal area, at the upper outer quadrant of buttocks; (g) epicondyle (lateral), 2 cm distal to the epicondyle; (h) greater trochanter, posterior to the trochanteric prominence; and (i) knee, at the medial fat pad, proximal to the articular line.

SECONDARY CLINICAL MANIFESTATIONS

"Musculoskeletal" symptoms. Individuals with fibromyalgia may report other musculoskeletal symptoms in addition to those included in the ACR criteria. These symptoms include morning stiffness, diffuse arthralgias and myalgias, subjective perceptions of joint and soft tissue swelling, and joint hypermobility (Goldman 1991; Littlejohn 1995). Patients frequently indicate that their symptoms vary with changes in the weather; Hagglund and colleagues (1994) reported higher functional impairment in weather-sensitive patients with fibromyalgia than in those who were not sensitive to changes in weather.

"Nonmusculoskeletal" symptoms. The most prominent "nonmusculoskeletal" manifestations associated with fibromyalgia are fatigue and sleep disturbances (Yunus 1994). The intensity of the fatigue described by patients with fibromyalgia tends to be variable. Fatigue generally is not the primary symptom that limits patients' activities of daily life. However, some patients experience both significant fatigue and pain. In fact, Aaron and colleagues (2000) recently reported that 64% of a sample of 22 patients with fibromyalgia also met standard criteria for chronic fatigue syndrome.

Sleep disturbances have been recognized for decades in patients with fibromyalgia. Two factors have been associated with sleep disturbance in these patients. Moldofsky and colleagues (1975) observed an abnormal pattern of alpha intrusion in the electroencephalographic (EEG) recordings of patients with fibromyalgia during slow-wave sleep. This abnormal EEG pattern is described in greater detail below in the section on the etiopathogenesis of fibromyalgia. Additionally, May and colleagues (1993) reported frequent occurrence of sleep apnea in men with fibromyalgia, and have suggested that fibromyalgia should be regarded as a marker for sleep apnea. It should be noted, however, that there are data indicating that the frequency of fibromyalgia in patients with sleep apnea is comparable to that observed in the general population (Alvarez-Lario et al. 1992).

Fibromyalgia tends to be associated with numerous other disorders characterized by pain or other unpleasant sensory phenomena such as migraine and tension headaches, irritable bowel syndrome, dysmenorrhea and urinary frequency, paresthesias or dysesthesias, photosensitivity, and Raynaud's phenomenon. With the possible exception of Raynaud's phenomenon, these manifestations cannot be corroborated by physical examination (Dinerman et al. 1986). Granges and Littlejohn (1993), however, found that reactive hyperemia and skin-fold tenderness can be objectively demonstrated in most patients with fibromyalgia. Similarly, cold-induced vasospasm, an infrequent event in normal adults, is present in nearly 40% of patients with fibromyalgia (Lapossy et al. 1994).

PATIENT SUBGROUPS

It is common practice to classify patients according to whether other medical conditions are associated with their fibromyalgia symptoms. Patients who meet ACR criteria for fibromyalgia but in whom an underlying or concomitant medical condition cannot be identified are classified as having *primary fibromyalgia*. Patients who develop fibromyalgia also may have suffered for a period of time from other rheumatic disorders such as RA or osteoarthritis. These patients are classified as having *secondary fibromyalgia*. The ACR Multicenter Committee recommended abolishing the use of the distinction between primary and secondary fibromyalgia for diagnostic purposes. Nevertheless, we believe the distinction is justifiable in both the research and clinical setting. With regard to the former, it is desirable to enter only patients with primary fibromyalgia in studies of etiopathogenesis so that any differences between patients and controls may be attributed to fibromyalgia per se and not to concomitant medical disorders. In addition, failure to differentiate primary fibromyalgia from secondary fibromyalgia may prevent investigators from identifying important biological abnormalities associated only with primary fibromyalgia, e.g., elevated cerebrospinal fluid (CSF) levels of nerve growth factor (NGF) (e.g., Giovengo et al. 1999).

Patients with fibromyalgia also can be classified according to whether the onset of symptoms is acute or insidious. Patients who report an acute onset often attribute their symptoms to the occurrence of a "precipitating" event such as a defined infectious process, physical and/or emotional trauma, or stressful life events. The precipitating events identified by patients are not necessarily recent. There is considerable controversy, however, regarding the extent to which some distal events, such as sexual or physical abuse, may be related to fibromyalgia symptoms (e.g., Boisett-Pioro 1995; McBeth et al. 1999). Evidence is conflicting regarding whether physical trauma prior to pain onset is associated with higher levels of pain and disability than those observed in patients with insidious pain onset (Turk et al. 1996b; Aaron et al. 1997a).

Finally, some evidence indicates that it is useful to classify patients with fibromyalgia on the basis of their responses to measures of psychosocial and behavioral responses to pain. A series of investigations using the Multidimensional Pain Inventory (Kerns et al. 1985) suggest that 87% of tertiary care clinic patients with this disorder may be classified into one of three groups using a set of empirically derived rules (e.g., Turk et al. 1996a). These groups were labeled (a) dysfunctional (23%), (b) interpersonally distressed (33%), and (c) adaptive copers (31%). An uncontrolled evaluation of an interdisciplinary pain treatment program found that the patients classified as dysfunctional or as adaptive copers experienced significant improvements in pain; only the dysfunctional patients also reported significant improvements in affective distress and disability (Turk et al. 1998a). It may be useful, then, to tailor treatment plans based on patients' psychosocial and behavioral responses to the experience of chronic pain.

EPIDEMIOLOGY

Fibromyalgia is diagnosed mainly in Caucasian women between the ages of 30 and 50, although it has been observed in children and older adults. Fibromyalgia is recognized primarily in persons from the middle and upper socioeconomic strata (e.g., Wolfe et al. 1995), although one Canadian population-based study suggests that relatively low levels of education are associated with increased risk for fibromyalgia (White et al. 1999). Studies in North America have not carefully examined ethnic group differences in the prevalence of fibromyalgia, although one population-based study in Wichita, Kansas revealed that non-whites comprised only 11% of persons identified as having fibromyalgia (Wolfe et al. 1995).

The incidence of fibromyalgia is unknown, but its prevalence has been estimated using population-based, primary-care-based, or referral-based data (e.g., Forseth and Gran 1993; Masi 1993). The prevalence estimates from various population-based studies are difficult to compare because different criteria have been used to define cases. However, using the ACR classification criteria, population-based studies in Wichita, Kansas and London, Ontario have found overall prevalence rates of 2% and 3%, respectively (Wolfe et al. 1995; White et al. 1999). Both of these studies revealed that nearly 90% of the identified FM cases were women.

Primary-care-based studies have confirmed that fibromyalgia is a disorder that predominantly affects women. The frequency of fibromyalgia among men and women in the primary care setting varies between 1.9% and 3.7%. However, fibromyalgia constitutes one of the most common diagnoses in referral-based rheumatology practices, where the frequency of this disorder varies from 3% to 20% (Masi 1993).

NATURAL HISTORY

Although fibromyalgia often is considered to be a relatively benign disorder, this view is not supported by the few longitudinal studies that have been performed. Three studies of the natural history of fibromyalgia in adults have been performed in the United States (Hawley et al. 1988; Felson and Goldenberg 1994; Waylonis and Perkins 1994). Each found that most patients' symptoms remained stable over periods ranging from 1 to 2 years. However, studies performed in Scandinavia indicate that between 50% and 75% of patients with fibromyalgia report that their symptoms became more severe over periods ranging from 4 to 5.5 years (e.g., Forseth et al. 1999).

ETIOPATHOGENESIS

Many studies have examined biological and psychological variables associated with fibromyalgia. These studies suggest that genetic factors, in combination with abnormal peripheral or central pain mechanisms, are involved in the development of the widespread and chronic pain experienced by patients with fibromyalgia (e.g., Pellegrino et al. 1989).

GENETIC FACTORS

Several studies have examined the relationship between family history and pain experiences in community-based samples (e.g., Lester et al. 1994, Fillingim et al. 2000). All have shown that a family history of pain is associated with increased pain complaints among the respondents. Indeed, two of these studies revealed that the relationship is stronger for women than men (Edwards et al. 1985, Fillingim et al. 2000). Similar findings recently have been produced in a small number of studies of persons with fibromyalgia.

Pellegrino and colleagues (1989) performed the first study of familial aggregation in fibromyalgia. They reported that 52% of a group of fibromyalgia patients' first-degree relatives (71% of women and 35% of men) had findings consistent with fibromyalgia. Buskila and associates (Buskila et al. 1996; Buskila and Neumann 1997) recently reported similar findings. Moreover, these investigators reported that only the female relatives showed significantly lower pain threshold levels than male and female controls at both a subset of the ACR tender points and a group of control points (Buskila and Neumann 1997). In addition, female relatives of the fibromyalgia patients reported poorer health status than did the male relatives of the patients and the controls (Neumann and Buskila 1997).

These findings suggest that a family history of pain may be a risk factor for the development of fibromyalgia. Indeed, Buskila and Neumann (1997) proposed that they indicate a sex-related, autosomal dominant genetic transmission of fibromyalgia. In response to these findings, Yunus and associates (1999) studied 39 women with fibromyalgia who had at least one first-degree relative diagnosed with the same disorder. They estimated that the human leukocyte antigen (HLA)-specific risk to a sister of a woman with fibromyalgia was 1.22. While this value was statistically significant, the strength of the genetic linkage of fibromyalgia to the HLA region was quite modest.

Offenbaecher and colleagues (1999) recently analyzed the genotypes of the promoter region of the serotonin transporter gene (5-HTT) in 59 women and 3 men with fibromyalgia as well as 110 controls (56 women and 54 men). They found that the fibromyalgia patients were significantly more likely than controls ($P = 0.046$) to show a functional polymorphism in the 5-HTT promoter region that has also been associated with affective disorders, anxiety-related traits, and migraine headaches. This relationship is modest in strength, but it is intriguing given the reliable evidence of low serotonin levels (see section "Central Mechanisms" below) and high frequencies of depression, anxiety, and headache among patients with fibromyalgia.

To summarize, a small number of studies suggest that familial factors may be related to the development of fibromyalgia. It should be noted that these preliminary findings are consistent with the evidence produced in animal studies of sex-related, familial differences in pain transmission or pain modulation (see Chapter 3). No relationships have yet been identified between sex-related genetic influences on pain transmission or modulation and the higher prevalence of fibromyalgia in women compared to men. However, we believe it is quite likely that these relationships will be documented in the future.

PERIPHERAL MECHANISMS

Both patients and their health care providers tend to describe the pain of fibromyalgia as muscular and articular in origin. It is not surprising, then, that many investigators have attempted to identify abnormalities in the muscle tissue of patients with fibromyalgia that might account for their pain. For example, Bengtsson and colleagues (1986) reported reductions in the levels of ATP and phosphocreatine, as well as the appearance of ragged red fibers, in the tender areas of the trapezius muscle of patients with fibromyalgia. This may reflect the sequelae of continuous muscle microtrauma, which might contribute to the postexertional pain and other painful symptoms experienced by these patients (Bennett 1993). Other investigators have suggested that prolonged muscle tension and ischemia may account for the painful symptoms of fibromyalgia (Bennett et al. 1989).

Despite these positive findings, no relationships have been found between muscle tension levels and pain in patients with fibromyalgia; moreover, electron microscopic evaluation of muscle biopsies has failed to reveal significant differences between tissue obtained from patients with fibromyalgia and healthy controls (Yunus et al. 1992a). Nevertheless, Park and colleagues (1998) recently used ^{31}P nuclear magnetic resonance spectroscopy to show that fibromyalgia patients, compared to controls, exhibit significantly lower phosphorylation potential and total oxidative capacity in the quadriceps muscle during rest and exercise. Patients also display significantly lower levels of phosphocreatine and ATP, as well as a lower phosphocreatine/inorganic phosphate ratio in this muscle at rest (Park et al. 1998). This represents the first strong evidence of metabolic abnormalities in muscle tissue that may contribute to the fatigue and weakness associated with fibromyalgia.

CENTRAL MECHANISMS

Numerous studies have found that patients with fibromyalgia display generalized tenderness in response to pressure stimulation of both tender points and a wide array of "control" points such as the mid-ulna, mid-tibia, and the thumb nail (e.g., Wolfe et al. 1990; Granges and Littlejohn 1993; Kosek et al. 1995). These patients also show relatively low pain threshold and tolerance levels in response to thermal and electrocutaneous stimulation (Arroyo et al. 1993; Gibson et al. 1994). Moreover, counterstimulation inhibits pain in pain-free controls but not in patients with fibromyalgia (Kosek and Hansson 1997; Lautenbacher and Rollman 1997). These findings suggest that the abnormalities in muscle tissue alone cannot account for the painful symptoms of fibromyalgia. Thus, attention has been directed to the identification of central mechanisms that may distinguish patients with fibromyalgia from healthy persons.

Nonrestorative sleep. Moldofsky and his colleagues (1975) were the first to observe an abnormal pattern in the electroencephalographic (EEG) recordings of patients with fibromyalgia during deep sleep. This abnormal pattern, termed the alpha EEG nonrapid eye movement (NREM) anomaly, is characterized by a relatively fast frequency alpha EEG wave superimposed on a slower frequency delta EEG. Indeed, induction of the alpha EEG NREM sleep anomaly by slow-wave sleep deprivation increases pain sensitivity among healthy men and women (Moldofsky et al. 1975; Lentz et al. 1999).

It should be emphasized that not all persons with fibromyalgia exhibit the alpha EEG NREM sleep anomaly (Carette et al. 1995). Moreover, this sleep disturbance is not specific to fibromyalgia, having been found in persons with RA and other painful disorders (Moldofsky et al. 1983, 1988). These findings suggest that slow-wave sleep disruption may contribute to the development of fibromyalgia symptoms, although the sleep disturbance is not necessary for the syndrome to occur.

Recent studies also indicate important clinical sequelae of sleep disruption in patients with fibromyalgia, such as slowed speed of performance on complex cognitive tasks, fatigue, and negative mood (Côte and Moldofsky 1997). In addition, an intensive longitudinal investigation revealed that, among fibromyalgia patients, a night of poor sleep is followed by increased pain ratings and greater attention to pain on the following day (Affleck et al. 1996). Thus, poor sleep may contribute to the hypervigilance for abnormal somatic perceptions that has been documented in this population (McDermid et al. 1996).

Neuroendocrine abnormalities. Patients with fibromyalgia exhibit several markers of dysregulation of the hypothalamic-pituitary-adrenal (HPA) axis, such as relatively low levels of 24-hour urine-free cortisol and low hypothalamic levels of corticotropin-releasing hormone (CRH) (e.g., McCain and Tilbe 1989; Crofford et al. 1994). They also exhibit impairments in autonomic nervous system functions, such as abnormal response to orthostatic stress and diminished sympathoadrenal responses to hypoglycemic challenge (Martinez-Lavin et al. 1997; Adler et al. 1999).

Abnormal CRH levels may be directly related to these impairments and to the painful symptoms of fibromyalgia (Lariviere and Melzack 2000). For example, CRH influences descending, antinociceptive pathways from the brain to the spinal dorsal horns through its effects on the sympathetic nervous system (Clauw and Chrousos 1997). CRH also may diminish pain through its facilitating effects on glucocorticoid production and opioid-secreting neurons in the hypothalamus that project to the brainstem and spinal cord (Chrousos and Gold 1992). Thus, abnormally low hypothalamic levels of CRH may disrupt the function of several biological systems involved in pain modulation.

There also is evidence of dysregulation of the hypothalamic-pituitary-thyroid (HPT) axis and the growth hormone (GH) axis in patients with fibromyalgia. For example, these patients display blunted secretion of thyroid-stimulating hormone and thyroid hormones in response to thyrotropin-releasing hormone, which suggests an impaired pituitary response (Neeck and Riedel

1992). Abnormalities in the GH axis also may contribute to the pain associated with fibromyalgia. GH has its peak secretion during stage 4 of REM sleep, and it is involved in the maintenance of muscle homeostasis. Bennett and colleagues (1992) have suggested that the alpha EEG NREM sleep anomaly documented in patients with fibromyalgia may lead to decreased GH secretion and subsequently to a vulnerability to muscle microtrauma and pain. Indeed, it has been shown that patients with fibromyalgia do show low basal levels of GH and insulin-like growth factor 1 (IGF-1) (e.g., Bennett et al. 1997). Furthermore, a recent placebo-controlled trial revealed that these patients display significant improvements in tender point scores and functional ability in response to GH injections (Bennett et al. 1998).

Finally, it is well known that sex hormones interact with peripheral and central pathways involved in pain modulation in multiple ways. For example, gonadal hormones influence the activity in the central nervous system (CNS) of neuromodulators involved in nociceptive processing such as substance P (Duval et al. 1996), amino acids such as GABA and glutamate, and other neurotransmitters (e.g., dopamine, serotonin, norepinephrine) (Smith 1994). As a result, some investigators have begun to examine the effects of menstrual-cycle-related hormonal events on symptom reports in women with fibromyalgia. For example, one retrospective study found that 72% of female patients with fibromyalgia reported increased symptom levels during the premenstrual phase (Ostensen et al. 1997). A subsequent prospective study showed that patients reported significantly higher levels of stiffness, fatigue, insomnia, depression, and anxiety during the luteal phase, relative to the follicular phase, of the menstrual cycle (Anderberg et al. 1998b). However, these investigators did not attempt to eliminate from their patient sample individuals who suffered from comorbid physical disorders, such as RA, in addition to fibromyalgia. Thus, the inclusion of these women with secondary fibromyalgia may have reduced the effect of menstrual cycle phase on reports of pain. Indeed, Anderberg and colleagues (1998a) recently reported that women with fibromyalgia, compared to controls, exhibit significantly lower levels of nociceptin, a neuropeptide similar in appearance to the opioid peptides, during the luteal phase of the menstrual cycle. The women with fibromyalgia also tended to show lower levels of nociceptin than controls across the menstrual cycle.

These findings, together with those described earlier regarding the HPA axis, suggest that in fibromyalgia, the pituitary release patterns of adrenocorticotropic hormone, thyroid-stimulating hormone, and growth hormone are altered substantially. The resulting abnormalities in hormone levels (e.g., cortisol, IGF-I), together with the influence of the menstrual cycle, may contribute to the pain, weakness, and fatigue experienced by patients with fibromyalgia. This evidence suggests that patients with fibromyalgia are characterized by multiple abnormalities of the neuroendocrine axes and the autonomic nervous system.

Neuropeptide abnormalities. Serotonin regulates the circadian fluctuations of the HPA axis (Krieger and Rizzo 1969) and probably plays a role in stimulating the release of CRH from the hypothalamus (Holmes et al. 1982). Moreover, it contributes to the activation of descending antinociceptive pathways from the brain to the spinal dorsal horns (Clauw and Chrousos 1997). Several investigators have reported that patients with fibromyalgia, compared to healthy persons, exhibit abnormal metabolism of serotonin and its precursor tryptophan, lower serum levels of serotonin, and lower CSF levels of 5-hydroxyindole acetic acid (5-HIAA, a product of serotonin metabolism) (Russell et al. 1992; Yunus et al. 1992b; Wolfe et al. 1997).

Patients with fibromyalgia also are characterized by elevated CSF levels of dynorphin A and calcitonin gene-related peptide (CGRP) (Vaeroy et al. 1989, 1991). Elevated levels of these neuropeptides and substance P are consistent with changes in CNS function that have been observed after tissue injury. Under these circumstances, a series of events can occur that produce allodynia, or abnormal pain sensitivity (Pillemer et al. 1997). One event is that new axon sprouts that are sensitive to stimulation often develop in the injured area of tissue. Spontaneous firings of these damaged nerves, as well as input from the dorsal horn ganglion, increase the neuronal barrage into the CNS and contribute to the perception of pain. Similarly, spinal dorsal horn neurons also show increased excitability after injury, which is characterized by enlargement of their peripheral receptive fields and enhanced responsiveness to mechanical, thermal, and chemical stimuli. This process of *central sensitization,* which also leads to increased neuronal input to the CNS, is mediated by activation of neurons with *N*-methyl-D-aspartate (NMDA) receptor sites by excitatory amino acids and is enhanced by neuropeptides such as dynorphin, substance P, and CGRP (Pillemer et al. 1997). There is no direct evidence of functional changes in peripheral or spinal dorsal horn neurons in patients with fibromyalgia. However, several recent laboratory studies of behavioral responses to noxious stimulation have shown that these patients display abnormal pain sensitivity consistent with the neuronal changes described above (e.g., Kosek et al. 1996). In addition, one recent study showed that patients with fibromyalgia, compared to controls, display significantly elevated plasma levels of nitric oxide during the vein distension test (Nicolodi et al. 1998). Furthermore, ketamine produced significant pain reductions in 13 of 19 patients with fibromyalgia. Both of these findings suggest that activation of NMDA-receptor sites may contribute to the abnormal pain sensitivity observed in persons with fibromyalgia.

Recent data suggest that stress may enhance the nociceptive effects of substance P release in persons with fibromyalgia. CNS activation by stress stimulates mammotroph cells in the anterior pituitary to secrete prolactin and NGF (Missole et al. 1996). Consistent with these findings, patients with primary fibromyalgia are characterized by elevated CSF levels of NGF (Giovengo et al. 1999). Given that NGF regulates substance P expression in sensory nerves and may inhibit the antinociceptive effects of substance P metabolites (Lindsay et al. 1989), stress may contribute to pain or allodynia in persons with fibromyalgia through its effects on NGF as well as on HPA axis function.

Abnormalities in brain function. Our research group used single photon emission computerized tomographic (SPECT) imaging to perform the first study of brain function in patients with fibromyalgia and healthy individuals during a resting state (Table I; Mountz et al. 1995). SPECT produces accurate, high-resolution images of regional cerebral blood flow (rCBF) that can be coregistered with magnetic resonance imaging (MRI) of brain structure. Alterations in rCBF, then, reflect changes in brain neuronal activity that may be produced by ongoing pathological pain conditions or other events (e.g., stress). Compared to healthy controls, patients with fibromyalgia exhibited significantly lower rCBF levels in the thalamus and caudate nucleus (Mountz et al. 1995). Dysregulation of thalamic activity may contribute to abnormalities that have been documented in HPA axis function and may be a cause of abnormal pain perception (Saade et al. 1999). Evidence from both human and animal studies shows that activation of the caudate nucleus is associated with pain modulation (Lineberry and Vierck 1975; Chudler et al. 1993). Thus, hypoperfusion of the caudate nucleus also may contribute to impaired pain modulation in persons with fibromyalgia.

We have replicated our finding of abnormal thalamic and caudate rCBF in an independent group of fibromyalgia patients (Bradley et al. 1999a). However, we observed that patients whose symptoms began with a physical

Table I
Mean (± SEM) regional cerebral blood flow (rCBF) in the thalamus and caudate nuclei of patients with fibromyalgia (FM) and healthy controls

Location of rCBF Measurement	FM Patients ($n = 10$)	Controls ($n = 7$)	P
Right thalamus	0.84 ± 0.04	1.05 ± 0.03	0.003
Left thalamus	0.87 ± 0.05	1.04 ± 0.03	0.01
Right caudate	0.77 ± 0.03	0.88 ± 0.02	0.02
Left caudate	0.77 ± 0.04	0.90 ± 0.02	0.01

Source: Reproduced with permission from Mountz et al. (1995).

trauma tended to show abnormal rCBF primarily in the thalamus, whereas patients whose symptoms had an insidious onset tended to be characterized by diminished rCBF in both the thalamus and the caudate nucleus. We also studied a small sample of community residents with fibromyalgia who had not yet sought medical care for painful symptoms with insidious onset. Similar to the patients with insidious onset of pain, these fibromyalgia "nonpatients" were characterized by low caudate rCBF. Finally, all of the fibromyalgia groups exhibited significantly higher CSF levels of substance P than the healthy controls. There were no differences among the fibromyalgia groups in pain threshold or clinical pain ratings, although the nonpatients reported lower levels of depression than the two patient groups. These findings indicate that abnormal brain function and CSF levels of substance P in persons with fibromyalgia are not due solely to the influence of psychological distress.

The cause of the thalamic and caudate rCBF abnormalities described above is not known. However, inhibition of thalamic activity may occur as a response to prolonged, excitatory nociceptive input (Iadarola et al. 1995). Indeed, we have proposed that the thalamic and caudate abnormalities in persons with fibromyalgia may be a marker for central sensitization (Pillemer et al. 1997; Weigent et al. 1998). Over time, the modulatory actions of these structures in nociceptive transmission become compromised, thereby contributing to the abnormal pain sensitivity exhibited by persons with fibromyalgia.

If these premises were valid, one would expect that persons with fibromyalgia would show abnormal changes in rCBF in the thalamus and other structures involved in pain processing during exposure to acute, painful stimuli. It should be noted that normal individuals respond to painful phasic stimulation with increases in rCBF in the contralateral thalamus, anterior cingulate (AC) cortex, primary and secondary somatosensory cortices (S1 and S2), and the insula (e.g., Coghill et al. 1994). Moreover, as stimulus intensity increases, bilateral activation occurs in the thalamus, AC cortex, S2, and insula, as well as in the putamen and cerebellum (Coghill et al. 1999). Preliminary findings in our laboratory indicate that fibromyalgia patients with an insidious onset of pain show a different pattern of brain activation than healthy controls during exposure to phasic, right-side, painful stimulation that was calibrated to subjects' pain threshold levels (Bradley et al. 1999b). Our controls showed significant increases in rCBF in the left S1 and left thalamus whereas our patients displayed significant activation of the left and right S1 and the right AC cortex. In addition, the patients' intensity ratings of the stimulation were twice as great as those of the controls, despite the fact that patients received significantly lower levels of stimulation than did the controls. Petzke and colleagues (1999) have used functional MRI (fMRI) to study brain response to noxious stimuli in fibromyalgia patients and have produced initial findings similar to ours.

The pattern of brain activation shown by the patients studied thus far is interesting for several reasons. First, the absence of significant thalamic activation in the fibromyalgia patients suggests that their low pain thresholds and clinical pain may be due, in part, to compromised pain modulation in this brain structure. Second, our patients' display of bilateral activation of S1 also occurs in patients with mononeuropathy and allodynia during brushing of the painful skin area (Petrovic et al. 1999). This pattern of cortical activation may be characteristic of patients with abnormal pain sensitivity (e.g., Pauli et al. 1999). It is still necessary to determine whether patients with fibromyalgia also show activation in the ipsilateral S1 and AC cortex during exposure to painful stimulation on the left side of the body.

PSYCHOLOGICAL DISTRESS AND PSYCHIATRIC MORBIDITY

Hudson and colleagues (1985, 1992) performed two studies in which patients with fibromyalgia were administered either the Diagnostic Interview Schedule (DIS) or the Structured Clinical Interview of the *Diagnostic and Statistical Manual of Mental Disorders III-Revised* (SCID-III-R). In the former study, patients with fibromyalgia more frequently met DIS criteria for lifetime diagnoses of major depression and anxiety disorders than patients with RA. The patients with fibromyalgia also were characterized by high familial prevalence of major affective disorders. The latter investigation involving the SCID-III-R replicated the finding of high familial rates of major affective disorders in fibromyalgia patients described above. These patients also were characterized by high frequencies of migraine headaches and irritable bowel syndrome. It was suggested that fibromyalgia, major affective disorder, panic disorder, and irritable bowel syndrome might represent a group of related conditions, which could be called affective spectrum disorder, that share a common pathophysiology (Hudson and Pope 1989; Hudson et al. 1992).

In contrast to the studies above, our group evaluated the frequencies of lifetime psychiatric diagnoses in three groups of individuals using a computerized version of the DIS (Aaron et al. 1996). These groups were (a) patients who met the ACR criteria for fibromyalgia, (b) community residents ("nonpatients") who also met ACR criteria for fibromyalgia but who had not sought treatment for their pain within the past 10 years, and (c) healthy community residents without any pain (controls). We found that patients with fibromyalgia met criteria for a significantly greater number of lifetime psychiatric diagnoses than either the nonpatients or the healthy controls.

However, we found no difference in psychiatric morbidity between the fibromyalgia nonpatients and healthy controls. These findings strongly suggest that high levels of psychological distress may contribute to the decision of individuals to seek health care for their fibromyalgia symptoms, but are not necessary factors in the etiopathogenesis of fibromyalgia.

We also have reported preliminary findings regarding the factors associated with health care seeking in a 30-month longitudinal study of our nonpatients (Aaron et al. 1997b). We found that the individuals who obtained medical care (i.e., became patients) for their fibromyalgia symptoms during the study period, relative to those who remained nonpatients, were more likely at baseline to report work-related stress, a psychiatric history of mood or substance abuse disorders, and use of prescription medication or medication for gastrointestinal disorders. However, the strongest predictor of seeking health care among these persons was the number of lifetime psychiatric diagnoses at baseline evaluation (Aaron et al. 1995).

MacFarlane and colleagues (1999) recently examined the relationship between psychiatric disorders, as measured by the General Health Questionnaire, and medical consultation in 88 men and 164 women community residents in the United Kingdom with chronic widespread pain and high levels of psychological distress. Across all residents, there was no difference in the risk for psychiatric illness between those who sought medical consultation and those who did not. Among women, however, the risk of psychiatric illness among the consulters was more than twice that of the nonconsulters.

In summary, abnormal pain sensitivity in fibromyalgia cannot be attributed solely to psychiatric illness (Aaron et al. 1996). We do acknowledge, however, that psychiatric illness and psychological distress may enhance perceptions of pain intensity (McDermid et al. 1996) and may motivate persons with fibromyalgia to consult health care providers for treatment.

FACTORS ASSOCIATED WITH SYMPTOM ONSET

Infectious illness. As many as 55% of patients with fibromyalgia report that their symptoms began suddenly during or after a flu-like febrile illness (Buchwald et al. 1987). Additionally, fibromyalgia has been reported to occur after infection with coxsackievirus or parvovirus (e.g., Berg et al. 1993), as well as with human immunodeficiency virus (Simms et al. 1992). However, it has not been possible to reliably identify any immunological abnormalities associated with fibromyalgia (see, e.g., Whelton et al. 1992).

Goldenberg (1993) has suggested that infection may be one of several events that promote a maladaptive behavior pattern leading to the development of fibromyalgia. For example, highly anxious individuals with chronic infections such as Lyme disease may experience sleep disturbance and increased muscle tension levels and avoid physical activity. The stress associated with the chronically high levels of anxiety, in combination with sleep disturbance and physical reconditioning, may then lead to the neuroendocrine abnormalities described earlier in this chapter and thus contribute to the development of fibromyalgia.

Physical trauma. Between 14% and 23% of patients with fibromyalgia report that their symptoms began following a physical injury or trauma such as surgery (e.g., Greenfield et al. 1992). Physical injury can lead to alterations in C-fiber substance P levels and to the development of centrally mediated pain syndromes (e.g., Coderre et al. 1993). However, a direct link between injury and chronic pain has not yet been demonstrated in patients with fibromyalgia.

Goldenberg (1993) has posited that, similar to infectious illness, physical injury or trauma among highly anxious persons may lead to development of fibromyalgia symptoms as a consequence of maladaptive behavior patterns. Indeed, patients who develop fibromyalgia following physical injury are characterized by significantly higher levels of disability, inactivity, or financial compensation than patients without "reactive" fibromyalgia (e.g., Turk et al. 1996b; Aaron et al. 1997a). It is possible therefore, that physical injury contributes to the development of fibromyalgia both directly, by means of changes in C-fiber substance P levels, and indirectly, through its association with financial compensation or other reinforcements (Coderre et al. 1993; Straaton et al. 1996).

Emotional trauma and stress. About 14% of patients with fibromyalgia who attend specialized rheumatology practices associate the onset of their symptoms with an emotionally traumatic event (Goldenberg 1993). We have shown that fibromyalgia patients with a history of sexual or physical abuse, compared to nonabused patients, report significantly higher levels of environmental stress, pain, fatigue, and functional disability (Alexander et al. 1998). In addition, these abused patients with fibromyalgia display a response bias toward perceiving a wide range of mechanical pressure stimuli as painful, regardless of their actual intensities. Studies from independent laboratories have suggested that the effects of abuse on pain and other physical symptoms are mediated by abnormalities in function of the HPA axis (Heim et al. 1998). However, evidence is conflicting regarding the possible role of adverse childhood experiences in the development of fibromyalgia (Boisset-Pioro et al. 1995; Alexander et al. 1998; McBeth et al. 1999).

A MODEL OF THE ETIOPATHOGENESIS OF ABNORMAL PAIN SENSITIVITY IN FIBROMYALGIA

Our group recently developed a model of the etiopathogenesis of abnormal pain sensitivity in fibromyalgia that is based on the literature described above (Fig. 1; Weigent et al. 1998). This model posits that both exogenous factors (e.g., physical trauma, environmental stressors) and endogenous abnormalities (e.g., in the neuroendocrine axes) in genetically predisposed individuals lead to a final common pathway, i.e., specific alterations in nociceptive transmission and neuropeptide production that underlie central sensitization. Activation of neurons with NMDA-receptor sites by excitatory amino acids, and the release of substance P, CGRP, and dynorphin (Russell 1998) cause functional alterations in the dorsal horn spinal neurons that greatly increase nociceptive transmission to the brain. The prolonged nociceptive input from the spinal cord to the brain produced by these alterations leads to functional abnormalities in brain structures, such as the thalamus, that process or modulate pain transmission. Moreover, there is a reciprocal interaction between structures in the brain's limbic system (e.g., the AC cortex) and the HPA axis such that alterations in the functioning of any of these systems may influence the other systems. Thus, the high level of

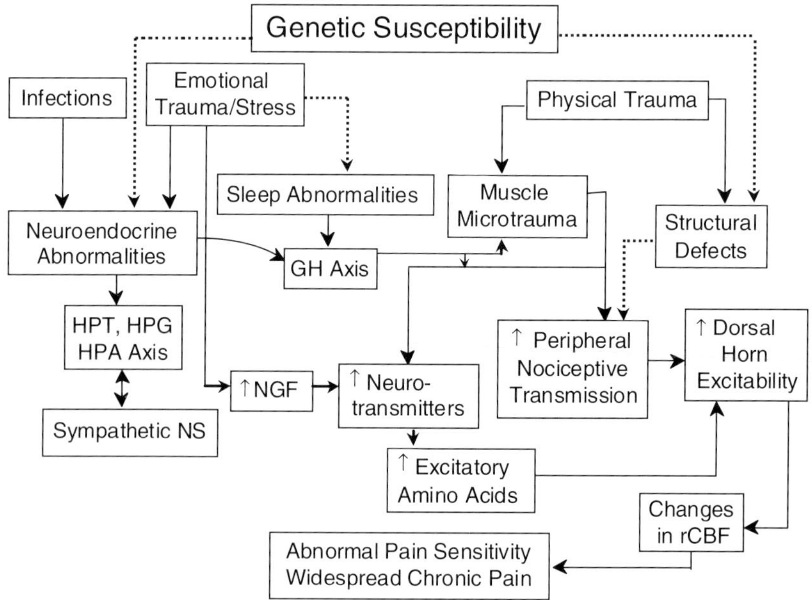

Fig. 1. Authors' model of the etiopathogenesis of fibromyalgia. Solid lines in this model represent established relationships and dotted lines represent relationships that are not yet well-established.

perceived aversiveness of fibromyalgia pain, which is largely processed by the limbic system (Rainville et al. 1997), may represent an emotional stressor that might contribute to and be influenced by the maintenance of HPA axis and related neuroendocrine abnormalities. The endpoints of all of these processes are the abnormal pain sensitivity and widespread, persistent pain that characterize fibromyalgia. Moreover, even after these abnormalities in pain processing have been established, exposure to environmental stressors may heighten perceptions of pain-related affect due to increases in limbic system activity that alter functional activity in the AC cortex, prefrontal cortex, and thalamus. Thus, psychiatric illness and other psychosocial factors may be involved in the development of abnormal pain sensitivity in some individuals and may influence individuals' pain experiences.

Our model is consistent with Melzack's (1996) recent revision of the gate control theory of pain transmission and modulation. The revised theory suggests that brain pathways linking the thalamus, cortex, and limbic system form a neuromatrix that generates patterns of neural activity. This activity underlies the awareness that one's body is distinct from the environment as well as perceptions of pain and pain behavior. Fig. 2 shows that multiple endogenous and exogenous factors may influence the functioning of the neuromatrix. Disorders characterized by chronic pain, such as fibromyalgia, may be produced by alterations in the neuromatrix that cannot be restored to normal function. However, any factor (e.g., change in sex-related hormones, treatment interventions) that alters the function of the pain transmission or

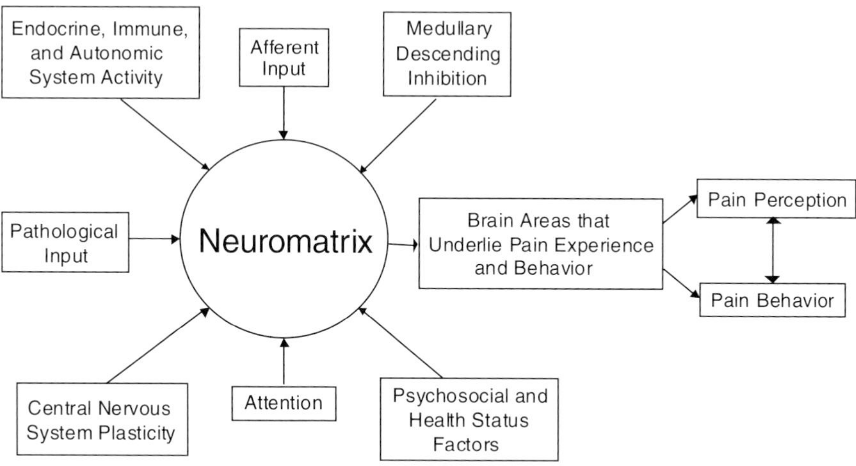

Fig. 2. Model of the neuromatrix. Chronic pain syndromes, such as fibromyalgia, may be produced by pathological alterations in the nervous system and neuromatrix that cannot be restored to normal functioning.

pain modulation pathways shown in our model and in the neuromatrix model may influence pain sensitivity.

TREATMENT

PHARMACOLOGICAL INTERVENTIONS

Amitriptyline and cyclobenzaprine. The first studies of pharmacological interventions for fibromyalgia focused on the efficacy of amitriptyline (a tricyclic antidepressant) and cyclobenzaprine (a tricyclic agent similar in structure to amitriptyline). It has been shown that amitriptyline is superior to placebo in decreasing patients' reports of pain intensity, sleep quality, and global symptom severity (e.g., Carette et al. 1986). There also is evidence that this medication is associated with improvements in pain threshold or tender point counts (e.g., Scudds et al. 1989). The outcomes produced by cyclobenzaprine are similar to those produced by amitriptyline (e.g., Bennett et al. 1988). Cyclobenzaprine appears to induce more consistent improvements in patients' ratings of sleep than in pain intensity, however. Nevertheless, there is strong evidence that the efficacy of these medications diminishes over time (e.g., Carette et al. 1994).

Other psychotropic medications. Anxiety and depression tend to amplify pain perception. Therefore, alprazolam, the selective serotonin reuptake inhibitors (SSRIs), and other psychotropic compounds have been used to modify the pain associated with fibromyalgia. Unfortunately, most of the outcome studies performed with these pharmacological agents have used small patient samples or have been characterized by important methodological weaknesses. Three major findings have been produced to date in this literature. First, Russell et al. (1991) demonstrated that alprazolam and ibuprofen together produce significantly greater reductions than placebo in the tender point index and patients' ratings of disease severity. The effects of these medications have not been assessed over prolonged follow-up periods, however.

Second, two trials suggest that sertraline hydrochloride and venlafaxine produce significant improvements in fibromyalgia symptoms (Alberts et al. 1998; Dwight et al. 1998). The sertraline study is especially noteworthy given that it was a double-blind, placebo-controlled trial. Patients in both the drug and placebo conditions reported significant improvement in pain and mood. However, only the patients who received sertraline showed significant increases in pain thresholds at tender and control points and increases in rCBF in the right and left frontal cortices (Alberts et al. 1998).

Finally, two controlled trials performed in Europe have evaluated the effectiveness of SAMe in patients with fibromyalgia (Tavoni et al. 1987; Jacobsen et al. 1991). SAMe is a methyl donor that exerts antidepressant, anti-inflammatory, and analgesic effects. These investigations demonstrated that SAMe is superior to placebo in improving patients' ratings of disease activity, pain, fatigue, and mood. However, the effects of SAMe over extended follow-up are not known.

Other pharmacological compounds. Generalists and specialists alike use numerous other agents to treat patients with fibromyalgia (Wolfe et al. 1997). The efficacy of these compounds, which include nonsteroidal anti-inflammatory agents (NSAIDs), non-narcotic and narcotic analgesics, and muscle relaxants, have not been rigorously evaluated in patients with fibromyalgia. In this group of drugs, only cyclobenzaprine and growth hormone are known to be superior to placebo in reducing fibromyalgia symptoms (Bennett et al. 1988, 1998).

Meta-analysis of pharmacological interventions. Rossy and colleagues (1999) performed a meta-analysis of the literature on treatment interventions for patient with fibromyalgia. The authors found that antidepressant medications produced significant reductions on measures of fibromyalgia symptoms (e.g., self-reports of pain) and muscle relaxants significantly reduced measures of symptoms and physical status (e.g., tender point counts). However, the positive effects of pharmacological interventions were found primarily in investigations with relatively weak experimental designs (see Bradley and Alarcón 2000).

BEHAVIORAL INTERVENTIONS

Aerobic exercise. McCain and associates (1988) compared the outcomes produced by a 20-week cardiovascular fitness training program with those produced by training in flexibility exercises. Cardiovascular fitness was superior to flexibility training in improving cardiovascular fitness indices, pain threshold, and subjective ratings of disease activity. Similar findings were reported by Burckhardt et al. (1994) and by Gowans et al. (1999). Rossy et al.'s (1999) meta-analysis revealed that aerobic exercise and other physically based interventions produced significant improvements on measures of fibromyalgia symptoms and physical status. Thus, it appears that a structured exercise program that emphasizes aerobic fitness training produces significant and sustained improvements in patients with fibromyalgia.

Cognitive-behavioral therapies. Numerous investigations have shown that cognitive-behavioral therapy (CBT) interventions significantly reduce fibromyalgia patients' ratings of pain, other clinical symptoms, functional disability, and pain thresholds or tender point counts (e.g., Turk et al. 1998a,b). A few of these studies reported that improvements in pain behavior and ratings of pain or functional ability were maintained for up to 30 months after treatment termination (e.g., White and Nielson 1995). In addition, one investigation showed that the effects of CBT were clinically as well as statistically significant (Turk et al. 1998b).

However, only three investigators have performed placebo-controlled studies of CBT interventions for fibromyalgia (Vlaeyen et al. 1996; Nicassio et al. 1997; Buckelew et al. 1998). Two of these groups found that CBT was no more effective than an attention-placebo condition (Vlaeyen et al. 1996; Nicassio et al. 1997). The third group compared the effects of CBT to an exercise intervention, a combination of CBT and exercise, and an attention-placebo condition (Buckelew et al. 1998). All three active treatments produced significantly better tender point index scores than the attention-placebo condition. Nevertheless, this effect was primarily produced by increased pain sensitivity among the attention-placebo patients over time. There were no significant CBT treatment effects on measures of pain or pain behavior. At present, then, CBT interventions cannot be considered to be superior to placebo for the treatment of fibromyalgia (Bradley and Alberts 1999).

TREATMENT RECOMMENDATIONS

There is no generally accepted clinical care pathway for the treatment of patients with fibromyalgia. However, most researchers agree that successful treatment plans should begin with patient education and reassurance that the disorder is neither life-threatening nor imaginary, or associated with development of joint deformities (Buckelew 1989).

There also is general agreement that, although pharmacological therapies do not eliminate pain, they may help patients better manage their pain. Our group tends to emphasize the use of medications such as amitriptyline and cyclobenzaprine. If these are ineffective, we often try SSRIs such as fluoxetine and sertraline, despite the inconsistent evidence regarding their efficacy. Alternatively, we may use anxiolytic medications such as alprazolam in patients who are highly anxious.

Finally, on very rare occasions, we have resorted to short courses of very small doses of corticosteroids for those patients with joint hypermobility in whom pain flares appear to be clearly related to physical trauma and who cannot take either the classical NSAIDs (COX-1-inhibitors) or the newer ones (COX-2 inhibitors).

Another key element in the treatment of fibromyalgia is physical exercise. We encourage our patients to engage in graduated aerobic exercise regimens led by physical therapists who are skilled in using learning principles to reward patients for meeting daily exercise quotas (Fordyce 1976). This approach to physical therapy may be supplemented by palliative interventions such as massage or tender point injections.

Finally, persons who are experienced in providing CBT interventions should administer these therapies to patients who require training in pain-coping skills and who appear able to practice and incorporate these skills in their daily routines. We are aware that, overall, the efficacy of CBT training for fibromyalgia has not been established in placebo-controlled trials. However, our experience is consistent with that of Turk et al. (1998a) in finding that there are subgroups of patients who do respond well to CBT training.

ACKNOWLEDGMENTS

Preparation of this chapter was supported by the National Institute of Arthritis, Musculoskeletal and Skin Disease (1 RO1 AR43136-01; P60 AR20164), and the National Center for Research Resources (5M0100032).

REFERENCES

Aaron LA, Bradley LA, Alexander MT, et al. Prediction of health-care seeking for fibromyalgia (FM) symptoms among community residents with FM. *Arthritis Rheum* 1995; 38:S230.

Aaron LA, Bradley LA, Alarcón GS, et al. Psychiatric diagnoses are related to health care seeking behavior rather than illness in fibromyalgia. *Arthritis Rheum* 1996; 39:436–445.

Aaron LA, Bradley LA, Alarcón GS, et al. Perceived physical and emotional trauma as precipitating events in fibromyalgia: association with health care seeking and disability status but not pain severity. *Arthritis Rheum* 1997a; 40:453–460.

Aaron LA, Bradley LA, Alexander MT, et al. Work stress, psychiatric history, and medication usage predict initial use of medical treatment for fibromyalgia symptoms: a prospective analysis. In: Jensen TS, Turner JA, Wiesenfeld-Hallin Z (Eds). *Proceedings of the 7th World Congress on Pain,* Progress in Pain Research and Management, Vol. 8. Seattle: IASP Press, 1997b, pp 683–691.

Aaron LA, Burke MM, Buchwald D. Overlapping conditions among patients with chronic fatigue syndrome, fibromyalgia, and temporomandibular disorder. *Arch Intern Med* 2000; 160:221–227.

Adler GK, Kinsley BT, Hurwitz S, Mosey CJ, Goldenberg DL. Reduced hypothalamic-pituitary and sympathoadrenal responses to hypoglycemia in women with fibromyalgia syndrome. *Am J Med* 1999; 106:534–543.

Affleck G, Urrows S, Tennen H, Higgins P, Abelis M. Sequential daily relations of sleep, pain intensity, and attention to pain among women with fibromyalgia. *Pain* 1996; 68:363–368.

Alberts KR, Bradley LA, Alarcón GS, et al. Sertraline hydrochloride alters pain threshold, sensory discrimination ability, and functional brain activity in patients with fibromyalgia (FM): a randomized, controlled trial (RCT). *Arthritis Rheum* 1998; 41:S259.

Alexander RW, Bradley LA, Alarcón GS, et al. Sexual and physical abuse in women with fibromyalgia: association with outpatient health care utilization and pain medication usage. *Arthritis Care Res* 1998; 11:102–115.

Alvarez-Lario B, Teran J, Alonso JL, et al. Lack of association between fibromyalgia and sleep apnoea syndrome. *Ann Rheum Dis* 1992; 51:108–111.

Anderberg UM, Liu Z, Berglund L, Nyberg F. Plasma levels of nociceptin in female fibromyalgia syndrome patients. *Z Rheumatol* 1998a; 57(Suppl 2):77–80.

Anderberg UM, Marteinsdottir I, Hallman J, Backstrom T. Variability in cyclicity affects pain and other symptoms in female fibromyalgia syndrome patients. *J Musculoskel Pain* 1998b; 6:5–22.

Arroyo JF, Cohen ML. Abnormal responses to electrocutaneous stimulation in fibromyalgia. *J Rheumatol* 1993; 20:1925–1931.

Bengtsson A, Henriksson KG, Larsson J. Muscle biopsy in primary fibromyalgia: light-microscopical and histochemical findings. *Scand J Rheumatol* 1986; 15:1–6.

Bennett RM. Fibromyalgia and the facts. Sense or nonsense. *Rheum Dis Clin North Am* 1993; 19:45–59.

Bennett RM, Gatter RA, Campbell SM, et al. A comparison of cyclobenzaprine and placebo in the management of fibrositis. A double-blind controlled study. *Arthritis Rheum* 1988; 31:1535–1542.

Bennett RM, Clark SR, Goldberg L, et al. Aerobic fitness in patients with fibrositis: a controlled study of respiratory gas exchange and ^{133}xenon clearance from exercising muscle. *Arthritis Rheum* 1989; 32:454–460.

Bennett RM, Clark SR, Campbell SM, Burckhardt CS. Low levels of somatomedin C in patients with the fibromyalgia syndrome: a possible link between sleep and muscle pain. *Arthritis Rheum* 1992; 35:1113–1116.

Bennett RM, Cook DM, Clark SR, et al. Hypothalamic-pituitary-insulin-like growth factor-I axis dysfunction in patients with fibromyalgia. *J Rheumatol* 1997; 24:1384–1389.

Bennett RM, Clark SR, Walczk J. A randomized, double-blind, placebo-controlled study of growth hormone in the treatment of fibromyalgia. *Am J Med* 1998; 104:227–231.

Berg AM, Naides SJ, Simms RW. Established fibromyalgia and Parvovirus B19 infection. *J Rheumatol* 1993; 20:1941–1943.

Boisset-Pioro MH, Esdaile JM, Fitzcharles MA. Sexual and physical abuse in women with fibromyalgia syndrome. *Arthritis Rheum* 1995; 38:235–241.

Bradley LA, Alarcón GS. Fibromyalgia. In: Koopman WJ (Ed). *Arthritis and Allied Conditions,* Vol. 14. Baltimore: Williams & Wilkins, 2000, in press.

Bradley LA, Alberts KR. Psychological and behavioral approaches to pain management for patient with rheumatic disease. *Rheum Dis Clin North Am* 1999; 25:215–232.

Bradley LA, Sotolongo A, Alberts KR, et al. Abnormal regional cerebral blood flow in the caudate nucleus among fibromyalgia patients and non-patients is associated with insidious symptom onset. *J Musculoskel Pain* 1999a; 7:285–292.

Bradley LA, Sotolongo A, Alarcón GS, Mountz JM, et al. Dolorimeter stimulation elicits abnormal pain sensitivity and regional cerebral blood flow (rCBF) in the right cingulate cortex (CC) as well as passive coping strategies in non-depressed patients with fibromyalgia (FM). *Arthritis Rheum* 1999b; 42:S342.

Buchwald D, Goldenberg DL, Sullivan JL, Komaroff AL. The "chronic, active Epstein-Barr virus infection" syndrome and primary fibromyalgia. *Arthritis Rheum* 1987; 30:1132–1136.

Buckelew SP. Fibromyalgia: a rehabilitation approach. *Am J Phys Med Rehabil* 1989; 68:37–42.

Buckelew SP, Conway R, Parker J, et al. Biofeedback/relaxation training and exercise interventions for fibromyalgia: a prospective trial. *Arthritis Care Res* 1998; 11:196–209.

Burckhardt CS, Mannerkorpi K, Hendenberg L, Bjelle A. A randomized, controlled clinical trial of education and physical training for women with fibromyalgia. *J Rheumatol* 1994; 21:714–720.

Buskila D, Neumann L. Fibromyalgia syndrome (FM) and non-articular tenderness in relatives of patients with FM. *J Rheumatol* 1997; 24:941–944.

Buskila D, Neumann L, Hozanov I, Carmi R. Familial aggregation in the fibromyalgia syndrome. *Semin Arthritis Rheum* 1996; 26: 605–611.

Carette S, McCain GA, Bell DA, Fam AG. Evaluation of amitriptyline in primary fibrositis: a double-blind, placebo-controlled study. *Arthritis Rheum* 1986; 29:655–659.

Carette S, Bell MJ, Reynolds WJ, et al. Comparison of amitriptyline, cyclobenzaprine, and placebo in the treatment of fibromyalgia: a randomized, double-blind clinical trial. *Arthritis Rheum* 1994; 37:32–40.

Carette S, Oakson G, Guimont C, Steriade M. Sleep electroencephalography and the clinical response to amitriptyline in patients with fibromyalgia. *Arthritis Rheum* 1995; 38:1211–1217.

Chrousos GP, Gold PW. The concepts of stress and stress symptom disorders. Overview of physical and behavioral homeostasis. *JAMA* 1992; 267:1244–1252.

Chudler EH, Swigiyama K, Dong WK. Nociceptive responses in the neostriatum and globus pallidus of the anesthetized rat. *J Neurophysiol* 1993; 69:1890–1903.

Clark S, Tindall E, Bennett RM. A double blind crossover trial of prednisone versus placebo in the treatment of fibrositis. *J Rheumatol* 1985; 12:980–983.

Clauw DJ, Chrousos GP. Chronic pain and fatigue syndromes: overlapping clinical and neuroendocrine features and potential pathogenic mechanisms. *Neuroimmunomodulation* 1997; 4:134–153.

Coderre TJ, Katz J, Vaccarino AL, Melzack R. Contribution of central neuroplasticity to pathological pain: review of clinical experimental evidence. *Pain* 1993; 52:259–285.

Coghill RC, Talbot JD, Evans AC, et al. Distributed processing of pain and vibration by the human brain. *J Neurosci* 1994; 14:4095–4108.

Coghill RC, Sang CN, Maisog JM, Iadarola MJ. Pain intensity processing within the human brain: a bilateral, distributed mechanism. *J Neurophysiol* 1999; 82:1934–1943.

Côte KA, Moldofsky H. Sleep, daytime symptoms, cognitive performance in patients with fibromyalgia. *J Rheumatol* 1997; 24:2014–2023.

Crofford LJ, Pillemer SR, Kalogeras KT, et al. Hypothalamic-pituitary-adrenal axis perturbations in patients with fibromyalgia. *Arthritis Rheum* 1994; 37:1583–1592.

Dinerman H, Goldenberg DL, Felson DT. A prospective evaluation of 118 patients with the fibromyalgia syndrome: prevalence of Raynaud's phenomenon, sicca symptoms, ANA, low complement, and Ig deposition at the dermal-epidermal junction. *J Rheumatol* 1986; 13:368–373.

Duval P, Lenoir V, Moussaoui C, et al. Substance P and neurokinin A variations throughout the rat estrous cycle: comparison with ovariectomized and male rats: II. Trigeminal nucleus and cervical spinal cord. *J Neurosci Res* 1996; 45:610–616.

Dwight MD, Arnold LM, O'Brien H, et al. An open clinical trial of venlafaxine treatment of fibromyalgia. *Psychosomatics* 1998; 39:14–17.

Edwards PW, Zeichner A, Kuczmierczyk AR, Boczowski J. Familial pain models: the relationship between family history of pain and current pain experience. *Pain* 1985; 21:379–384.

Felson DT, Goldenberg DL. The natural history of fibromyalgia. *Arthritis Rheum* 1994; 29:1522–1526.

Fillingim RB, Edwards RR, Powell T. Sex-dependent effects of reported familial pain history on clinical and experimental pain responses. *Pain* 2000; 86:87–94.

Fordyce WE. *Behavioral Methods for Chronic Pain and Illness.* St Louis: CV Mosby, 1976.

Forseth KO, Gran JT. The occurrence of fibromyalgia-like syndromes in a general female population. *Clin Rheumatol* 1993; 12:23–27.

Forseth DO, Forre O, Gran JT. A 5.5 year prospective study of self-reported musculoskeletal pain and of fibromyalgia in a female population: significance and natural history. *Clin Rheumatol* 1999; 18:114–121.

Gibson JJ, Littlejohn GO, Gorman MM, Helme RD, Granges G. Altered heat pain thresholds and cerebral event-related potentials following painful CO_2 laser stimulation in subjects with fibromyalgia syndrome. *Pain* 1994; 58:185–193.

Giovengo SL, Russell IJ, Larson AA. Increased concentrations of nerve growth factor in cerebrospinal fluid of patients with fibromyalgia. *J Rheumatol* 1999; 26:1564–1569.

Goldenberg DL. Do infections trigger fibromyalgia? *Arthritis Rheum* 1993; 36:1489–1492.

Goldman JA. Hypermobility and deconditioning: important links to fibromyalgia/fibrositis. *South Med J* 1991; 84:1192–1196.

Gowans SE, deHuerck A, Voss S, Richardson M. A randomized, controlled trial of exercise and education for individuals with fibromyalgia. *Arthritis Care Res* 1999; 12:120–128.

Granges G, Littlejohn G. Pressure pain threshold in pain-free subjects, in patients with chronic regional pain syndromes, and in patients with fibromyalgia syndrome. *Arthritis Rheum* 1993; 36:642–646.

Greenfield S, Fitzcharles MA, Esdaile JM. Reactive fibromyalgia syndrome. *Arthritis Rheum* 1992; 35:678–681.

Hagglund KJ, Deuser WE, Buckelew SP, Hewett J, Kay DR. Weather, beliefs about weather, and disease severity among patients with fibromyalgia. *Arthritis Care Res* 1994; 7:130–135.

Hawley DJ, Wolfe F, Cathey MA. Pain, functional disability, and psychological status: a 12-month study of severity in fibromyalgia. *J Rheumatol* 1988; 15:1551–1556

Heim C, Ehlert V, Hander JP, Hellhammer DH. Abuse-related posttraumatic stress disorder and alterations of the hypothalamic-pituitary-adrenal axis in women with chronic pelvic pains. *Psychosom Med* 1998; 60:309–318.

Holmes MC, DiRentzy G, Giliam B et al. Role of serotonin in the control of secretion of corticotrophin releasing factor. *J Endocrinol* 1982; 93:151–160.

Hudson JI, Pope HG. Fibromyalgia and psychopathology: is fibromyalgia a form of "affective spectrum disorder." *J Rheumatol* 1989; 16:15–22.

Hudson JI, Hudson MS, Pliner LF, et al. Fibromyalgia and major affective disorder: a controlled phenomenology and family history study. *Am J Psychiatry* 1985; 142:441–446.

Hudson JI, Goldenberg DL, Pope HG, et al. Comorbidity of fibromyalgia with medical and psychiatric disorders. *Am J Med* 1992; 92:363–367.

Iadarola MJ, Max MD, Berman KF, et al. Unilateral decrease in thalamic activity observed with position emission tomography in patients with chronic neuropathic pain. *Pain* 1995; 63:55–64.

Jacobsen S, Danneskiold-Samsøe B, Andersen RB. Oral S-adenosylmethionine in primary fibromyalgia: double-blind clinical evaluation. *Scand J Rheumatol* 1991; 20:294–302.

Kerns RD, Turk DC, Audy TE. The West Haven-Yale Multidimensional Pain Inventory (WHYMPI). *Pain* 1985; 23:345–356.

Kosek E, Hansson P. Modulatory influence on somatosensory perception from vibration and heterotopic noxious conditioning stimulation (HNCS) in fibromyalgia patients with healthy subjects. *Pain* 1997; 70:41–51.

Kosek E, Ekholm J, Hansson P. Increased pressure pain sensibility in fibromyalgia patients is located deep to the skin, but not restricted to muscle tissue. *Pain* 1995; 63:33–39.

Kosek E, Ekholm J, Hansson P. Sensory dysfunction in fibromyalgia patients with implications for pathogenic mechanisms. *Pain* 1996; 68:375–383.

Krieger DT, Rizzo F. Serotonin mediation of circadian periodicity of plasma 17-hydroxycorticosteroids. *Am J Physiol* 1969; 217:1703–1707.

Lapossy E, Gasser P, Hrycaj P, et al. Cold-induced vasospasm in patients with fibromyalgia and chronic low back pain in comparison to healthy subjects. *Clin Rheumatol* 1994; 13:442–445.

Lariviere WR, Melzack R. The role of corticotrophin-releasing factor in pain and analgesia. *Pain* 2000; 84:1–12.

Lautenbacher S, Rollman GB. Possible deficiencies of pain modulation in fibromyalgia. *Clin J Pain* 1997; 13:189–196.

Lentz MJ, Landis CA, Rathermel J, Shaver JLF. Effects of selective slow wave sleep disruption on musculoskeletal pain and fatigue in middle aged women. *J Rheumatol* 1999; 26:1586–1592.

Lester N, Lefebvre JC, Keefe FJ. Pain in young adults: I. Relationship to gender and family pain history. *Clin J Pain* 1994; 10:282–289.

Lindsay RM, Lockett C, Sternberg J, Winter J. Neuropeptide expression in cultures of adult sensory neurons: modulation of substance P and calcitonin gene-related peptide levels by nerve growth factor. *Neuroscience* 1989; 33:53–65.

Lineberry CG, Vierck CJ. Attenuation of pain reactivity by caudate nucleus stimulation in monkeys. *Brain Res* 1975; 9:119–134.

Littlejohn GO. A database for fibromyalgia. *Rheum Dis Clin N Am* 1995; 21:527–557.

MacFarlane GJ, Morris S, Hunt IM, et al. Chronic widespread pain in the community: the influence of psychological symptoms and mental disorder on healthcare seeking behavior. *J Rheumatol* 1999; 26:413–419.

Martin L, Nutking A, McIntosh BR, Edworthy SM, Butterwick D, Cook J. An exercise program in the treatment of fibromyalgia. *J Rheumatol* 1996; 23:1050–1053.

Martinez-Lavin M, Hermosillo AG, Mendoza C, et al. Orthostatic sympathetic derangement in subjects with fibromyalgia. *J Rheumatol* 1997; 24:714–718.

Masi AT. Review of the epidemiology and criteria of fibromyalgia and myofascial pain syndromes: concepts of illness in populations as applied to dysfunctional syndromes. In: Jacobsen S, Danneskiold-Samsøe B, Lund B (Eds). *Musculoskeletal Pain, Myofascial Pain Syndrome, and the Fibromyalgia Syndrome.* New York: Haworth Medical Press, 1993, pp 113–136.

May KP, West SG, Baker MR, Everett DW. Sleep apnea in male patients with the fibromyalgia syndrome. *Am J Med* 1993; 94:505–508.

McBeth J, MacFarlane GJ, Benjamin J, Morris S, Silman AJ. The association between tender points, psychological distress, and adverse childhood experiences: a community-based study. *Arthritis Rheum* 1999; 42:1397–1404.

McCain GA, Tilbe KS. Diurnal hormone variation in fibromyalgia syndrome. A comparison with rheumatoid arthritis. *J Rheumatol* 1989; 16:154–157.

McCain GA, Bell DA, Mai FM, Halliday PD. A controlled study of the effects of a supervised cardiovascular fitness training program on the manifestations of primary fibromyalgia. *Arthritis Rheum* 1988; 31:1135–1141.

McDermid AJ, Rollman GB, McCain GA. Generalized hypervigilance in fibromyalgia: evidence of perceptual amplification. *Pain* 1996; 66:133–144.

Melzack R. Gate control theory: on the evolution of pain concepts. *Pain Forum* 1996; 5:125–128.

Missole C, Toroni F, Sigala S, et al. Nerve growth factor in the anterior pituitary: localization in mammotroph cells and cosecretion with prolactin by a dopamine-regulated mechanism. *Proc Natl Acad Sci USA* 1996; 93:4240–4245.

Moldofsky H, Scarisbrick P, England R, et al. Musculoskeletal symptoms and non-REM sleep disturbances in patients with fibrositis syndrome and healthy subjects. *Psychosom Med* 1975; 37:341–351.

Moldofsky H, Lue FA, Smythe HA. Alpha EEG sleep and morning symptoms in rheumatoid arthritis. *J Rheumatol* 1983; 10:373–379.

Moldofsky H, Saskin P, Lue FA. Sleep and symptoms in fibrositis syndrome after a febrile illness. *J Rheumatol* 1988; 15:1701–1704.

Mountz JM, Bradley LA, Modell JG, et al. Fibromyalgia in women. Abnormalities of regional cerebral blood flow in the thalamus and the caudate nucleus are associated with low pain threshold levels. *Arthritis Rheum* 1995; 38:926–938.

Neeck G, Riedel W. Thyroid function in patients with fibromyalgia syndrome. *J Rheumatol* 1992; 18:1120–1122.

Neumann L, Buskila D. Quality of life and physical functioning of relatives of fibromyalgia patients. *Semin Arthritis Rheum* 1997; 26:834–839.

Nicassio PM, Radojevic V, Weisman MH, et al. A comparison of behavioral and educational interventions for fibromyalgia. *J Rheumatol* 1997; 24:2000–2007.

Nicolodi M, Volpe AR, Sicuteri F. Fibromyalgia and headache. Failure of serotonergic analgesia and N-methyl-D-aspartate-mediated neuronal plasticity: their common clues. *Cephalalgia* 1998; 18(Suppl 21):41–44.

Offenbaecher M, Bondy B, de Jonge S, et al. Possible association of fibromyalgia with a polymorphism in the serotonin transporter gene regulatory region. *Arthritis Rheum* 1999; 42:2482–2488.

Ostensen M, Rugelsjoen A, Wigers SH. The effects of reproductive events and alterations of sex hormone levels on the symptoms of fibromyalgia. *Scand J Rheumatol* 1997; 26:355–360.

Park JH, Phothimat P, Oates C, et al. Use of p31 magnetic resonance spectroscopy to detect metabolic abnormalities in muscles of patients with fibromyalgia. *Arthritis Rheum* 1998; 41:406–413.

Pauli P, Wiedemann G, Nickola M. Pain sensitivity, cerebral laterality, and negative affect. *Pain* 1999; 80:359–364.

Pellegrino MJ, Waylonis GW, Sommer A. Familial occurrence of primary fibromyalgia. *Arch Phys Med Rehabil* 1989; 70:61–63.

Petrovic P, Ingvar M, Stone-Elander S, et al. A PET activation study of dynamic mechanical allodynia in patients with mononeuropathy. *Pain* 1999; 83:459–470.

Petzke F, Wolf JM, Clauw DJ, et al. FMRI evaluation of pressure pain in patients with fibromyalgia. *Abstracts: 9th World Congress on Pain.* Seattle: IASP Press, 1999, p 44.

Pillemer SR, Bradley LA, Crofford LJ, Moldofsky H, Chrousos G. The neuroscience and endocrinology of fibromyalgia. *Arthritis Rheum* 1997; 40:1928–1937.

Rainville P, Duncan GH, Price DD, Carrier B, Bushnell MC. Pain affect encoded in human anterior cingulate but not somatosensory cortex. *Science* 1997; 277:968–971.

Rossy LA, Buckelew SP, Dorr N, et al. A meta-analysis of fibromyalgia treatment interventions. *Ann Behav Med* 1999; 21:180–191.

Russell IJ. Advances in fibromyalgia: possible role for central neurochemicals. *Am J Med Sci* 1998; 315:377–384.

Russell IJ, Fletcher EM, Michalek JE, et al. Treatment of primary fibrositis/fibromyalgia syndrome with ibuprofen and alprazolan. *Arthritis Rheum* 1991; 34:552–560.

Russell IJ, Michalek JE, Vipario GA, et al. Platelet ^{3}H-imipramine uptake receptor density and serum serotonin levels in patients with fibromyalgia/fibrositis syndrome. *J Rheumatol* 1992; 19:104–109.

Saade WE, Kafroumi AI, Saab CY, et al. Chronic thalamotomy increases pain-related behavior in rats. *Pain* 1999; 83:401–410.

Scudds RA, McCain GA, Rollman GB, Harth M. Improvements in pain responsiveness in patients with fibrositis after successful treatment with amitriptyline. *J Rheumatol* 1989; 16(Suppl 19):98–103.

Simms RW, Zerbini CA, Ferrante N, et al. Fibromyalgia syndrome in patients infected with human immunodeficiency virus. The Boston City Hospital Clinical AIDS Team. *Am J Med* 1992; 92:368–374.

Smith SS. Female sex steroid hormones: from receptors to networks to performance-actions on the sensorimotor system. *Prog Neurobiol* 1994; 44:55–86.

Straaton KV, Maisiak R, Wrigley JM, et al. Barriers to return to work among persons unemployed due to arthritis and musculoskeletal disorders. *Arthritis Rheum* 1996; 39:101–109.

Tavoni A, Vitali C, Bombardieri S, Pasero G. Evaluation of S-adenosylmethionine in primary fibromyalgia: a double-blind crossover study. *Am J Med* 1987; 83(Suppl 5A):107–110.

Turk DC, Okifuji A, Sinclair JD, Starz TW. Pain, disability, and physical functioning in subgroups of patients with fibromyalgia. *J Rheumatol* 1996a; 23:1255–1262.

Turk DC, Okifuji A, Starz TW, Sinclair JD. Effects of type of symptom onset on psychological distress and disability on fibromyalgia syndrome patients. *Pain* 1996b; 68:423–430.

Turk DC, Okifuji A, Sinclair JD, Starz TW. Differential responses by psychosocial subgroups of fibromyalgia syndrome patients to an interdisciplinary treatment. *Arthritis Care Res* 1998a; 11:397–404.

Turk DC, Okifuji A, Sinclair JD, et al. Interdisciplinary treatment for fibromyalgia syndrome: clinical and statistical significance. *Arthritis Care Res* 1998b; 11:186–195.

Vaeroy H, Sakurda T, Forre O, Kass E, Terenius L. Modulation of pain in fibromyalgia (fibrositis syndrome): cerebrospinal fluid (CSF) investigation of pain-related neuropeptides with special reference to calcitonin gene-related peptide (CGRP). *J Rheumatol* 1989; 19:94–97.

Vaeroy H, Nyberg F, Terenius L. No evidence for endorphin deficiency in fibromyalgia following investigation of cerebrospinal fluid (CSF) dynorphin A and Met-enkephalin-Arg6-Phe7. *Pain* 1991; 46:139–143.

Vlaeyen JWS, Teeken-Gruben NJG, Boosens MEJB, et al. Cognitive-educational treatment of fibromyalgia: a randomized clinical trial. I. Clinical effects. *J Rheumatol* 1996; 23:1237–1245.

Waylonis GW, Perkins RH. Post-traumatic fibromyalgia. A long-term follow-up. *Am J Phys Med Rehab* 1994; 73:403–412.

Weigent DA, Bradley LA, Blalock JE, Alarcón GS. Current concepts in the pathophysiology of abnormal pain perception in fibromyalgia. *Am J Med Sci* 1998; 315:405–412.

Whelton CL, Salit I, Moldofsky H. Sleep, Epstein-Barr virus infection, musculoskeletal pain, and depressive symptoms in chronic fatigue syndrome. *J Rheumatol* 1992; 19:939–943.

White KP, Nielson WR. Cognitive-behavioral treatment of fibromyalgia syndrome: a follow-up assessment. *J Rheumatol* 1995; 22:717–721.

White KC, Speechly M, Harth M, Ostliye T. The London fibromyalgia epidemiology study: the prevalence of fibromyalgia syndrome in London, Ontario. *J Rheumatol* 1999; 26:1570–1576.

Wolfe F, Smythe HA, Yunus MB, et al. The American College of Rheumatology 1990 criteria for the classification of fibromyalgia. Report of the multicenter criteria committee. *Arthritis Rheum* 1990; 33:160–172.

Wolfe F, Ross K, Anderson J, Russell IJ, Hebert L. The prevalence and characteristics of fibromyalgia in the general population. *Arthritis Rheum* 1995; 38:19–28.

Wolfe F, Russell IJ, Vipraio G, Ross K, Anderson J. Serotonin levels, pain threshold, and fibromyalgia symptoms in the general population. *J Rheumatol* 1997; 24:555–559.

Yunus MB. Fibromyalgia syndrome: clinical features and spectrum. In: Pillemer SR (Ed). *The Fibromyalgia Syndrome: Current Research and Future Directions in Epidemiology, Pathogenesis, and Treatment*. New York: Haworth Medical Press, 1994, pp 5–21.

Yunus MB, Kalyan-Raman UP, Masi AT. Electron microscopic studies of muscle biopsy in primary fibromyalgia syndrome: a controlled and blinded study. *J Rheumatol* 1992a; 16:97–101.

Yunus MB, Dailey JW, Aldag JC, Masi AT, Jobe PC. Plasma tryptophan and other amino acids in primary fibromyalgia: a controlled study. *J Rheumatol* 1992b; 19:90–94.

Yunus MB, Khan MA, Rawlings KK, et al. Genetic linkage analysis of multicase families with fibromyalgia syndrome. *J Rheumatol* 1999; 26:408–412.

Correspondence to: Laurence A. Bradley, PhD, Division of Clinical Immunology and Rheumatology, University of Alabama at Birmingham, School of Medicine, 475 Boshell Diabetes Building, 1808 7th Avenue South, Birmingham, AL 35294, USA. email: larry.bradley@ccc.uab.edu.

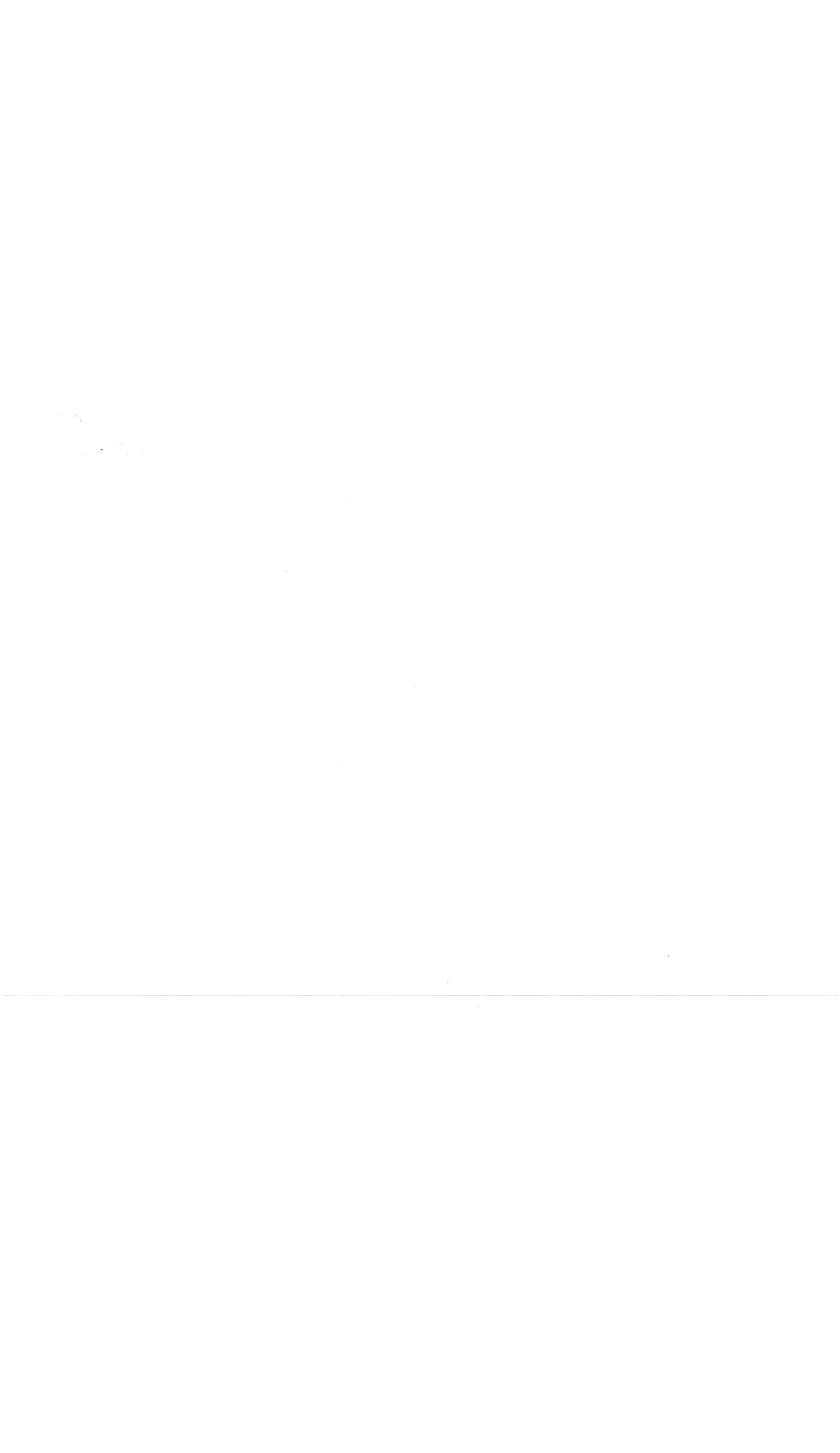

Sex, Gender, and Pain, Progress in Pain Research and Management, Vol. 17, edited by R.B. Fillingim, IASP Press, Seattle, © 2000.

15

Sex-Related Factors in Temporomandibular Disorders

Roger B. Fillingim[a] and William Maixner[b]

[a]*Departments of Psychology and Orthodontics, University of Alabama, Birmingham, Alabama, USA;* [b]*Department of Endodontics and Pharmacology, University of North Carolina, Chapel Hill, North Carolina, USA*

Temporomandibular disorders (TMD) represent a group of conditions characterized by pain and dysfunction in the temporomandibular joint (TMJ) and the surrounding muscles (Dworkin and LeResche 1992). Signs and symptoms of TMD include joint sounds such as clicking and crepitus during mandibular motion, limited mouth opening, pain on palpation of masticatory muscles, and pain on function. These disorders are common, with a prevalence of approximately 12% in the U.S. population (Dworkin et al. 1990; LeResche 1997a). Conceptualizations of the etiology of TMD abound, but these notions are often based on "clinical wisdom" rather than science, and there is little agreement among them. Dworkin (1999) has noted that TMD patients display many similarities to patients with other chronic pain syndromes with regard to the following: low correspondence between subjective symptoms and objective pathophysiological findings; maladaptive behaviors that negatively impact symptoms (e.g., clenching and other parafunctions); clinically significant psychological distress; pain that interferes with occupational, social, and/or interpersonal function; excessive use of the health care system by a proportion of patients.

Thus, TMD is a common and potentially debilitating chronic pain disorder. Several recent reviews have expertly presented information regarding TMD from both epidemiologic and psychosocial perspectives (LeResche 1997b; Dworkin 1999; Rollman and Gillespie 2000). This chapter examines the influence of sex-related factors in TMD, beginning with a review of epidemiologic data regarding sex differences in the prevalence of these disorders. We will discuss sex differences in TMD-related physical and psychosocial symptomatology. Next, we will present experimental findings related to enhanced pain sensitivity in patients with TMD, and discuss several sex-related mechanisms that may help explain why the disorder is more common among females. Finally, we will discuss future directions for the study of sex-related factors in TMD.

EPIDEMIOLOGY OF TMD

Before discussing the epidemiology of TMD, a brief description of diagnostic classification schemes is important. Multiple classification systems for the TMD have been used in the last 30 years. Dworkin et al. (1992) evaluated the methodological and clinical aspects of nine different taxonomic systems. One commonality among these systems is that each distinguishes joint pain (arthralgia) from muscle pain (myalgia). The most recently developed and widely accepted classification system is the Research Diagnostic Criteria (RDC) for TMD (Dworkin and LeResche 1992). The RDC employs a dual-axis system, coding physical conditions on Axis I and psychological status on Axis II. Physical diagnoses are subdivided into three nonexclusive categories: muscle pain (with or without limited opening of the jaw), disk displacements (reducing and nonreducing, with or without limited opening of the jaw), and joint conditions (arthralgia, osteoarthritis, and osteoarthrosis). Specific criteria are described for each diagnosis based on physical examination. Axis II assesses disability and psychological symptoms of depression and somatization using questionnaire methods. Based on their responses to these questions, patients can be placed into one of five graded chronic pain severity classifications. The RDC has shown adequate reliability and validity (Turk and Rudy 1995; Wahlund et al. 1998), and the development of this taxonomy provides the opportunity to standardize diagnoses, which will allow comparisons of research findings from different settings.

The epidemiology of TMD has been thoroughly reviewed in recent years by several investigators (Dworkin et al. 1990; LeResche 1997b; Drangsholt and LeResche 1999), and we will briefly summarize their findings. Given the historically wide variability in diagnostic schemes for TMD, it is important to note that most population-based studies of TMD prevalence use pain in the temporomandibular region as their case definition. This seems justified because pain accounts for most of the suffering associated with TMD, and pain is the predominant factor motivating TMD patients to seek treatment (Dworkin et al. 1990). For ambient TMD conditions present in the adult general population, prevalence rates range from 3.7% to 12%, and the female to male ratio ranges from 1.2 to 2.6, with an average of 2 (Drangsholt and LeResche 1999). Drangsholt and LeResche (1999) also presented data related to treatment seeking in TMD patients, reporting that one-quarter to one-third of TMD patients seek treatment each year, with a female to male ratio of 2.5. For children and adolescents, prevalence rates for TMD pain were generally clustered between 2% and 6%, with no obvious sex difference. However, a more recent survey indicated significantly higher prevalence and greater need for treatment in girls than in boys (List et al. 1999). Another important finding regarding the prevalence of TMD pain is that prevalence peaks between ages 25 and 44 and decreases with age (LeResche 1999). One research group reported that between the ages of 17 and 28, the proportion of women reporting TMD symptoms did not change, while the proportion of men reporting symptoms decreased (Wanman 1996); these findings indicate sex differences in the longitudinal course of TMD in young adults. Also, female patients with acute TMD were more likely than males to continue to have pain 6 months later, which suggests that sex is a risk factor for development of chronic TMD (Garofalo et al. 1998). These epidemiologic data indicate that TMD is a common pain condition associated with greater treatment demand among females, and that it is most prevalent in women during their reproductive years.

SEX DIFFERENCES IN PAIN AND PSYCHOSOCIAL SYMPTOMS AMONG TMD PATIENTS

Research examining sex differences in the severity of TMD-related pain has been limited by the relatively small number of males seeking treatment for this disorder. Bush and colleagues (1993) reported no consistent differences between women and men with TMD on measures of clinical pain, experimental pain sensitivity, personality, or illness behavior. Levitt and McKinney (1994) reported more severe physical and psychological symptoms in female compared to male patients with TMD; however, a greater percentage of male than female patients showed clinically significant psychological and stress-related symptoms. In another study, female TMD patients scored significantly higher on the Present Pain Intensity Scale of the McGill Pain Questionnaire (MPQ), but there were no sex differences on other pain or psychosocial measures (Krogstad et al. 1996). Interestingly, female patients showed reductions on scales of the MPQ 2 years after conservative multidisciplinary treatment, while male patients' pain reports did not change. Von Korff et al. (1990) reported that females were over-represented in Grades 3 and 4 of chronic pain severity, which are characterized by high levels of pain and disability. More recently, in a group of patients who had TMD and other forms of facial pain, reports of clinical pain were similar for men and women (Vickers et al. 1998). These data present a conflicting picture of differences in pain severity for women and men with TMD, which is consistent with findings from studies examining other chronic pain populations (see Chapter 4, this volume; Robinson et al. 1998).

In addition to investigating sex differences in the painful symptoms of TMD, it is important to determine whether TMD-related psychosocial symptoms differ for women compared to men. Psychosocial factors are a significant component of the clinical presentation of TMD. Higher levels of negative affectivity, somatization, stress, depression, and anxiety have been reported in TMD patients compared to healthy controls (see Rollman and Gillespie 2000). Gatchel and colleagues (1996) reported that patients with acute or chronic TMD show higher rates of psychopathology than the general population, and in a more recent study these investigators noted that psychopathology was most strongly associated with a diagnosis of muscle pain (Kight et al. 1999). While few studies have reported on sex differences in the relationship of psychological disorders to TMD, it is notable that some of the psychological disorders frequently reported in TMD patients are more common in females than males (e.g., depression and anxiety).

Another psychosocial variable with relevance to TMD pain is a history of sexual abuse or trauma. We (Fillingim et al. 1997) and others (Riley et al. 1998) have reported that nearly half of TMD patients report a history of sexual or physical abuse. Abuse history was associated with higher levels of depression, anxiety, and somatization in one study (Riley et al. 1998); however, we failed to observe any association between abuse history and clinical or psychosocial variables in our sample (Fillingim et al. 1997). This may be due to our smaller sample and its nonclinical nature, compared to Riley et al.'s larger clinical sample. Certainly, studies of abuse history in other chronic pain populations are more consistent with the findings of Riley's group in that abuse history is typically associated with increased physical and psychological symptoms in chronic pain patients (Domino and Haber 1987; Goldberg 1994; Scarinci et al. 1994; Leserman et al. 1996; Alexander et al. 1998). Indeed, even in nonclinical samples, self-reported abuse history has been related to increased pain complaints and psychological disturbance (Linton 1997; Fillingim et al. 1999c). Linton (1997) found that self-reported sexual abuse was associated with increased risk of pronounced musculoskeletal pain for females but not males; however, we (Fillingim et al. 1999c) found that abuse history was associated with increased pain complaints for both sexes. However, females are more often victims of abuse; thus, the effects of abuse on pain responses are more likely to be experienced by females than males.

STUDIES OF EXPERIMENTAL PAIN SENSITIVITY IN TMD

Maixner et al. (1995b) have previously proposed that TMD may be associated with impairments in the functional integrity of inhibitory systems in the central nervous system (CNS). They theorized that a dysregulation of CNS inhibition systems produces exaggerated responses to both aversive somatosensory and psychosocial stimuli. In support of this hypothesis, patients with myofascial pain in the temporomandibular region have demonstrated lower electrical and mechanical pain thresholds compared to pain-free controls (Molin et al. 1973; Malow et al. 1980). In addition, we have reported several findings suggesting enhanced pain sensitivity among patients with TMD. First, we compared responses to experimental pain in 52 TMD patients and 23 age- and sex-matched controls (Maixner et al. 1995a). The experimental pain protocol included assessment of pain threshold and tolerance both for thermal pain and for ischemic pain induced by the submaximal effort tourniquet procedure. The TMD group showed lower thermal pain threshold and lower ischemic pain threshold and tolerance relative to the controls. In a subsequent report, we examined the clinical relevance of the tourniquet procedure by comparing clinical pain and psychosocial variables in two groups of TMD patients who had high and low ischemic pain tolerance, respectively (Fillingim et al. 1996b). The only difference identified between the groups was that the low-tolerance patients also reported more clinical pain at the time of testing and for the week preceding the experimental session. Thus, greater ischemic pain sensitivity was associated with enhanced clinical pain. More recently, we reported that TMD patients showed more pronounced temporal summation of thermal pain compared to controls (Maixner et al. 1998). Taken together, these findings provide strong evidence that TMD is characterized by enhanced sensitivity to painful stimuli.

As described above, dysfunctional CNS inhibitory systems may not only contribute to increases in pain sensitivity, but may also enhance physiological and behavioral responses to psychosocial stressors. Several investigators have reported enhanced stress-related responses among TMD patients. For example, TMD patients reported greater physical and psychological symptoms of stress than controls (Beaton et al. 1991). Flor et al. (1991) also found that TMD patients reported greater stress than healthy controls. In addition, Flor's group examined electromyographic (EMG) responses to laboratory stress. TMD patients exhibited greater EMG reactivity in the masseter muscle during recall of a personally relevant stressor. Another study failed to find group differences in masseter activity, but reported slower habituation of temporalis muscle activity during stress in TMD patients (Katz et al.

1989). Another group of investigators reported enhanced EMG responses to stress in the frontalis muscles (Kapel et al. 1989). Curran et al. (1996) showed no differences in masseter muscle or cardiovascular responses to mental arithmetic or painful stimulation, but TMD patients reported more negative emotions in response to these stressors. These studies demonstrate consistently that TMD patients report greater subjective responses to stress compared to healthy controls, and provide some evidence of enhanced psychophysiological responses among individuals with TMD.

SEX-RELATED FACTORS CONTRIBUTING TO TMD

HORMONAL FACTORS

Ovarian hormones constitute an important set of sex-related factors that may contribute to symptomatology in TMD. Several recent reports have implicated ovarian hormones in this chronic pain condition, in part because its peak prevalence occurs in women during their reproductive years, when ovarian steroids are most active (LeResche 1997c). More direct evidence comes from a large-scale epidemiologic study by LeResche et al. (1997b), who demonstrated that oral contraceptive (OC) use and estrogen replacement therapy in pre- and postmenopausal women, respectively, were associated with significantly increased risk for TMD. In another study of TMD patients, those not using OC exhibited slightly more variance in pain reports across the menstrual cycle compared to OC users, with peak pain occurring during the menstrual and premenstrual phases (Dao et al. 1997). Moreover, females with premenstrual symptoms are more likely to report TMD than are women without premenstrual symptoms (LeResche et al. 1997a), and a recent study suggested increased premenstrual symptoms among TMD patients versus controls (Carlson et al. 1998).

The mechanisms whereby sex steroids produce their effects are unknown; however, as reviewed elsewhere in this volume and in other sources (Fillingim and Ness 2000), sex hormones can alter nociceptive processing in the periphery and in the CNS. Of particular relevance to TMD is the finding that estrogen treatments can alter receptive field properties of primary afferents in the trigeminal nerve (Bereiter et al. 1980). Also, estrogen receptors have been identified in the TMJ in nonhuman animals (Aufdemorte et al. 1986), although contradictory findings have been reported in human studies (Abubaker et al. 1993; Campbell et al. 1993). However, the function of these receptors, if present in the TMJ, remains unclear.

PSYCHOSOCIAL FACTORS

Psychosocial factors, whose importance in TMD has been reviewed by several authors (Dworkin 1999; Rollman and Gillespie 2000), represent another sex-related mechanism that may influence TMD. For example, psychological symptoms such as depression and anxiety are more prevalent among females than males in the general population, and are associated with increased pain and other physical symptoms (Moldin et al. 1993; Rajala et al. 1995; Kroenke and Spitzer 1998). In addition, affective distress has been related to greater experimental pain sensitivity (Graffenried et al. 1978; Dougher et al. 1987; Cornwall and Donderi 1988; Zelman et al. 1991). Therefore, greater emotional distress among females may predispose them to both increased clinical pain and enhanced experimental pain responses, both of which are characteristic of TMD. Another psychological variable, catastrophizing, has been associated with poorer adjustment to clinical pain (Lester et al. 1996; Kashikar-Zuck et al. 1997; Keefe et al. 1997) as well as decreased tolerance of laboratory pain (Geisser et al. 1992). We (Fillingim et al. 1999c) and others (Lefebvre et al. 1994) have reported higher levels of catastrophizing among healthy females relative to males, which could create an increased risk of experiencing clinical pain, including TMD-related pain. Recently, Kuttila et al. (1998) reported that female TMD patients had a more pronounced need for treatment, which seemed to be correlated with higher self-reported symptoms of stress.

In addition to increasing risk for experiencing pain, psychosocial factors may influence pain differently in women and men who already have TMD pain. Support for this view comes primarily from studies of non-TMD pain populations. For example, Haley and colleagues (1985) reported that depression was associated with pain severity among female patients with chronic pain, while depression related more to activity impairment among male patients. Weir and colleagues (1996) found that the predictors of adjustment varied for women and men in a heterogeneous chronic pain sample. Specifically, women's adjustment was accounted for primarily by cognitive variables, such as the meaning they attributed to their pain, whereas for males social support was the strongest predictor of adjustment. In addition, psychosocial adjustment was related to health expenditures for women, but not men. More recently, a self-reported history of traumatic events was associated with poorer affective adjustment among male patients with chronic musculoskeletal pain, but trauma history was not related to adjustment among female patients (Spertus et al. 1999). High levels of anxiety were associated with increased pain severity and greater pain-related disability among men, but not women, in a sample of patients with primarily musculoskeletal pain

(Edwards et al. 2000). These findings suggest that the predictors of adjustment to chronic pain may be sex-dependent; however, additional research is needed to determine whether these effects are present in patients with TMD.

CENTRAL PAIN MODULATION

As discussed above, we (Maixner et al. 1995a, 1998; Fillingim et al. 1996b) and others (Molin et al. 1973; Malow et al. 1980) have reported greater sensitivity to noxious stimuli in TMD patients compared to healthy controls. This finding supports the possibility that disturbances in CNS pain regulation contribute to the development and maintenance of TMD. Previous findings indicate that healthy females exhibit enhanced sensitivity to experimental pain relative to males (see Chapter 9). The greater sensitivity to pain among healthy females, which may result from sex differences in endogenous pain modulation, could thus be associated with increased risk for developing TMD. Indeed, we have previously reported greater sensitivity to thermal and ischemic pain among females compared to males (Fillingim et al. 1996, 1999a,b; Fillingim and Maixner 1996). Also, females demonstrated greater temporal summation of thermal pain than their male counterparts (Fillingim et al. 1998). These findings parallel the results from studies of TMD patients versus controls. Also, pain-free females developed greater jaw pain than males after two sessions of experimental jaw clenching (Plesh et al. 1998).

Recent studies have noted that the qualitative and quantitative nature of pain-regulatory systems that regulate ischemic muscle pain may differ between men and women. One endogenous system that regulates pain perception is influenced by resting arterial blood pressure. Several investigators have shown a relationship between resting arterial blood pressure and pain sensitivity (Bruehl et al. 1999; France 1999). Arterial blood pressure may influence pain sensitivity by activating baroreceptor afferents, which in turn activate central pain-inhibitory networks. In general, the relationship between blood pressure and pain sensitivity is readily observed in men, is less evident in females, and is not present in females with TMD (Fillingim and Maixner 1996; Maixner et al. 1997; E.E. Bragdon, unpublished observation). The ability of the endogenous opioid system to regulate pain perception may also show gender-specificity. We have recently observed that resting plasma levels of the endogenous opioid β-endorphin are positively correlated with ischemic pain tolerance in pain-free males, are not correlated with ischemic pain tolerance in pain-free females, and are negatively correlated in females with TMD. These data suggest that there may be both qualitative and quantitative differences in pain-regulatory systems in females and males, and that female TMD patients may have impairments in multiple pain-inhibitory systems. Whether these deficits represent predisposing risk factors that enable the development of TMD is an interesting question that only longitudinal prospective studies can answer.

COMORBIDITY WITH OTHER CLINICAL SYNDROMES

High rates of comorbidity have been reported between TMD and other clinical disorders that are also more common in women than men. For example, fibromyalgia (FM) is more common in patients with TMD than in the general population. Plesh and associates (1996) reported that 18.4% of TMD patients met the criteria for FM, while 75% of FM patients satisfied the criteria for TMD. Recently, Raphael and colleagues (2000) found that 23.5% of TMD patients also reported a history of FM; patients with comorbid FM had more severe physical and psychosocial symptoms of TMD. In addition, irritable bowel syndrome appears more common in TMD patients (Korszun et al. 1998), and depression is more common in TMD than in the general population (Gallagher et al. 1991; Dohrenwend et al. 1999). As noted above, there also appears to be comorbidity between TMD and premenstrual syndrome (LeResche et al. 1997a). Thus, it is possible that TMD is one of a cluster of stress-related disorders characterized by pain, hypothalamic-pituitary-adrenal axis dysfunction, and psychosocial symptoms for which women are at greater risk (Gruber et al. 1996; Crofford 1998).

FAMILIAL FACTORS

Familial factors have been demonstrated to influence several pain disorders. For example, in a heterogeneous group of chronic pain patients, 59.5% reported having a first-degree relative with chronic pain (Katon et al. 1985). Several studies indicate familial aggregation of fibromyalgia (FM) (Pellegrino et al. 1989; Buskila et al. 1996; Buskila and Neumann 1997), and Schanberg and associates (1998) reported that the parents of children with juvenile primary fibromyalgia syndrome had multiple chronic pain conditions. Also, a retrospective community survey found that a family history of headache was a significant predictor of developing this disorder, and that a family history of neck pain was the best predictor of whether subjects had experienced neck pain themselves (Schrader et al. 1996). Additional results have demonstrated the importance of family history in several headache conditions (Messinger et al. 1991; Ottman et al. 1993), and a recent study reported that a history of headache in family members, especially the mother, predicted the occurrence of headache in children (Aromaa et al. 1998).

Regarding familial influences on TMD, Hartrick and associates (1986) examined parent-child pairs in which both parent and child had been treated at the pain clinic for various pain conditions. Of 13 such pairs, 11 were mother-daughter pairs, and while none of the 11 mothers had TMD, 6 (55%) of the daughters had this disorder. Raphael and colleagues (1990) found that TMD patients reported significantly higher rates of illness in their children compared to controls. These studies indirectly suggest that familial factors may be involved in TMD; however, another investigation found that only 7% of a large group of non-neuropathic facial pain patients reported a family history of facial pain (Rasmussen 1990). More recently, Morrow and colleagues (1996) reported a higher rate of TMD among family members of TMD patients with anterior disk displacement compared to TMD patients without disk displacement. Conversely, Raphael and colleagues (1999) found no evidence of familial aggregation of myofascial TMD.

Thus, familial factors appear important in several chronic pain states, but the evidence supporting familial effects in TMD is inconsistent. However, familial factors may play a nonspecific role in TMD as well as other pain conditions by contributing to increased pain reports and potentially to enhanced pain sensitivity. Several community-based studies have reported that a familial pain history is associated with increased pain complaints (Edwards et al. 1985; Sternbach 1986; Lester et al. 1994; Koutantji et al. 1998). Some evidence indicates that the influence of family history on pain may be sex-related. For instance, Edwards et al. (1985) found that the relationship between family history and pain complaints was stronger for females than males. Also, Neumann and Buskila (1997) found that first-degree relatives of FM patients were characterized by higher tender-point counts than controls, regardless of gender; however, only female relatives exhibited lower pressure pain thresholds, and female relatives of FM patients had poorer health status than did male relatives of FM patients and controls. We have recently shown that a self-reported familial pain history is associated with increased recent pain complaints and enhanced experimental pain sensitivity among females, but not males (Fillingim et al. 2000). Thus, it seems plausible that a familial pain history may increase risk for TMD (and possibly other pain conditions) by producing enhanced pain sensitivity and greater likelihood of experiencing clinical pain, and this effect may be stronger for females than males.

TREATMENT OF TMD

Clinical management of TMD takes on many forms, including surgery, pharmacotherapy, occlusal interventions, oral splints, physical therapy, and psychosocial interventions. A review of the efficacy of these forms of treatment is outside the scope of this chapter, and the reader is referred to several recent reviews for more information (Dolwick and Dimitroulis 1994; Dworkin 1996; Ash and Ramfjord 1998; Brazeau et al. 1998; Dao and Lavigne 1998). While multiple treatment modalities are available, prevailing opinions favor conservative, reversible treatment due to the unknown pathogenesis of TMD and its generally self-limiting nature (McNeill 1997; Stohler and Zarb 1999). Oral splints are the most frequently used treatment option, and they appear to be effective; however, the mechanisms of action remain unknown and the therapeutic benefits may be nonspecific (Dao and Lavigne 1998). Cognitive-behavioral therapies are generally effective, although the treatment effects may be modest (Dworkin 1996, 1997, 1999). Interestingly, combinations of therapies may prove more effective than either treatment alone. For example, Turk and colleagues (1993) reported that biofeedback and intraoral appliance therapies were equally effective; however, the two treatments combined provided significantly better results than either treatment alone.

There are important potential sex differences in the delivery and effectiveness of treatment for TMD. Treatment need is higher in women, and the female to male ratio is much higher in clinical populations than in the community (Carlsson and LeResche 1995). The reasons for increased treatment seeking among females are not known; however, in general women seek more health care than men (Verbrugge 1989; Kandrack et al. 1991). Also, TMD patients with higher levels of pain, disability, and somatization seek treatment more often than those with milder symptoms (Dworkin 1994), and women are over-represented in the higher grades of chronic pain severity (Von Korff et al. 1990). Indeed, von Korff (1991) reported that the greater health care use among TMD patients was not accounted for by gender alone; rather, female patients sought care more frequently because they had more severe pain. The type of treatment provided may also differ for women and men. For example, Marbach and colleagues (1997) reported that female patients are treated more often by surgical intervention than males. The reasons for this discrepancy are unclear, but the authors point out that it may result from patient self-selection or an increased likelihood that a clinician would recommend surgery for a female. To our knowledge only one study provides data on sex differences in treatment outcomes for TMD. These investigators reported that females showed significant decreases in pain 2 years after conservative multidisciplinary treatment, while male patients' pain reports remained unchanged (Krogstad et al. 1996). Clearly, additional research is needed to determine whether various treatments are differentially effective for women and men.

CONCLUSIONS AND FUTURE DIRECTIONS

The information presented in this chapter indicates that sex-related factors may contribute to TMD in important ways. Population-based studies indicate that women are twice as likely as men to experience TMD, and the sex ratio in the clinic is far more disproportionate, suggesting much greater treatment seeking among women. Various factors could account for these sex differences, including hormonal factors, psychosocial considerations, sex differences in pain perception and central pain modulation, and social factors such as family history. Complex interactions among these and other factors are probably responsible for the sex differences in the prevalence and impact of TMD. Several important questions related to sex-related contributions in TMD must be addressed. Additional research is needed into the influence of ovarian hormones in TMD. How do these hormones influence symptoms of TMD, and what is the function of estrogen receptors in the TMJ? Also, a better understanding of sex differences in treatment seeking for TMD is required. What are the factors that create this difference? Should public health advocates encourage males to seek more treatment or females to seek less? Another important issue is the role of enhanced pain sensitivity in TMD risk. Does enhanced pain sensitivity predispose individuals to TMD, or does TMD produce greater pain sensitivity after it develops? Longitudinal prospective studies of pain-free individuals are needed to determine whether premorbid pain sensitivity is a risk factor for the development of TMD. Theories of the pathogenesis of TMD must take sex-related factors into account, and further research on these issues will enhance our understanding of this complex disorder and will ultimately lead to improved diagnosis and treatment.

ACKNOWLEDGMENTS

This work was supported in part by NIH/NIDCR grants DE12261 (R.B. Fillingim), DE07509 (W. Maixner), and 1-P60-DE13079 (W. Maixner).

REFERENCES

Abubaker AO, Raslan WF, Sotereanos GC. Estrogen and progesterone receptors in temporomandibular joint discs of symptomatic and asymptomatic persons: a preliminary study. *J Oral Maxillofac Surg* 1993; 51:1096–1100.

Alexander RW, Bradley LA, Alarcon GS, et al. Sexual and physical abuse is associated with outpatient health care utilization and pain medication usage in women with fibromyalgia. *Arthritis Care Res* 1998; 11:102–115.

Aromaa M, Rautava P, Helenius H, Sillanpaa ML. Factors of early life as predictors of headache in children at school entry. *Headache* 1998; 38:23–30.

Ash MMJ, Ramfjord SP. Reflections on the Michigan splint and other intraocclusal devices. *J Mich Dent Assoc* 1998; 80:32–35.

Aufdemorte TB, Van Sickels JE, Dolwick MF, et al. Estrogen receptors in the temporomandibular joint of the baboon (*Papio cynocephalus*): an autoradiographic study. *Oral Surg Oral Med Oral Pathol Oral Radiol Endodot* 1986; 61:307–314.

Beaton RD, Egan KJ, Nakagawa Kogan H, Morrison KN. Self-reported symptoms of stress with temporomandibular disorders: comparisons to healthy men and women. *J Prosthet Dent* 1991; 65:289–293.

Bereiter DA, Stanford LR, Barker DJ. Hormone-induced enlargement of receptive fields in trigeminal mechano-receptive neurons. II. Possible mechanisms. *Brain Res* 1980; 184:411–423.

Brazeau GA, Gremillion HA, Widmer CG, et al. The role of pharmacy in the management of patients with temporomandibular disorders and orofacial pain. *J Am Pharm Assoc* 1998; 38:354–361.

Bruehl S, McCubbin JA, Harden RN. Theoretical review: altered pain regulatory systems in chronic pain. *Neurosci Biobehav Rev* 1999; 23:877–890.

Bush FM, Harkins SW, Harrington WG, Price DD. Analysis of gender effects on pain perception and symptom presentation in temporomandibular joint pain. *Pain* 1993; 53:73–80.

Buskila D, Neumann L. Fibromyalgia syndrome (FM) and nonarticular tenderness in relatives of patients with FM. *J Rheumatol* 1997; 24:941–944.

Buskila D, Neumann L, Hazanov I, Carmi R. Familial aggregation in the fibromyalgia syndrome. *Semin Arthritis Rheum* 1996; 26:605–611.

Campbell JH, Courey MS, Bourne P, Odziemiec C. Estrogen receptor analysis of human temporomandibular disc. *J Oral Maxillofac Surg* 1993; 51:1101–1105.

Carlson CR, Reid KI, Curran SL, et al. Psychological and physiological parameters of masticatory muscle pain. *Pain* 1998; 76:297–307.

Carlsson GE, LeResche L. Epidemiology of temporomandibular disorders. In: Sessle BJ, Bryant PS, Dionne RA (Eds). *Temporomandibular Disorders and Related Pain Conditions,* Progress in Pain Research and Management, Vol. 4. Seattle: IASP Press, 1995, pp 211–226.

Cornwall A, Donderi DC. The effect of experimentally induced anxiety on the experience of pressure pain. *Pain* 1988; 35:105–113.

Crofford LJ. Neuroendocrine abnormalities in fibromyalgia and related disorders. *Am J Med Sci* 1998; 315:359–366.

Curran SL, Carlson CR, Okeson JP. Emotional and physiologic responses to laboratory challenges: patients with temporomandibular disorders versus matched control subjects. *J Orofac Pain* 1996; 10:141–150.

Dao TT, Lavigne GJ. Oral splints: the crutches for temporomandibular disorders and bruxism? *Crit Rev Oral Biol Med* 1998; 9:345–361.

Dao TTT, Knight K, Ton-That V. Modulation of myofascial pain patterns by oral contraceptives: a preliminary report. *J Am Dent Assoc* 1997; 76:148.

Dohrenwend BP, Raphael KG, Marbach JJ, Gallagher RM. Why is depression comorbid with chronic myofascial face pain? A family study test of alternative hypotheses. *Pain* 1999; 83:183–192.

Dolwick MF, Dimitroulis G. Is there a role for temporomandibular joint surgery? *Br J Oral Maxillofac Surg* 1994; 32:307–313.

Domino JV, Haber JD. Prior physical and sexual abuse in women with chronic headache: clinical correlates. *Headache* 1987; 27:310–314.

Dougher MJ, Goldstein D, Leight KA. Induced anxiety and pain. *J Anxiety Disord* 1987; 1:259–264.

Drangsholt M, LeResche L. Temporomandibular disorder pain. In: Crombie IK, Croft PR, Linton SJ, LeResche L, Von Korff M (Eds). *Epidemiology of Pain.* Seattle: IASP Press, 1999, pp 203–233.

Dworkin SF. Perspectives on the interaction of biological, psychological and social factors in TMD. *J Am Dent Assoc* 1994; 125:856–863.

Dworkin SF. The case for incorporating biobehavioral treatment into TMD management. *J Am Dent Assoc* 1996; 127:1607–1610.

Dworkin SF. Behavioral and educational modalities. *Oral Surg Oral Med Oral Path Oral Radiol Endodont* 1997; 83:128–133.

Dworkin SF. Temporomandibular disorders: a problem in oral health. In: Gatchel RJ, Turk DC (Eds). *Psychosocial Factors in Pain.* New York: Guilford Press, 1999, pp 213–226.

Dworkin SF, LeResche L. Research diagnostic criteria for temporomandibular disorders. *J Craniomandib Disord* 1992; 6:302–355.

Dworkin SF, Huggins KH, LeResche L, et al. Epidemiology of signs and symptoms in temporomandibular disorders: clinical signs in cases and controls. *J Am Dent Assoc* 1990; 120:273–281.

Edwards PW, Zeichner A, Kuczmierczyk AR. Boczkowski J. Familial pain models: the relationship between family history of pain and current pain experience. *Pain* 1985; 21:379–384.

Edwards RR, Augustson E, Fillingim RB. Sex-specific effects of pain-related anxiety on adjustment to chronic pain. *Clin J Pain* 2000; 16:46–53.

Fillingim RB, Maixner W. The influence of resting blood pressure and gender on pain responses. *Psychosom Med* 1996; 58:326–332.

Fillingim RB, Ness TJ. Sex–related hormonal influences on pain and analgesic responses. *Neurosci Biobehav Rev* 2000; 24:485–501.

Fillingim RB, Keefe FJ, Light KC, Booker DK, Maixner W. The influence of gender and psychological factors on pain perception. *J Gender Cult Health* 1996a; 1:21–36.

Fillingim RB, Maixner W, Kincaid S, Sigurdsson A, Harris MB. Pain sensitivity in patients with temporomandibular disorders: relationship to clinical and psychosocial factors. *Clin J Pain* 1996b; 12:260–269.

Fillingim RB, Maixner W, Sigurdsson A, Kincaid S. Sexual and physical abuse history in subjects with temporomandibular disorders: relationship to clinical variables, pain sensitivity, and psychologic factors. *J Orofac Pain* 1997; 11:48–57.

Fillingim RB, Maixner W, Kincaid S, Silva S. Sex differences in temporal summation but not sensory-discriminative processing of thermal pain. *Pain* 1998; 75:121–127.

Fillingim RB, Edwards RR, Powell T. The relationship of sex and clinical pain to experimental pain responses. *Pain* 1999a; 83:419–425.

Fillingim RB, Maddux V, Shackelford JM. Sex differences in heat pain thresholds as a function of assessment method and rate of rise. *Somatosens Motor Res* 1999b; 16:57–62.

Fillingim RB, Wilkinson CS, Powell T. Self-reported abuse history and pain complaints among healthy young adults. *Clin J Pain* 1999c; 15:85–91.

Fillingim RB, Edwards RR, Powell T. Sex-dependent effects of reported familial pain history on clinical and experimental pain responses. *Pain* 2000; 86:87–94.

Flor H, Birbaumer N, Schulte W, Roos R. Stress-related electromyographic responses in patients with chronic temporomandibular pain. *Pain* 1991; 46:145–152.

France CR. Decreased pain perception and risk for hypertension: considering a common physiological mechanism. *Psychophysiology* 1999; 36:683–692.

Gallagher RM, Marbach JJ, Raphael KG, Dohrenwend BP, Cloitre M. Is major depression comorbid with temporomandibular pain and dysfunction syndrome? A pilot study. *Clin J Pain* 1991; 7:219–225.

Garofalo JP, Gatchel RJ, Wesley AL, Ellis E. Predicting chronicity in acute temporomandibular joint disorders using the research diagnostic criteria. *J Am Dent Assoc* 1998; 129:438–447.

Gatchel RJ, Garofalo JP, Ellis E, Holt C. Major psychological disorders in acute and chronic TMD: an initial examination. *J Am Dent Assoc* 1996; 127:1365–1370.

Geisser ME, Robinson ME, Pickren WE. Differences in cognitive coping strategies among pain-sensitive and pain-tolerant individuals on the cold pressor test. *Behav Ther* 1992; 23:31–42.

Goldberg RT. Childhood abuse, depression, and chronic pain. *Clin J Pain* 1994; 10:277–281.

Graffenried BV, Adler R, Abt K, Nuesch E, Spiegel R. The influence of anxiety and pain sensitivity on experimental pain in man. *Pain* 1978; 4:253–263.

Gruber AJ, Hudson JI, Pope HZ Jr. The management of treatment-resistant depression in disorders on the interface of psychiatry and medicine. Fibromyalgia, chronic fatigue syndrome, migraine, irritable bowel syndrome, atypical facial pain, and premenstrual dysphoric disorder. *Psychiatr Clin North Am* 1996; 19:351–369.

Haley WE, Turner JA, Romano JM. Depression in chronic pain patients: relation to pain, activity, and sex differences. *Pain* 1985; 23:337–343.

Hartrick CT, Dobritt DW, Eckstein L. Clinical impression that familial models are an important influence in the development and expression of chronic pain and pain behavior. *Pain* 1986; 25:279–280.

Kandrack MA, Grant KR, Segall A. Gender differences in health related behaviour: some unanswered questions. *Soc Sci Med* 1991; 32:579–590.

Kapel L, Glaros AG, McGlynn FD. Psychophysiological responses to stress in patients with myofacial pain-dysfunction syndrome. *J Behav Med* 1989; 12:397–406.

Kashikar-Zuck S, Keefe FJ, Kornguth P, et al. Pain coping and the pain experience during mammography: a preliminary study. *Pain* 1997; 73:165–172.

Katon W, Egan K, Miller D. Chronic pain: lifetime psychiatric diagnoses and family history. *Am J Psychiatry* 1985; 142:1156–1160.

Katz JO, Rugh JD, Hatch JP, et al. Effect of experimental stress on masseter and temporalis muscle activity in human subjects with temporomandibular disorders. *Arch Oral Biol* 1989; 34:393–398.

Keefe FJ, Kashikar-Zuck S, Robinson E, et al. Pain coping strategies that predict patients' and spouses' ratings of patients' self-efficacy. *Pain* 1997; 73:191–199.

Kight M, Gatchel RJ, Wesley L. Temporomandibular disorders: evidence for significant overlap with psychopathology. *Health Psychol* 1999; 18:177–182.

Korszun A, Papadopoulos E, Demitrack M, Engleberg C, Crofford L. The relationship between temporomandibular disorders and stress-associated syndromes. *Oral Surg Oral Med Oral Path Oral Radiol Endodont* 1998; 86:416–420.

Koutantji M, Pearce SA, Oakley DA. The relationship between gender and family history of pain with current pain experience and awareness of pain in others. *Pain* 1998; 77:25–31.

Kroenke K, Spitzer RL. Gender differences in the reporting of physical and somatoform symptoms. *Psychosom Med* 1998; 60:150–155.

Krogstad BS, Jokstad A, Dahl BL, Vassend O. The reporting of pain, somatic complaints, and anxiety in a group of patients with TMD before and 2 years after treatment: sex differences. *J Orofac Pain* 1996; 10:263–269.

Kuttila M, Niemi PM, Kuttila S, Alanen P, Le Bell Y. TMD treatment need in relation to age, gender, stress, and diagnostic subgroup. *J Orofac Pain* 1998; 12:67–74.

Lefebvre JC, Lester N, Keefe FJ. Gender differences in pain location and pain coping strategy use in a college sample. *Proceedings of the American Pain Society* 1994; 13:A-81.

LeResche L. Epidemiology of temporomandibular disorders: implications for the investigation of etiologic factors. *Crit Rev Oral Biol Med* 1997; 8:291–305.

LeResche L, Dworkin SF, Truelove EL, Mancl L. Relationship of premenstrual symptoms to TMD and other pain problems. *J Am Dent Assoc* 1997a; 76:148.

LeResche L, Saunders K, Von Korff MR, Barlow W, Dworkin SF. Use of exogenous hormones and risk of temporomandibular disorder pain. *Pain* 1997b; 69:153–160.

LeResche L. Gender considerations in the epidemiology of chronic pain. In: Crombie IK, Croft PR, Linton SJ, LeResche L, Von Korff M (Eds). *Epidemiology of Pain.* Seattle: IASP Press, 1999, pp 43–52.

Leserman J, Drossman DA, Li Z, et al. Sexual and physical abuse history in gastroenterology practice: how types of abuse impact health status. *Psychosom Med* 1996; 58:4–15.

Lester N, Lefebvre JC, Keefe FJ. Pain in young adults. I: Relationship to gender and family pain history. *Clin J Pain* 1994; 10:282–289.

Lester N, Lefebvre JC, Keefe FJ. Pain in young adults. III: Relationships of three pain-coping measures to pain and activity interference. *Clin J Pain* 1996; 12:291–300.

Levitt SR, McKinney MW. Validating the TMJ scale in a national sample of 10,000 patients: demographic and epidemiologic characteristics. *J Orofac Pain* 1994; 8:25–35.

Linton SJ. A population-based study of the relationship between sexual abuse and back pain: establishing a link. *Pain* 1997; 73:47–53.

List T, Wahlund K, Wenneberg B, Dworkin SF. TMD in children and adolescents: prevalence of pain, gender differences, and perceived treatment need. *J Orofac Pain* 1999; 13:9–20.

Maixner W, Fillingim R, Booker D, Sigurdsson A. Sensitivity of patients with painful temporomandibular disorders to experimentally evoked pain. *Pain* 1995a; 63:341–351.

Maixner W, Sigurdsson A, Fillingim R, Lundeen T, Booker D. Regulation of acute and chronic orofacial pain. In: Fricton JR, Dubner RB (Eds). *Orofacial Pain and Temporomandibular Disorders*. New York: Raven Press, 1995b, pp 85–102.

Maixner W, Fillingim R, Kincaid S, Sigurdsson A, Harris MB. Relationship between pain sensitivity and resting arterial blood pressure in patients with painful temporomandibular disorders. *Psychosom Med* 1997; 59:503–511.

Maixner W, Fillingim R, Sigurdsson A, Kincaid S, Silva S. Sensitivity of patients with temporomandibular disorders to experimentally evoked pain: evidence for altered temporal summation of pain. *Pain* 1998; 76:71–81.

Malow RM, Grimm L, Olson RE. Differences in pain perception between myofascial pain dysfunction patients and normal subjects: a signal detection analysis. *J Psychosom Res* 1980; 24:303–309.

Marbach JJ, Ballard GT, Frankel MR, Raphael KG. Patterns of TMJ surgery: evidence of sex differences. *J Am Dent Assoc* 1997; 128:609–614.

McNeill C. Management of temporomandibular disorders: concepts and controversies. *J Prosthet Dent* 1997; 77:510–522.

Messinger HB, Spierings EL, Vincent AJ, Lebbink J. Headache and family history. *Cephalalgia* 1991; 11:13–18.

Moldin SO, Scheftner WA, Rice JP, et al. Association between major depressive disorder and physical illness. *Psychol Med* 1993; 23:755–761.

Molin C, Edman G, Schalling D. Psychological studies of patients with mandibular pain dysfunction syndrome. *Swed Dent J* 1973; 66:15–23.

Morrow D, Tallents RH, Katzberg RW, Murphy WC, Hart TC. Relationship of other joint problems and anterior disc position in symptomatic TMD patients and in asymptomatic volunteers. *J Orofac Pain* 1996; 10:15–20.

Neumann L, Buskila D. Quality of life and physical functioning of relatives of fibromyalgia patients. *Semin Arthritis Rheum* 1997; 26:834–839.

Ottman R, Hong S, Lipton RB. Validity of family history data on severe headache and migraine. *Neurology* 1993; 43:1954–1960.

Pellegrino MJ, Waylonis GW, Sommer A. Familial occurrence of primary fibromyalgia. *Arch Phys Med Rehab* 1989; 70:61–63.

Plesh O, Wolfe F, Lane N. The relationship between fibromyalgia and temporomandibular disorders: prevalence and symptom severity. *J Rheumatol* 1996; 23:1948–1952.

Plesh O, Curtis DA, Hall LJ, Miller A. Gender difference in jaw pain induced by clenching. *J Oral Rehab* 1998; 25:258–263.

Rajala U, Keinanen-Kiukaanniemi S, Uusimaki A, Kivela SL. Musculoskeletal pains and depression in a middle-aged Finnish population. *Pain* 1995; 61:451–457.

Raphael KG, Dohrenwend BP, Marbach JJ. Illness and injury among children of temporomandibular pain and dysfunction syndrome (TMPDS) patients. *Pain* 1990; 40:61–64.

Raphael KG, Marbach JJ, Gallagher RM, Dohrenwend BP. Myofascial TMD does not run in families. *Pain* 1999; 80:15–22.

Raphael KG, Marbach JJ, Klausner J. Myofascial face pain—clinical characteristics of those with regional vs. widespread pain. *J Am Dent Assoc* 2000; 131:161–171.

Rasmussen P. Facial pain. I. A prospective survey of 1052 patients with a view of: definition, delimitation, classification, general data, genetic factors, and previous diseases. *Acta Neurochir* 1990; 107:112–120.

Riley JL, Robinson ME, Kvaal SA, Gremillion HA. Effects of physical and sexual abuse in facial pain: direct or mediated? *Cranio* 1998; 16:259–266.

Robinson ME, Wise EA, Riley JLI. Sex differences in clinical pain: a multi-sample study. *J Clin Psychol Med Settings* 1998; 5:413–423.

Rollman GB, Gillespie JM. The role of psychosocial factors in temporomandibular disorders. *Curr Rev Pain* 2000; 4:71–81.

Scarinci IC, McDonald Haile J, Bradley LA, Richter JE. Altered pain perception and psychosocial features among women with gastrointestinal disorders and history of abuse: a preliminary model. *Am J Med* 1994; 97:108–118.

Schanberg LE, Keefe FJ, Lefebvre JC, Kredich DW, Gil KM. Social context of pain in children with juvenile primary fibromyalgia syndrome: parental pain history and family environment. *Clin J Pain* 1998; 14:107–115.

Schrader H, Obelieniene D, Bovim G, et al. Natural evolution of late whiplash syndrome outside the medicolegal context. *Lancet* 1996; 347:1207–1211.

Spertus IL, Burns J, Glenn B, Lofland K, McCracken L. Gender differences in associations between trauma history and adjustment among chronic pain patients. *Pain* 1999; 82:97–102.

Sternbach RA. Survey of pain in the United States: the Nuprin Pain Report. *Clin J Pain* 1986; 2:49–53.

Stohler CS, Zarb GA. On the management of temporomandibular disorders: a plea for a low-tech, high-prudence therapeutic approach. *J Orofac Pain* 1999; 13:255–261.

Turk DC, Rudy TE. A dual-diagnostic approach assesses TMD patients. *J Mass Dent Soc* 1995; 44:16–19.

Turk DC, Zaki HS, Rudy TE. Effects of intraoral appliance and biofeedback/stress management alone and in combination in treating pain and depression in patients with temporomandibular disorders. *J Prosthet Dent* 1993; 70:158–164.

Verbrugge LM. The twain meet: empirical explanations of sex differences in health and mortality. *J Health Soc Behav* 1989; 30:282–304.

Vickers ER, Cousins MJ, Woodhouse A. Pain description and severity of chronic orofacial pain conditions. *Aust Dent J* 1998; 43:403–409.

Von Korff M, Dworkin SF, Le Resche L. Graded chronic pain status: an epidemiologic evaluation. *Pain* 1990; 40:279–291.

Von Korff M, Wagner EH, Dworkin SF, Saunders KW. Chronic pain and use of ambulatory health care. *Psychosom Med* 1991; 53:61–79.

Wahlund K, List T, Dworkin SF. Temporomandibular disorders in children and adolescents: reliability of a questionnaire, clinical examination, and diagnosis. *J Orofac Pain* 1998; 12:42–51.

Wanman A. Longitudinal course of symptoms of craniomandibular disorders in men and women. A 10-year follow-up study of an epidemiologic sample. *Acta Odontol Scand* 1996; 54:337–342.

Weir R, Browne G, Tunks E, Gafni A, Roberts J. Gender differences in psychosocial adjustment to chronic pain and expenditures for health care services used. *Clin J Pain* 1996; 12:277–290.

Zelman DC, Howland EW, Nichols SN, Cleeland CS. The effects of induced mood on laboratory pain. *Pain* 1991; 46:105–111.

Correspondence to: Roger B. Fillingim, PhD, Department of Operative Dentistry, Public Health Services and Research, University of Florida, P.O. Box 100404, 1600 SW Archer Road, D8-37, Gainesville, FL 32610-0404, USA. Email: RFillingim@ufl.edu.

Sex, Gender, and Pain, Progress in Pain Research and Management, Vol. 17, edited by R.B. Fillingim, IASP Press, Seattle, © 2000.

16

Sex and Gender in Irritable Bowel Syndrome

Bruce D. Naliboff,[a,b,e] Margaret M. Heitkemper,[f] Lin Chang,[a,c] and Emeran A. Mayer [a,c,d]

[a]CURE Digestive Diseases Research Center, Neuroenteric Disease Program, [b]Department of Psychiatry and Behavioral Sciences, and [c]Departments of Medicine and [d]Physiology, School of Medicine, University of California, Los Angeles, California, USA; [e]Psychophysiology Research, VA Medical Center, Greater Los Angeles Healthcare System, Los Angeles, California, USA; [f]Department of Biobehavioral Nursing and Health Systems, University of Washington, Seattle, Washington, USA

It has long been recognized that symptoms from the gastrointestinal (GI) tract, including pain, bloating, urgency, nausea, constipation, diarrhea, and difficult passage of food, urine, or stool, are common, and often occur without a specific detectable lesion. These symptoms range from mild and occasional in many individuals to frequent, severe, and chronic in a small but significant minority of the population. In the last 25 years there has been an accelerating interest in and understanding of these complaints, now labeled *functional gastrointestinal disorders*. A symptom-based classification and diagnostic system for such disorders, developed over the past 15 years and recently revised, includes five site-related diagnostic groups (gastroduodenal, bowel, abdominal pain, biliary, and anorectal; Thompson et al. 1999). Several disorders may be identified within each site category depending on the independence of cardinal symptoms. Irritable bowel syndrome (IBS), probably the most common and best studied of the functional GI disorders, is characterized by abdominal pain or discomfort associated with defecation or altered bowel habit. It is distinct from other functional bowel disorders (such as functional constipation or diarrhea and chronic abdominal pain) by the presence of both sensory and bowel habit disturbance. While this chapter will focus on IBS, many of the psychological and biological mechanisms presented may well apply to these other disorders. The suggestion that sex- and gender-linked factors may play an important role in IBS stems primarily from epidemiologic data indicating that IBS (like many but not all of the functional GI disorders) occurs with greater frequency in women than men. In addition, intriguing findings have recently suggested a sex-specific therapeutic response to a promising new drug for IBS (Northcutt et al. 1998).

IBS SYMPTOMS, PREVALENCE, AND COST

IBS is characterized by abdominal pain or discomfort associated with defecation or a change in bowel habit or stool composition (diarrhea or constipation). The most recent consensus diagnosis defines IBS as abdominal pain and/or discomfort for at least 12 weeks in the preceding 12 months that is associated with at least two of three bowel habit features: pain or discomfort relieved with defecation, onset associated with a change in frequency of stool, and/or onset associated with a change in stool form (Thompson et al. 1999). Like all functional GI disorders, IBS is only diagnosed in the absence of a structural or biochemical explanation for the symptoms. Surveys in developed countries point to a prevalence of IBS of between 15% and 20% of the adult and adolescent population (Drossman et al. 1997). Symptoms may range from very mild to severe and disabling; it is estimated that only a fraction of persons with IBS-type symptoms seek medical care for this problem (Talley et al. 1995). Rates of health care utilization among persons meeting the IBS symptom criteria vary from 25% to 70%, depending in part on health care coverage (with lower rates in the United States and much higher rates in countries with universally accessible health care) (Talley et al. 1997).

Despite the heterogeneity of presentation, IBS is estimated to account for 3.5 million physician visits in the United States annually and is the most common reason for referral to a gastroenterologist (about 25% of all patients) (Everhart and Renault 1991). Patients with IBS have increased absenteeism from work, make more doctor visits for GI- and non-GI-related problems, and report significantly reduced well-being or quality of life (Everhart and Renault 1991; Gralnek et al. 1999). Whitehead et al. (1990a) noted that 21% of their female IBS sample had undergone hysterectomies for treatment of their GI symptoms; this rate is much higher than the national average of 5.5%. In this sample the GI symptoms persisted after surgery.

GENDER DIFFERENCES IN IBS PREVALENCE

Female to male IBS prevalence ratios for the general population vary from 1:1 to over 2:1 across a variety of studies (Camilleri and Choi 1997). A greater female predominance is typically seen in medical clinic and tertiary care populations. Some of this variability can be explained by cultural factors, as in the frequently cited increased male prevalence in a clinic population in India (Jain et al. 1991). Some is also undoubtedly due to a generally higher rate of medical consulting among women, given that the gender differences are more pronounced in clinic compared to community samples. The differences seen even in community samples may reflect a differential response bias in women toward reporting any physical discomfort (Fillingim and Maixner 1995). One of the few prospective approaches to studying IBS etiology is to follow patients after a bout of acute gastroenteritis. A significant percentage of individuals with acute gastroenteritis will develop more chronic, IBS-like symptoms. Several studies have found that significant life stress occurring either before or immediately after the acute infection is the strongest predictor of IBS development. It is interesting to note that the development of post-infectious IBS also shows a female predominance. In one study examining equal numbers of men and women with gastroenteritis, IBS symptoms were present at 3 months in 77% of women and only 36% of men (Gwee 1999).

Although the adult IBS diagnostic criteria cannot be applied directly to young children, several conditions such as recurrent abdominal pain and certain forms of chronic functional constipation or diarrhea may well represent functional bowel spectrum conditions in prepuberty. Such functional GI disorders occur about equally in boys and girls, which suggests that psychosocial or biological changes with puberty may lead to differential rates of IBS in adults (Walker 1999).

There has been some discussion that gender differences in the prevalence of IBS symptoms may be related to gender differences in symptom profiles. Two criteria are commonly used to diagnose IBS: the Manning criteria (Manning et al. 1978) and more recently, the Rome criteria (Thompson et al. 1999). Both criteria include similar symptoms, e.g., abdominal pain associated with looser and more frequent stools as well as altered stool frequency, form, passage, and bloating. Using a mixed gender sample, Smith et al. (1991) found that the Manning criteria were positively correlated with an IBS diagnosis in women but negatively in men. Thompson (1997) reported that in a sample of 156 IBS patients (17% male), women were more likely than men to meet either the Manning or Rome criteria. However, patients of both genders reported similar levels of abdominal pain that was relieved by defecation and was associated with changes in stool frequency and consistency. Gender-related differences thus may be due in part to differences in symptom profiles or to the fact that the criteria were based on clinical experiences with a predominately female population.

OVERLAP OF IBS WITH OTHER VISCERAL AND SOMATIC PAIN DISORDERS

An important feature of the epidemiology of IBS is its high co-occurrence with other GI disorders and with non-GI pain disorders. Other GI syndromes such as functional dyspepsia (upper abdominal pain that is not associated with ulcers) may be present in 30–60% of the IBS population (Talley et al. 1998a), and nausea and vomiting occur in 25–50% of IBS patients. Increased urinary frequency and urgency affect approximately 65% of female patients with IBS and are often associated with abnormal urodynamic test results (Oddsson et al. 1978). Fibromyalgia and other rheumatological symptoms may occur in over 60% of female IBS patients. Hypertension, low back pain, headaches, nonspecific fatigue, insomnia, and palpitations are reported more commonly in patients with IBS than in the general population (Whitehead et al. 1982; Whorwell et al. 1986). There is also an important overlap of chronic pelvic pain and other gynecological symptoms in female patients with IBS. Walker et al. (1996) report a 35% prevalence of chronic pelvic pain in women with IBS compared to 14% of patients with inflammatory bowel disease. Women with both pelvic pain and IBS had a higher frequency of lifetime dysthymic disorder and panic disorder as well as a history of sexual abuse and hysterectomy compared to women with IBS alone.

In summary, IBS is more prevalent among women (about 2:1), with increasing female predominance in clinic populations. Gender differences in IBS prevalence are influenced by cultural factors, symptom criteria used for diagnosis, and global male/female differences in symptom reporting. Many, but not all, of the functional GI disorders have similar gender ratios, and the gender differences appear to be present in adolescents but not in children, which suggests that sex- and/or gender-based mechanisms may emerge during puberty. IBS patients, and particularly female IBS patients, have a greater risk for various other functional and pain disorders.

GENDER DIFFERENCES IN IBS SYMPTOMS

Research on differential symptom expression between males and females with IBS has focused on both GI and extra-intestinal symptoms, and on the fluctuation of symptoms based on the female menstrual cycle. We have recently reported that women with IBS recruited by community advertising and through clinic referrals showed significantly different symptom patterns compared to men, even after controlling for overall IBS severity, chronicity, and psychological distress (Lee et al. 1999). While men and women with IBS have similar incidence of a predominant bowel habit of diarrhea and alternating diarrhea and constipation, constipation is seen much less frequently in men. In addition, women show greater frequency of extra-intestinal symptoms such as headache and other chronic pain, and self-reported sensitivity to medications and foods. We speculated that these differences were not hormonally mediated because they were similar in a sample of pre- and postmenopausal women, but differed in age-matched males.

Talley (1991) found that in a community sample, women with IBS reported more symptoms of constipation and abdominal discomfort (bloating), while men with IBS reported more diarrhea. Corney and Stanton (1990), using a 7-day symptom diary, reported that women had longer pain episodes and more bloating, nausea, and vomiting, while in a relatively small sample of men, 91% reported having diarrhea. In a large survey of college students (Taub et al. 1995), women reported significantly more GI symptoms than men, including abdominal pain relieved by bowel movements and pain associated with looser and more frequent stools, bloating, and constipation. It remains to be studied whether differences in predominant symptoms and symptom intensity are due to gender-related pain expression, differences in reporting style, and/or factors that exacerbate symptoms. Despite these differences in symptom expression, factor analysis revealed a common set of core IBS symptoms across both males and females (Taub et al. 1995), suggesting that IBS gender differences may be quantitative, rather than qualitative.

SEXUAL TRAUMA AND SEXUAL ABUSE IN IBS

A history of major traumatic events (i.e., physical and/or sexual abuse) or major losses (i.e., the loss of a parent) during childhood was found more frequently in IBS patients than in healthy controls (Scarinci et al. 1994; Talley et al. 1994, 1998b). In a study of women at the University of North

Carolina, 53% of women with IBS had a history of abuse, compared to 37% of women with structural GI diagnoses (Drossman et al. 1990). History of sexual trauma may be a specific or nonspecific risk factor for development of IBS. In a large cross-sectional population study, Talley et al. (1998b) examined the role of sexual trauma in predicting IBS, either directly or as mediated through a personality variable of neuroticism. The findings support increased trauma history in IBS patients, but this relationship could be completely explained by levels of neuroticism. Interestingly, this relationship did not interact with gender, which implies a similar role for abuse in both men and women with IBS. Sexual abuse or other trauma may thus be an important mechanism leading to stress reactivity (neuroticism), but may not be specific to IBS or perhaps even to gender (except that abuse is more common among women). This view is supported by the findings of increased risk for a variety of physical and emotional symptoms following childhood trauma (Walker et al. 1999).

SEXUAL DYSFUNCTION IN IBS

IBS and other functional disorders are often associated with changes in non-GI vital functions such as sleep, energy level, and sexual activity. Reported levels of sexual dysfunction range from 24% to 83% (Dotevall et al. 1982; Whorwell et al. 1986; Guthrie et al. 1987), and dyspareunia (painful intercourse) has been emphasized as a specific problem in women with IBS. We recently examined the prevalence of several categories of sexual dysfunction in men and women with IBS compared to both controls and patients with non-ulcer dyspepsia (NUD) (Fass et al. 1998). Surprisingly, only about 14% of female IBS patients (and almost none of the women with NUD) reported dyspareunia. However, a large percentage of both patient groups (43%) reported some sexual dysfunction, compared to 16% of the controls. By far the most commonly reported dysfunction for all groups and for both men and women was decreased sexual drive. Interestingly, reported sexual dysfunction was associated with severity of GI symptoms, but not with psychological symptoms (as measured by the Symptom Checklist 90). While IBS overlaps significantly with pelvic pain, it appears that visceral hyperalgesia is not a primary cause of sexual dysfunction, even in women with IBS. Decreased libido, perhaps linked to altered central stress responses (such as enhanced stress-induced secretion of corticotropin-releasing factor), may account for the high rates of sexual dysfunction in both men and women with IBS as well as those with overlapping conditions such as chronic fatigue syndrome and fibromyalgia.

MENSTRUAL-CYCLE-RELATED VARIATION IN IBS SYMPTOMS

Several investigators have reported variations in GI symptoms during different phases of the menstrual cycle, which suggest altered motility and/or enhanced visceral sensitivity to normal GI events. Heitkemper and Jarrett (1992) stated that more women, both with and without GI symptoms, reported stomach pains during the perimenstrual phase compared to the nonmenses phases of their cycle. Stomach pain, pelvic cramping, nausea, and diarrhea, but not back pain, were rated higher during menses in the IBS group than in the control group, suggesting enhanced visceral sensitivity during the perimenstrual period. Women with IBS also reported higher levels of perimenstrual symptoms on six of the eight Menstrual Distress Questionnaire subscales. Whitehead et al. (1990a) reported similar findings. Neither study found a significant effect of menstrual cycle on self-reports of anxiety or depression, although Heitkemper and Jarrett did find an effect of cycle and group on the negative affect scale of the Menstrual Distress Questionnaire. As in other studies that have failed to demonstrate a direct correlation between plasma levels of ovarian hormones and perimenstrual symptoms (Schmidt et al. 1991), the authors failed to show a group difference in plasma estradiol and progesterone levels between women with and without IBS symptoms.

In addition to the higher prevalence of visceral pain in women during the perimenstrual phase, Crowell et al. (1994) have shown that a diagnosis of IBS was three times more common in women with dysmenorrhea (painful menstruation) than in those without. A similar comorbidity between dysmenorrhea and fibromyalgia has been suggested (Giamberardino et al. 1995).

PSYCHOPATHOLOGY AND IBS

As with other functional disorders, IBS has long been associated with altered psychological functioning, and the syndrome has been seen as a manifestation of stress, depression, anxiety, somatization, or as a product of learned illness behavior (for reviews see Olden 1996). There is also a significant comorbidity of IBS in mental health clinic populations, with recent reports of a 60% prevalence of IBS in patients seeking help for dysthymia and 46% for panic disorder (Kaplan et al. 1996; Masand et al. 1997). Despite these findings, the importance of psychological factors in IBS has been questioned due to several studies comparing the psychological profiles of IBS patients with individuals who fulfill the IBS criteria but have not sought medical care for their symptoms (IBS "non-patients"; Drossman et al. 1988;

Whitehead et al. 1988). These studies, conducted in the United States, suggest that "non-patients" with IBS may show much less psychological disturbance than those who consult physicians and specialists, indicating that many of the psychological findings reported in clinic samples may be associated with seeking health care and not with functional GI symptoms per se. However, this hypothesis has been challenged recently by a study in Australia (a country with universal health care). This population study showed a much higher consulting rate (up to 70%) for IBS symptoms, and neuroticism, psychological comorbidity, and a history of abuse did not explain this high rate (Talley et al. 1997). In contrast, severity and duration of abdominal pain had statistically significant and independent effects on the likelihood that persons with IBS would seek care for their GI problems. It is unknown whether gender interacts with these variables.

Creed (1999) recently summarized published data on the proportion of IBS clinic patients with psychiatric diagnoses. This analysis of studies using adequate patient numbers and a standardized research psychiatric interview showed that 50–60% of patients with IBS seen in gastroenterology clinics have psychiatric disorders. The proportion of patients entering treatment trials who have psychiatric disorders is similar (Creed 1999). The high prevalence of affective disorders in clinic samples of IBS patients could reflect a high comorbidity in all affected patients, could be explained by a "self-selection hypothesis" (Drossman and Thompson 1992), or could result from a combination of both phenomena. Population-based studies of persons with psychiatric disorders also shed some light on the role of psychiatric symptoms in IBS. Lydiard et al. (1994) reported the prevalence of GI symptoms (including an IBS "composite" of such symptoms) in individuals with panic disorder and other psychiatric disorders in a national community survey of 13,537 respondents (NIMH Epidemiologic Catchment Area [ECA] study). Persons with panic disorder had the highest rate of unexplained GI symptoms (7.2%) compared with the other diagnostic categories. The risk for IBS symptoms was nearly five-fold higher for persons with panic disorder compared with persons without this disorder. Walker et al. (1992) reviewed structured psychiatric interviews from nearly 19,000 subjects from the NIMH ECA study for prevalence of GI distress symptoms and selected psychiatric disorders. The prevalence of unexplained GI symptoms in this sample of the general population ranged between 6% and 25%. Subjects who reported two GI symptoms had significantly higher lifetime prevalence rates for depression, panic, and agoraphobia compared to those who reported no GI symptoms. Thus, while the ECA surveys were not specifically designed to determine affective comorbidity rates of those experiencing IBS symptoms, they strongly suggest an association of affective disorders with functional GI symptoms, even in those not seeking health care for their abdominal symptoms. Gender differences in the overlap between IBS and psychiatric symptoms has not been well studied, although one of the most prominent overlap syndromes is panic disorder, which has a significant female predominance (Lydiard and Falsetti 1999).

In addition to having psychiatric symptoms, patients with IBS often report that stressful life events preceded the onset or exacerbation of their GI symptoms. In a questionnaire study of 135 IBS patients and 654 controls, 73% of the patients and 54% of the control group reported that stress led to abdominal pain (Drossman et al. 1982). Stress also correlates with the number of bowel symptoms, disability days, and physician visits (Whitehead et al. 1992). A prospective study in IBS patients found that more than 90% of the variance in IBS symptoms over a 16-month period was explained by prolonged, threatening stressors (Bennett et al. 1998). Stress was measured as the presence of significant, threatening life events (such as divorce or loss of a job) rather than as a subjective response to typical events. This difference is important because it minimizes the influence of anxiety and depression on the perceived severity and frequency of life stressors. Another recent study (Gwee 1999) demonstrated that more patients who developed IBS symptoms following an acute enteric infection had experienced a life event involving disruption of personal relationships. In addition, the post-infectious IBS group had experienced significant life events in the 3 months following the acute gastroenteritis. One reason for the greater susceptibility of IBS patients to certain types of environmental stressors may be related to differences in somatic threat appraisal, poor coping skills, and inadequate belief systems regarding management of life stresses and symptoms (Whitehead et al. 1988). Another reason may involve differences in central responses to perceived threat, i.e., alterations in the different outputs of the central stress response.

In summary, the data continue to support a significant role for life stress and affective disturbance in IBS that is probably related to both symptom generation and consulting behavior. As yet the evidence is insufficient to determine whether these relationships are different between men and women.

PERIPHERAL AND CENTRAL MECHANISMS OF IBS

The cause, or more likely causes, of IBS and the other functional GI disorders remain unknown. However, recent research has suggested various possible mechanisms to explain the chronic sensory and motor symptoms of these disorders. A fuller understanding of these mechanisms will necessarily enhance our understanding of the gender differences in IBS epidemiology and presentation. We have recently proposed a model that emphasizes the importance of the emotional motor system (EMS) of the central nervous system (CNS) in mediating characteristic IBS symptoms of abdominal pain and discomfort and autonomic dysregulation of the gut (Mayer 2000). The term EMS refers to a specific set of parallel motor pathways governing somatic, autonomic, antinociceptive, and endocrine responses of an organism when its homeostasis is threatened or perceived to be threatened (Holstege et al. 1996). EMS activation is a part of the central stress response and may be associated with both acute and learned (conditioned) fear. The following paragraphs will briefly describe research on the autonomic, neuroendocrine, and antinociceptive outputs of this network and outline possible gender differences that may be relevant for IBS and other functional syndromes.

Role of the locus ceruleus. Neuroanatomical models derived from animal studies suggest a plausible role for the locus ceruleus (LC) complex as an integrative brain region that receives peripheral sensory (visceral) impulses, participates in autonomic nervous system (ANS) arousal, modifies gastric and colonic motor activity, and plays a role in endogenous pain inhibition. In the rat, connections between the LC and Barrington's nucleus, and thence to parasympathetic pontine and spinal nuclei (dorsal vagal complex and sacral parasympathetic nucleus), form the mechanism by which anxiety is linked to the characteristic responses for the GI tract: inhibition of gastric emptying and enhanced parasympathetic output to the left colon (Valentino et al. 1999). Gender and hormonal variations in morphology and activity of the LC suggest a possible neurophysiological basis for differences between the sexes in symptoms and levels of physiological arousal (Guillanon et al. 1988).

ANS modulation of colonic motility. The role of autonomic dysregulation of the gut or other organs in IBS symptom generation is incompletely understood. While fairly good evidence supports a role of altered ANS regulation of gut function in the development of diarrhea and certain forms of constipation, a role of ANS dysfunction in the development of abdominal pain and discomfort has not been established. Increases and decreases in the frequency of both propagating and nonpropagating contractions have been found in patients with diarrhea- and constipation-predominant IBS, respectively (Bazzocchi et al. 1990; Gorard et al. 1994). Colonic motility is also significantly influenced by stress in both IBS and healthy subjects (Almy et al. 1949; Welgan et al. 1988; Ditto et al. 1998). Even though distinct motility changes have been poorly associated with IBS symptoms, in particular pain and discomfort (Quigley 1992), altered motility clearly is a proximate cause of diarrhea and certain forms of constipation (slow transit) (Mertz et al. 1999). Compared to men, women have slower gut transit times, generally less frequent stools, and a higher incidence of constipation (Metcalf et al. 1987; Everhart et al. 1989). Since colonic motor activity is controlled by the ANS through modulation of circuits of the enteric nervous system, the role of altered ANS activity in IBS has recently been more carefully investigated.

A small number of preliminary studies indicate altered ANS function in IBS as well as ANS differences across IBS subgroups based on gender and bowel habit, but the findings have not been completely consistent. It has been difficult to quantitatively study ANS activity in the GI tract, so evaluation of non-GI autonomic function in IBS patients is based on the notion that tests of ANS function will provide indirect information about the extrinsic ANS innervation to the GI tract. Recent evidence has demonstrated correlations between gut-specific measures such as colonic mucosal blood flow and cardiovagal tone (Emmanuel and Kamm 1999).

ANS regulation of extracolonic functions. ANS responsivity can be determined in the laboratory using heart rate and blood pressure responses to Valsalva's maneuver, the sudomotor axon test, blood pressure response to supine and standing positions, heart rate response to deep breathing, and sympathetically mediated sweat gland activity (skin conductance). In addition, measures of heart rate variability (HRV) may serve as tools for evaluating the balance between the parasympathetic nervous system (PSNS) and sympathetic nervous system (SNS) (Akselrod et al. 1981; DeBoer et al. 1984).

Aggarwal et al. (1994) found that sympathetic dysfunction (assessed by postural change) was present in diarrhea-predominant IBS, while parasympathetic dysfunction (HRV during deep breathing) was present in constipation-predominant IBS. Other studies have examined overall ANS function in IBS with mixed findings, including lower vagal tone (Hausken et al. 1993; Heitkemper et al. 1998) and altered sympathetic activity (Camilleri and Fealey 1990). Using laboratory tests of ANS function, Lindgren et al. (1991) and Smart and Atkinson (1987) respectively found that 36% and 26% of IBS patients had autonomic dysfunction. Lee et al. (1997) reported increased PSNS tone and lower SNS/PSNS ratio in diarrhea-predominant IBS patients (men and women) using 24-hour ambulatory heart rate monitoring.

Gender differences in autonomic responses. Greater sympathetic responses to somatic pain have been reported for males compared to females (Maixner et al. 1995). Cowan et al. (1994) reported that basal vagal tone does not differ between men and women, but that men have heightened SNS activation. Jensen-Urstad et al. (1997) obtained similar results in a large study of gender differences using a stratified sample of men and women across age cohorts 20–29 years to 60–69 years. Across all age groups, women had significantly lower sympathetic predominance compared to men. Few studies have used ANS measures to compare male and female IBS patients, and most of the studies discussed above used predominantly female samples. Adeyemi et al. (1999) found decreased sympathetic responses in his mostly male IBS sample compared to controls. In a recent study (Lee et al. 1999) we also found that male IBS patients had higher sympathetic and lower vagal activation as indexed by skin conductance and HRV during balloon distension, compared to women with IBS and both male and female controls. Unfortunately, no menstrual cycle data were available.

Menstrual cycle and hormonal influences on ANS activity. Menstrual cycle and gender differences may modify ANS activity, as shown in studies using HRV measures. Sato et al. (1995) studied changes in HRV in menstruating women who were asked to perform a complex tracing task while supine. The authors found an increase in parasympathetic tone in the follicular (high estrogen) compared to the luteal phase (estrogen plus progesterone). Saeki et al. (1997) found that parasympathetic tone was greatest in the follicular phase compared to the ovulatory, luteal, premenstrual, and menses phases, but the difference was significant only in the menses phase.

Catecholamines (CA). Several studies have shown that CA levels tend to be higher in IBS patients relative to controls or other patient groups (Esler and Goulston 1973; Jorgensen et al. 1986; Heitkemper et al. 1996). In samples of female IBS patients, IBS "non-patients," and asymptomatic controls, urine norepinephrine and epinephrine (measured in nanograms per milligram creatinine) were higher in morning and evening samples in women with IBS than in the other two groups (Heitkemper et al. 1996). In healthy women, norepinephrine but not epinephrine levels increased significantly from the follicular to luteal phase (Goldstein et al. 1983; Davidson et al. 1985), although these studies used small samples and some tested different women in the follicular and luteal phases. Men aged 25–35 years showed a nonsignificant variability in urinary CA release from day to day (Curtin et al. 1996, 1997).

Neuroendocrine responses in IBS patients. Jorgensen et al. (1993) found no differences in adrenocorticotropic hormone (ACTH) or cortisol levels among controls or patients with duodenal ulcers or functional abdominal pain. In contrast, Heitkemper et al. (1996) found that urine cortisol levels obtained immediately upon rising were significantly higher in IBS women as compared to control women. Using a different approach, Fukudo et al. (1999) found that IBS patients had an exaggerated ACTH response to corticotropin-releasing hormone (CRH) compared to controls. Studies comparing urinary cortisol levels in men and women show that men excrete higher levels of urinary cortisol than women (Lamb et al. 1994; Fraser et al. 1999). Using a stressful challenge, Kirschbaum et al. (1999) showed that women excreted higher levels, similar to men, of salivary free cortisol during the luteal phase when compared to the follicular phase, although baseline levels did not differ. The role of altered hypothalamic-pituitary-adrenal (HPA) axis responses in IBS symptom generation is unknown, but preliminary data suggest differences in HPA axis responses in IBS patients that may reflect altered stress responses, which may be moderated by gender and menstrual cycle.

ROLE OF GONADAL STEROIDS IN IBS

Emerging evidence indicates that the gonadal steroids may influence a variety of pain-related experiences. Mechanisms by which gonadal steroids might work to modulate the abdominal pain associated with IBS are complex and may involve influences on central pain processing (as discussed in Chapters 5 and 10 of this volume) and direct effects on GI motility. Evidence suggests that estrogen and progesterone modify GI function. Hutson et al. (1989) argued that sex steroids inhibit gastric emptying, and reported that both premenopausal women and postmenopausal women taking ovarian hormones had slower gastric emptying of solids compared both with men and with postmenopausal women not on hormone replacement. Wald et al. (1981) reported that GI transit was significantly prolonged in the luteal compared with the follicular phase. Walsh et al. (1996) showed that acute progesterone administration, particularly in combination with estrogen, was associated with bradygastria in nonpregnant cycling adult women. Hence, one model would be an association of low or decreasing ovarian hormone levels with more rapid or vigorous motility and amplified experience of symptoms.

Men, under the influence of testosterone, may not have cyclic changes in symptoms or in GI motor activity. Limited research in rat models has demonstrated that testosterone has no influence on gastric emptying or GI transit, while estrogen and progesterone slow gastric emptying (Chen et al. 1995). However, Girma et al. (1997) showed that estradiol and testosterone both influence gastric acid secretion in rats. A recent study by Houghton et al. (1999) showed that men's level of discomfort with rectal balloon distension was negatively correlated with testosterone levels.

In summary, clinical evidence shows that in menstruating women, cycle variations contribute to GI symptoms, with the greatest reporting of GI symptoms at menses. However, more research is needed to determine whether gonadal hormone changes related to the menstrual cycle influence IBS symptoms via alterations in GI motility or by their impact on endogenous pain modulation systems.

VISCERAL SENSITIVITY IN IBS

Altered function of GI tract sensory nerves has emerged as an important theme in functional GI research that has yielded significant new data regarding several categories of functional disorders (IBS, NUD, noncardiac chest pain) (Richter et al. 1986; Mayer and Raybould 1990; Mertz et al. 1998). Perhaps most important, the study of sensory hypersensitivity has pointed to common mechanisms for what were often viewed as separate disorders, albeit with significant comorbidity. A more centralized hypersensitivity hypothesis provides a unifying neurophysiological model for functional disorders involving different target organ systems. The initial clinical observations that led to the hypothesis of visceral hypersensitivity in IBS included recurring abdominal pain and excessive pain during endoscopic examinations of the sigmoid colon. More recent experimental evidence from studies assessing visceral sensitivity suggests that a variety of perceptual abnormalities in relation to GI stimuli may be more frequent in IBS patients (Kellow et al. 1991; Bradette et al. 1994; Mertz et al. 1995). For example, Mertz et al. (1995) found that IBS patients had a significantly lower median discomfort threshold for a 30-second rectal balloon stimulus compared to a normal population. When lowered threshold and two other perceptual abnormalities were considered (an abnormal area of sensory referral or increased intensity of rectal sensations during balloon distension), 95% of IBS patients had at least one abnormality. Only 7% of a control population had at least one of these three sensory findings. Other studies have also found significant perceptual alterations in IBS populations, including lowered discomfort thresholds for balloon distension of the small intestine and colon (Ritchie 1973; Whitehead et al. 1990b; Kellow et al. 1991; Prior et al. 1993; Bradette et al. 1994; Trimble et al. 1995). Similar findings of hypersensitivity have been reported for patients with functional dyspepsia (Bradette et al. 1991; Mearin et al. 1991; Mertz et al. 1998) and noncardiac chest pain (Cannon and Benjamin 1993; Richter and Bradley 1993). These results are paralleled by similar findings of target system hypersensitivity in other disorders such as fibromyalgia and myofascial pain disorder. Evidence from various studies confirms perceptual differences in IBS. Some of the relevant findings are as follows: (1) IBS is associated with hypersensitivity in the upper GI tract as well as the colon (Constantini et al. 1993; Trimble et al. 1995); (2) IBS is associated with a heightened perception of normal intestinal contractions (Kellow et al. 1991); (3) IBS (unlike fibromyalgia) is not associated with a generalized hypersensitivity to noxious somatic stimulation (Cook et al. 1987; Whitehead et al. 1990b); and (4) the perception of colonic distensions is modifiable by attention, anxiety, and relaxation (Ford et al. 1995; Accarino et al. 1997).

We have previously suggested that these findings point to two overlapping perceptual abnormalities in IBS—increased hypervigilance to expected aversive visceral events, and a hyperalgesia that is inducible by sustained noxious visceral stimulation (Naliboff et al. 1997). Hypervigilance is a critical component of the response to threat and has been demonstrated in IBS patients in both experimental and clinical studies; IBS patients are more hypersensitive to predictably increasing stimuli compared to randomly presented stimuli, show greater affective responses to visceral distension, and give increased ratings of GI descriptors as compared to non-IBS controls (Naliboff et al. 1997).

Studies have not shown significant gender differences in pain or discomfort thresholds to rectal balloon distension in either controls or IBS patients (Whitehead et al. 1990b; Mertz et al. 1995; Jackson et al. 1997; Naliboff et al. 1997). However, most visceral distension studies have not directly addressed potential gender differences or have lacked an adequate gender mix to allow for meaningful post hoc comparisons. Also, none of the studies have directly manipulated expectation so as to assess gender differences in vigilance or response bias. In addition, these studies offer no information about the hormonal status of the women, and fail to mention whether they are menstruating, taking birth control pills, or using postmenopausal hormone replacement. Thus it is unclear whether there are meaningful differences in visceral hypersensitivity between men and women with IBS (or men and women in general), despite differences in IBS symptom presentation.

A few preliminary studies have shown potential effects of menstrual cycle hormonal changes on visceral perception. Jackson et al. (1994, 1997) reported that female IBS patients, but not healthy controls, show menstrual-cycle-related changes in perceptual sensitivity to rectal distension, with greater sensitivity during the perimenstrual period. Delechenaut et al. (1991) found that the tolerance to vaginal (but not rectal) distension was lower during the luteal phase of the cycle. We have attempted to further test visceral sensory processes by using a train of repetitive high-pressure distensions of the sigmoid colon as a conditioning stimulus. We have recently demonstrated the development of rectal hyperalgesia in response to sigmoid stimulation in menopausal and hormone-controlled women with IBS (Munakata et al. 1997). Sensitization seems to develop to a lesser extent in male IBS patients and does not occur in healthy controls of either gender (Lee et al. 1999). Repetitive mechanical activity is characteristic of the viscera, in particular of the sigmoid colon and uterus, and such activity could play a role in inducing visceral hyperalgesia and cramping pain in predisposed individuals. Repetitive distension of the feline gallbladder has been shown to result in "wind-up," and the degree of spinal sensitization was modulated by descending pain inhibitory systems (Cervero et al. 1992). Such findings could be explained by an alteration in the balance of endogenous pain modulation systems, activated by the noxious repetitive stimulus, which in turn modulates spinal cord excitability (Mayer and Gebhart 1993, 1994). Gender-related differences in the counter-regulation of such central sensitization could be responsible for the gender differences in perception of visceral pain. Indeed, females exhibit greater wind-up in response to cutaneous heat pain than do males (Fillingim et al. 1998); whether this sex difference extends to repetitive visceral stimuli remains to be determined.

GENDER IN IBS TREATMENT

Until recently the medical treatment for IBS was focused on a combination of: (1) reassurance to the patient that the symptoms did not result from a serious illness, (2) dietary change (e.g., high fiber, low fat), (3) use of symptomatic medications (for constipation, diarrhea, and/or pain), and often (4) for more severe cases or more distressed patients, use of a tricyclic antidepressant (Camilleri and Choi 1997; Drossman et al. 1997). For the most part these interventions are not gender specific and have limited effectiveness. A small but growing literature describes psychological treatment approaches, including multimodal cognitive-behavioral interventions (Lynch and Zamble 1989; Blanchard et al. 1992; Dulmen et al. 1996), hypnosis (Whorwell et al. 1987; Harvey et al. 1989), relaxation therapy (Blanchard et al. 1993), and group and individual psychotherapy (Svedlund et al. 1983; Guthrie et al. 1991). The generally similar results obtained by these varied approaches indicate that the critical factor addressed is the patient's belief system, his or her understanding of the disorder, and an enhanced sense of control. This is clearly illustrated in two behavioral treatment studies that included an active placebo control condition (Blanchard et al. 1992). In both studies, Blanchard and colleagues compared two conditions: a multimodal behavioral treatment that included education, biofeedback-assisted relaxation, and cognitive stress-coping training, and a placebo condition consisting of "pseudomeditation" and EEG alpha suppression (suppressed alpha is associated with an alert, not a relaxed state). Both the active and placebo treatments led to similar expectations of treatment success and outcome, and both led to greater positive changes than did a symptom-monitoring control condition. Interestingly, some evidence indicates that a treatment that focuses only on changing beliefs (cognitive therapy) may be superior to these other approaches. In two small studies, cognitive therapy resulted in a very high success rate and was superior to a support group condition with equal expectations of efficacy (Greene and Blanchard 1994; Payne and Blanchard 1995).

The psychological treatment literature thus supports a central role for patients' beliefs in perpetuating functional GI disorders by maintaining vigilance and arousal and avoiding situations in which conditioned stress-related GI responses might be extinguished. Given this conclusion, other groups as well as our own have begun to explore psychoeducational programs for IBS treatment. These treatments directly target patients' beliefs and their resulting behaviors by providing clear and convincing information on IBS as a biobehavioral disorder (including the role of stress and coping in IBS symptom maintenance), and by teaching positive self-management strategies, while discouraging health care seeking. Self-management strategies include relaxation training, stress management, self-hypnosis, and proper use of diet, exercise, and medications. Like the cognitive therapy approach, the goal of these interventions is not to provide patients with any specific "magic bullet" strategy to cure their IBS, but instead to change their beliefs and understanding so that they are more likely to benefit from a variety of approaches, both psychological and physiological, which in combination can help their symptoms. Outcomes from these cost-effective treatments have been positive. Colwell et al. (1998) report significant symptomatic improvement from a six-session educational group treatment program. We have also reported significant changes from an 8-week psychoeducational group in overall symptom severity, abdominal pain, and quality of life (Balice et al. 1998). Our intervention emphasized providing patients with a neurobiological model to explain the interactions between chronic stress, GI symptoms, and affective disorders, by pointing out the self-healing mechanisms of the organism and the plasticity of the nervous system in response to chronic stress and the potential for reversal of these changes by regular relaxation exercises. In addition, patients were trained to differentiate between ineffective, emotional coping styles and effective, rational strategies. Interestingly, the changes we observed were not predicted by or associated with changes in psychiatric symptoms. This is important because these interventions are targeted for IBS sufferers in general, most of whom have no significant psychiatric comorbidity. Further studies will be needed to compare educationally oriented treatments with more intense cognitive-behavioral approaches and to examine how these interventions may work for subpopulations of IBS patients.

Discussion has been limited on the role of gender-related issues in psychological treatment for IBS. Toner (1994), in a discussion of cognitive-behavioral therapy for this syndrome, recommended attention to gender-specific themes of possible sexual and physical abuse, gender role socialization, gender role conflict, public embarrassment and humiliation (related to GI symptoms such as belching, gas, frequent trips to the bathroom, and soiling), perfectionistic views of bodily function, and the need to balance personal interests versus supportive roles. However, none of the psychological treatment trials have yet addressed differential outcome based on gender.

The role of gender has also emerged in the search for new IBS-specific medications. In initial studies, a promising new medication for nonconstipated IBS patients (a 5-HT_3 antagonist, Alosetron) showed efficacy only in female subjects (Northcutt et al. 1998). Glaxo Wellcome has taken the unusual step of asking for approval for the drug only as a treatment for women with IBS. As yet there is no clear physiological explanation for the drug's gender-specific effects, however, these findings will surely encourage further research to clarify this issue.

BIOBEHAVIORAL IBS MODEL AND THE USE OF BRAIN IMAGING

As discussed above, we have recently presented a biobehavioral model that integrates central autonomic, pain-modulatory, and cognitive mechanisms underlying the symptoms of IBS and other functional disorders (Mayer and Naliboff 1999; Naliboff et al. 1999; Mayer 2000). At the neurophysiological level, the model supports the concept that the organism's response to stress is generated by a integrated network involving subcortical structures such as subregions of the hypothalamus—the paraventricular nucleus (PVN), amygdala, and periaqueductal gray (PAG). These structures receive peripheral input from visceral and somatic afferents and cortical input from subregions of the cingulate and prefrontal cortices and the anterior insula. In turn, the output from this network (the emotional motor system) modulates activity in medullary pontine nuclei such as the locus ceruleus complex, dorsal vagal complex, and rostral ventral medulla. These networks are concerned with processing of different aspects of pain and visceral sensations, recall of past visceral pain and unpleasant visceral sensations, vigilance toward expected pain, autonomic responses, and antinociception. At the psychological level the model incorporates the contributions of attitudes, beliefs, interoceptive conditioned responses, and coping skills. The model takes into account a variety of potentially important mechanisms by which sex and gender may influence IBS presentation. These range from possible cognitive differences in body awareness based on gender roles to neurobiological differences in autonomic, antinociceptive, or attentional systems in the brain.

We and others have recently begun to use brain imaging (combined with visceral stimuli and simultaneous measurement of autonomic and perceptual responses) as a paradigm to study CNS networks. Initial studies have been performed using $H_2{}^{15}O$ positron emission tomography (PET) (Silverman et al. 1997; Mayer et al. 1998; Naliboff et al. 1998). Taken together, the findings suggest that in healthy controls, rectosigmoid distension is associated with activation of brain regions that are part of the central fear circuits (perigenual cingulate cortex, PAG, insula, and medulla). IBS patients show less activation of these circuits but greater activity in the rostral mid-cingulate, posterior cingulate, and retrosplenial cortex brain regions that are associated with processing of emotionally charged and unpleasant information.

Preliminary evidence also suggests that activation of central networks involved in the processing of visceral afferent input may differ between male and female IBS patients (Derbyshire et al. 1999; Berman et al. 2000). In the first PET study to evaluate this distinction in IBS patients (Berman et al. 2000), male but not female IBS patients showed bilateral activation of the insula, a brain region that receives extensive visceral information (noxious and non-noxious, spinal and vagal) and also plays an important role in autonomic responses (Cechetto and Saper 1990; Yasui et al. 1991) and emotional processing (Casey et al. 1994; Augustine 1996). The use of imaging techniques to study gender differences in pain is a recent development that has not yet generated consistent results. In particular, insula activation by a painful somatic stimulus has recently been reported to show no gender difference (Derbyshire et al. 1998), to be greater in women (Paulson et al. 1998), *and* to be greater in men (Becerra et al. 1998). However, the distension stimulus used in our studies may be more similar to studies of the pelvic region, where gender differences in pain perception have been most consistent (Unruh 1996; Berkley 1997a,b).

SUMMARY

Substantial evidence demonstrates that gender differences in IBS prevalence and symptom presentation exist in both clinic samples and the large group of IBS sufferers outside the medical system. IBS seems to occur at about twice the rate in women as men, and women with IBS report more constipation and bloating, as well as more non-GI symptoms such as somatic pain. Despite these variations in presentation, the current data do not support the concept of a different syndrome for men and women, since the core symptoms and natural history are similar irrespective of gender. Various mechanisms have been proposed to explain the symptoms of IBS as well as the gender differences observed. Psychological factors clearly play a role in IBS, but no specific psychopathology (e.g., depression, anxiety, or somatization) has a close enough association with IBS in the general population to be a primary cause of the disorder. Some aspects of psychological functioning (e.g., depression or health beliefs) may directly influence health care seeking, while others (such as life stress or phobic anxiety regarding symptoms) are more likely to be associated with symptom maintenance and exacerbation. Gender differences in these relationships clearly need further study. The ANS plays a crucial role in IBS through both visceromotor responses and effects on pain modulation. Gender-specific differences in ANS responses are beginning to emerge, and ongoing research in gastroenterology and other fields may provide important mechanistic explanations for the heterogeneity of IBS symptoms as well as for gender-specific effects such as the decreased prevalence of constipation-predominant IBS in men. The role of neuroendocrine and sex-linked hormones in ANS functioning and pain modulation is another important area, and initial findings point to mechanisms for understanding the variation in IBS symptoms (such as increased symptoms in women during menses). Finally, it is becoming increasingly clear that an understanding of brain-gut interactions is essential for future progress in understanding and treating IBS. Few studies have directly examined gender differences in IBS from this biobehavioral perspective, so this chapter may seem to offer more questions than answers. However, potential targets of new research integrating central and peripheral mechanisms have been identified, and technologies for investigating these targets are rapidly becoming available. Thus we expect rapid progress toward a better understanding of IBS and of the gender-specific aspects of this and other functional disorders.

ACKNOWLEDGMENTS

The authors would like to thank Teresa Olivas for her assistance with this manuscript. Financial support was provided by NIH grant NR 04881 (B.D. Naliboff) and DK 48351 (E.A. Mayer).

REFERENCES

Accarino A, Azpiroz F, Malagelada JR. Attention and distraction: effects on gut perception. *Gastroenterology* 1997; 113:415–422.

Adeyemi EOA, Desai KD, Towsey M, Ghista D. Characterization of autonomic dysfunction in patients with irritable bowel syndrome by means of heart rate variability studies. *Am J Gastroenterol* 1999; 94:816–823.

Aggarwal A, Cutts TF, Abell TL, et al. Predominant symptoms in irritable bowel syndrome correlate with specific autonomic nervous system abnormalities. *Gastroenterology* 1994; 106:945–950.

Akselrod S, Gordon D, Ubel FA, et al. Power spectrum analysis of heart rate fluctuation: a quantitative probe of beat to beat cardiovascular control. *Science* 1981; 213:220–222.

Almy TP, Kern F, Tulin M. Alterations in colonic function in man under stress. II: Experimental production of sigmoid spasm in healthy persons. *Gastroenterology* 1949; 12:425–436.

Augustine JR. Circuitry and functional aspects of the insular lobe in primates including humans. *Brain Res Brain Res Rev* 1996; 22:229–244.

Balice G, Raeen H, Liu C, et al. Effect of a short term cognitive behavioral group intervention on symptoms and quality of life (QOL) in patients with functional bowel disorders (FBD). *Gastroenterology* 1998; 114:716.

Bazzocchi G, Ellis J, Villanueva-Meyer J, et al. Postprandial colonic transit and motor activity in chronic constipation. *Gastroenterology* 1990; 98:686–693.

Becerra L, Comite A, Breiter H, Gonzalez RG, Borsook D. Differential CNS activation following a noxious thermal stimulus in men and women: an fMRI study. *Soc Neurosci Abstracts* 1998; 241:136.

Bennett EJ, Tennant CC, Piesse C, Badcock C-A, Kellow JE. Level of chronic life stress predicts clinical outcome in irritable bowel syndrome. *Gut* 1998; 43:256–261.

Berkley KJ. Female vulnerability to pain and the strength to deal with it. *Behav Brain Sci* 1997a; 20:473–479.

Berkley KJ. Sex differences in pain. *Behav Brain Sci* 1997b; 20:371–380.

Berman S, Munakata J, Naliboff B, et al. Gender differences in regional brain response to visceral pressure in IBS patients. *Eur J Pain* 2000; in press.

Blanchard EB, Schwarz SP, Suls, et al. Two controlled evaluations of multicomponent psychological treatment of irritable bowel syndrome. *Behav Res Ther* 1992; 30:175–189.

Blanchard EB, Green B, Scharff L, Schwarz-McMorris SP. Relaxation training as a treatment for irritable bowel syndrome. *Biofeedback Self-Regulation* 1993; 18:125–132.

Bradette M, Pare P, Douville P, Morin A. Visceral perception in health and functional dyspepsia. Crossover study of gastric distension with placebo and domperidone. *Dig Dis Sci* 1991; 36:52–58.

Bradette M, Delvaux M, Staumont G, et al. Evaluation of colonic sensory thresholds in IBS patients using a barostat. *Dig Dis Sci* 1994; 39:449–457.

Camilleri M, Choi M-G. Review article: irritable bowel syndrome. *Aliment Pharmacol Ther* 1997; 11:3–15.

Camilleri M, Fealey RD. Idiopathic autonomic denervation in eight patients presenting with functional gastrointestinal disease. A causal association? *Dig Dis Sci* 1990; 35:609–616.

Cannon RO, Benjamin SB. Chest pain as a consequence of abnormal visceral nociception. *Dig Dis Sci* 1993; 38:193–196.

Casey KL, Minoshima S, Berger KL, et al. Positron emission tomographic analysis of cerebral structures activated specifically by repetitive noxious heat stimuli. *J Neurophysiol* 1994; 71:802–807.

Cechetto DF, Saper CB. Role of the cerebral cortex in autonomic function. In: Anonymous. *Central Regulation of Autonomic Function.* New York: Oxford University Press, 1990, pp 208–223.

Cervero F, Laird JMA, Pozo MA. Selective changes of receptive field properties of spinal nociceptive neurons induced by noxious visceral stimulation in the cat. *Pain* 1992; 51:335–342.

Chen TS, Doong ML, Chang FY, Lee SD, Wang PS. Effects of sex steroid hormones on gastric emptying and gastrointestinal transit in rats. *Am J Physiol* 1995; 268:G171–G176

Colwell LJ, Prather CM, Phillips SF, Zinsmeister AR. Effects of an irritable bowel syndrome educational class on health-promoting behaviors and symptoms. *Am J Gastroenterol* 1998; 93:901–905.

Constantini M, Sturniolo GC, Zaninotto G, et al. Altered esophageal pain threshold in irritable bowel syndrome. *Dig Dis Sci* 1993; 38:206–212.

Cook IJ, Van Eeden A, Collins SM. Patients with irritable bowel syndrome have greater pain tolerance than normal subjects. *Gastroenterology* 1987; 93:727–733.

Corney RH, Stanton R. Physical symptom severity, psychological and social dysfunction in a series of outpatients with irritable bowel syndrome. *J Psychosom Res* 1990; 34(5):483–491.

Cowan MJ, Pike K, Burr RL. Effects of gender and age on heart rate variability in healthy individuals and in persons after sudden cardiac arrest. *J Electrocardiol* 1994; 27(Suppl):P1–9.

Creed F. The relationship between psychosocial parameters and outcome in the irritable bowel syndrome. *Am J Med* 1999; (Suppl) 107:74S–80S.

Crowell MD, Dubin NH, Robinson JC, et al. Functional bowel disorders in women with dysmenorrhea. *Am J Gastroenterol* 1994; 89:1973–1977.

Curtin F, Walker JP, Schulz P. Day-to-day intraindividual reliability and interindividual differences in monoamines excretion. *J Affect Disord* 1996; 38:173–178.

Curtin F, Walker JP, Peyrin L, et al. Reward dependence is positively related to urinary monoamines in normal men. *Biol Psychiatry* 1997; 42:275–281.

Davidson L, Rouse IL, Vandongen R, Beilin LJ. Plasma noradrenaline and its relationship to plasma oestradiol in normal women during the menstrual cycle. *Clin Exp Pharmacol Physiol* 1985; 12:489–493.

DeBoer RW, Karemaker JM, Strackee J. Comparing spectra of a series of point events, particularly for heart rate variability spectra. *IEEE Trans Biomed Eng BME* 1984; 31:384–387.

Delechenaut P, Weber J, Ducrotte P, et al. Rectal and vaginal maximum tolerable volumes during menstrual cycle. *Eur J Gastroenterol Hepatol* 1991; 3:847–849.

Derbyshire SWG, Jones AKP, Townsend D. Gender differences in the central response to pain controlled for stimulus intensity. *Soc Neurosci Abstracts* 1998; 24:528.

Derbyshire SWG, Naliboff BD, Munakata J, et al. Gender differences in the central response to visceral pain and anticipation of pain in irritable bowel syndrome (IBS). *Gastroenterology* 1999; 116:A1038.

Ditto B, Miller SB, Barr RG. A one-hour active coping stressor reduces small bowel transit time in healthy young adults. *Psychosom Med* 1998; 60:7–10.

Dotevall G, Svedlund J, Sjodin I. Symptoms in irritable bowel syndrome. *Scand J Gastroenterol Suppl* 1982; 79:16–19.

Drossman DA, Thompson WG. Irritable bowel syndrome: a graduated multicomponent treatment approach. *Ann Intern Med* 1992; 118:1001–1008.

Drossman DA, Sandler RS, McKee DC. Bowel patterns among subjects not seeking health car. *Gastroenterology* 1982; 83:529–534.

Drossman DA, McKee DC, Sandler RS, et al. Psychosocial factors in the irritable bowel syndrome. a multivariate study of patients and nonpatients with irritable bowel syndrome. *Gastroenterology* 1988; 95:701–708.

Drossman DA, Leserman J, Nachman G, et al. Sexual and physical abuse in women with functional or organic gastrointestinal disorders. *Ann Intern Med* 1990; 113(11):828–833.

Drossman DA, Whitehead WE, Camilleri M. Irritable bowel syndrome: a technical review for practice guideline development. *Gastroenterology* 1997; 112:2120–2137.

Dulmen AM, Fennis MD, Bleijenberg G. Cognitive-behavioral group therapy for irritable bowel syndrome: effects and long-term follow-up. *Psychosom Med* 1996; 58:508–514.

Emmanuel AV, Kamm MA. Laser Doppler measurement of rectal mucosal blood flow. *Gut* 1999; 45:64–69.

Esler MD, Goulston KJ. Levels of anxiety in colonic disorders. *N Engl J Med* 1973; 288:16–20.

Everhart JE, Renault PF. Irritable bowel syndrome in office-based practice in the United States. *Gastroenterology* 1991; 100(4):998–1005.

Everhart JE, Go VLW, Johannes RS, et al. A longitudinal survey of self-reported bowel habits in the United States. *Dig Dis Sci* 1989; 34:1153–1162.

Fass R, Fullerton S, Naliboff B, Hirsh T, Mayer EA. Sexual dysfunction in patients with irritable bowel syndrome and non-ulcer dyspepsia. *Digestion* 1998; 59:79–85.

Fillingim RB, Maixner W. Gender differences in the responses to noxious stimuli. *Pain Forum* 1995; 4:209–221.

Fillingim RB, Maixner W, Kincaid S, Silva S. Sex differences in temporal summation but not sensory-discriminative processing of thermal pain. *Pain* 1998; 75:121–127.

Ford MJ, Camilleri M, Zinsmeister AR, Hanson RB. Psychosensory modulation of colonic sensation in the human transverse and sigmoid colon. *Gastroenterology* 1995; 109:1772–1780.

Fraser R, Ingram MC, Anderson NH, et al. Cortisol effects on body mass, blood pressure, and cholesterol in the general population. *Hypertension* 1999; 33:1364–1368.

Fukudo S, Nomura T, Hongo M. Impact of corticotropin-releasing hormone on gastrointestinal motility and adrenocorticotropic hormone in normal controls and patients with irritable bowel syndrome. *Gut* 1999; 42:845–849.

Giamberardino MA, Berkley KJ, Iezzi S, deBigonlina P, Vecchiet L. Changes in skin and muscle sensitivity in dysmenorrheic vs. normal women as a function of body site and monthly cycle. *Soc Neurosci Abstracts* 1995; 21:1638.

Girma K, Janczewska I, Segal HL, et al. Twenty-four-hour basal and repetitive pentagastrin-stimulated gastric acid secretion in normal and sham-operated rats and in rats after gonadectomy or treatment with estradiol or testosterone. *Scand J Gastroenterol* 1997; 32:669–675.

Goldstein DS, Levinson P, Keiser HR. Plasma and urinary catecholamines during the human ovulatory cycle. *Am J Obstet Gynecol* 1983; 146:824–829.

Gorard DA, Libby GW, Farthing MJ. Ambulatory small intestinal motility in diarrhoea predominant irritable bowel syndrome. *Gut* 1994; 35:203–210.

Gralnek IM, Hays RD, Kilbourne A, Mayer EA. Impact of irritable bowel syndrome on health-related quality of life (HRQOL). *Gastroenterology* 1999; 116:A1038.

Greene B, Blanchard EB. Cognitive therapy for irritable bowel syndrome. *J Consult Clin Psychol* 1994; 62:576–582.

Guillanon A, deBlas MR, Segovia S. Effects of sex steroids on the development of the locus coeruleus in the rat. *Brain Res* 1988; 468:306–310.

Guthrie E, Creed FH, Whorwell PJ. Severe sexual dysfunction in women with the irritable bowel syndrome: comparison with inflammatory bowel disease and duodenal ulceration. *BMJ* 1987; 295:577–578.

Guthrie E, Creed F, Dawson D, Tomenson B. A controlled trial of psychological treatment for the irritable bowel syndrome. *Gastroenterology* 1991; 100:450–457.

Gwee KA. The role of psychological and biological factors in postinfective gut dysfunction. *Gut* 1999; 44:400–406.

Harvey RF, Hinton RA, Gunary RM, Barry RE. Individual and group hypnotherapy in treatment of refractory irritable bowel syndrome. *Lancet* 1989; 1:424–425.

Hausken T, Svebak S, Wilhelmsen I, et al. Low vagal tone and antral dysmotility in patients with functional dyspepsia. *Psychosom Med* 1993; 55:12–22.

Heitkemper MM, Jarrett M. Patterns of gastrointestinal and somatic symptoms across the menstrual cycle. *Gastroenterology* 1992; 102:505–513.

Heitkemper M, Jarrett M, Cain K, et al. Increased urine catecholamines and cortisol in women with irritable bowel syndrome. *Am J Gastroenterol* 1996; 91:906–913.

Heitkemper M, Burr RL, Jarrett M. Evidence for autonomic nervous system imbalance in women with irritable bowel syndrome. *Dig Dis Sci* 1998; 43:2093–2098.

Holstege G, Bandler R, Saper CB. The emotional motor system. In: Holstege G, Bandler R, Saper CB (Eds). *Progress in Brain Research.* Amsterdam: Elsevier, 1996, pp 3–6.

Houghton LA, Jackson NA, Whorwell PJ, Morris J. Do male sex hormones protect from irritable bowel syndrome? *Gastroenterology* 1999; 116:G4381.

Hutson WR, Roehrkasse RL, Wald A. Influence of gender and menopause on gastric emptying and motility. *Gastroenterology* 1989; 96:11–17.

Jackson NA, Houghton LA, Whorwell PJ, Currer B. Does the menstrual cycle affect anorectal physiology? *Dig Dis Sci* 1994; 39:2607–2611.

Jackson NA, Houghton LA, Whorwell PJ. The menstrual cycle affects rectal visceral sensitivity in patients with irritable bowel syndrome (IBS) but not healthy volunteers. *Gastroenterology* 1997; 112:A1132.

Jain AP, Gupta OP, Jajoo UN, Sieber WJ. Clinical profile of irritable bowel syndrome at a rural based teaching hospital in central India. *J Assoc Physicians India* 1991; 39:385–386.

Jensen-Urstad K, Storck N, Bouvier F. Heart rate variability in healthy subjects is related to age and gender. *Acta Physiol Scand* 1997; 160:235–241.

Jorgensen LS, Bonlokke NJ, Christensen NJ. Life strain, life events, and autonomic response to a psychological stressor in patients with chronic upper abdominal pain. *Scand J Gasterenterol* 1986; 21:605–613.

Jorgensen LS, Christiansen P, Raundahl U. Autonomic nervous system function in patients with functional abdominal pain. *Scand J Gastroenterol* 1993; 28:63–68.

Kaplan DS, Masand PS, Gupta S. The relationship of irritable bowel syndrome (IBS) and panic disorder. *Ann Clin Psychiatry* 1996; 8:81–88.

Kellow JE, Eckersley CM, Jones MP. Enhanced perception of physiological intestinal motility in the irritable bowel syndrome. *Gastroenterology* 1991; 101(6):1621–1627.

Kirschbaum C, Kudielka BM, Gaab J, Schommer NC, Helhammer DH. Impact of gender, menstrual cycle phase, and oral contraceptives on the activity of the hypothalamus-pituitary-adrenal axis. *Psychosom Med* 1999; 61:154–162.

Lamb EJ, Noonan KA, Burrin JM. Urine-free cortisol excretion: evidence of sex-dependence. *Ann Clin Biochem* 1994; 31:455–458.

Lee KT, Rhee PL, Kim J, et al. Assessment of autonomic tone over a 24-hour period in patients with irritable bowel syndrome. *Gastroenterology* 1997; 112:A773.

Lee OY, Schmulson M, Mayer EA, Chang L, Naliboff BD. Gender related differences in irritable bowel syndrome symptoms. *Gastroenterology* 1999; 116:A1026.

Lindgren S, Lilja B, Rosen I, Sundkvist G. Disturbed autonomic nerve function in patients with Crohn's disease. *Scand J Gastroenterol* 1991; 26:361–366.

Lydiard RB, Falsetti SA. Experience with anxiety and depression treatment studies: implication for designing IBS clinical trials. *Am J Med* 1999; (Suppl) 107:65S–73S.

Lydiard RB, Greenwald S, Weissman MM, et al. Panic disorder and gastrointestinal symptoms: findings from the NIMH Epidemiologic Catchment Area Project. *Am J Psychiatry* 1994; 151:64–70.

Lynch PM, Zamble E. A controlled behavioral treatment study of irritable bowel syndrome. *Behav Ther* 1989; 20:509–523.

Maixner W, Fillingim R, Booker D, Sigurdson A. Sensitivity of patients with painful temporomandibular disorders to experimentally evoked pain. *Pain* 1995; 63:341–351.

Manning AP, Thompson WD, Heaton KW, Morris AF. Towards positive diagnosis in the irritable bowel syndrome. *BMJ* 1978; 2:653–654.

Masand PS, Kaplan DS, Gupta S, Bhandary AN. Irritable bowel syndrome and dysthymia. Is there a relationship? *Psychosomatics* 1997; 38:63–69.

Mayer EA. The neurobiology of stress and gastrointestinal disease. *Gut* 2000; in press.

Mayer EA, Gebhart GF. Functional bowel disorders and the visceral hyperalgesia hypothesis. In: Mayer EA, Raybould HE (Eds). *Basic and Clinical Aspects of Chronic Abdominal Pain.* New York: Elsevier, 1993, pp 3–28.

Mayer EA, Gebhart GF. Basic and clinical aspects of visceral hyperalgesia. *Gastroenterology* 1994; 107:271–293.

Mayer EA, Naliboff B. Supraspinal modulation of visceral afferent input. *Falk Symposium* 1999.

Mayer EA, Raybould HE. Role of visceral afferent mechanisms in functional bowel disorders. *Gastroenterology* 1990; 99:1688–1704.

Mayer EA, Liu M, Munakata J, et al. Regional brain activity before and after visceral sensitization. *Soc Neurosci Abstracts* 1998; 24:529.

Mearin F, Cucala M, Azpiroz F, Malagelada J-R. The origin of symptoms on the brain-gut axis in functional dyspepsia. *Gastroenterology* 1991; 101:999–1006.

Mertz H, Naliboff B, Munakata J, Niazi N, Mayer EA. Altered rectal perception is a biological marker of patients with irritable bowel syndrome. *Gastroenterology* 1995; 109:40–52.

Mertz H, Fullerton S, Naliboff B, Mayer EA. Symptoms and visceral perception in severe functional and organic dyspepsia. *Gut* 1998; 42:814–822.

Mertz H, Naliboff B, Mayer EA. Symptoms and physiology in severe chronic constipation. *Am J Gastroenterol* 1999; 94:131–138.

Metcalf AM, Phillips SF, Zinsmeister AR, et al. Simplified assessment of segmental colonic transit. *Gastroenterology* 1987; 92:40–47.

Munakata J, Naliboff B, Harraf F, et al. Repetitive sigmoid stimulation induces rectal hyperalgesia in patients with irritable bowel syndrome. *Gastroenterology* 1997; 112:55–63.

Naliboff BD, Munakata J, Fullerton S, et al. Evidence for two distinct perceptual alterations in irritable bowel syndrome. *Gut* 1997; 41:505–512.

Naliboff B, Silverman DHS, Munakata J, et al. Altered regional brain activity to rectal distension following repetitive sigmoid stimulation in IBS. *Gastroenterology* 1998; 114:809.

Naliboff B, Chang L, Munakata J, Mayer EA. Towards an integrative model of irritable bowel syndrome. In: Mayer EA, Saper CB (Eds). *The Biological Basis for Mind Body Interactions.* Amsterdam: Elsevier, 1999.

Northcutt AR, Camilleri M, Mayer EA. Alosetron, a 5-HT_3-receptor antagonist, is effective in the treatment of female irritable bowel syndrome patients. *Gastroenterology* 1998; 114:812.

Oddsson E, Rask-Madsen J, Krag E. A secretory epithelium of the small intestine with increased sensitivity to bile acids in irritable bowel syndrome associated with diarrhea. *Scand J Gastroenterol* 1978; 13:409–416.

Olden KW. *Handbook of Functional Gastrointestinal Disorders.* New York: Marcel Dekker, 1996.

Paulson PE, Minoshima S, Morrow TJ, Casey KL. Gender differences in pain perception and patterns of cerebral activation during noxious heat stimulation in humans. *Pain* 1998; 76:223–229.

Payne A, Blanchard EB. A controlled comparison of cognitive therapy and self-help support groups in the treatment of irritable bowel syndrome. *J Consult Clin Psychol* 1995; 63:779–786.

Prior A, Sorial E, Sun W-M, Read NW. Irritable bowel syndrome: differences between patients who show rectal sensitivity and those who do not. *Eur J Gastroenterol Hepatol* 1993; 5:343–349.

Quigley EMM. Intestinal manometry—technical advances, clinical limitations. *Dig Dis Sci* 1992; 37:10–13.

Richter JE, Bradley LA. The irritable esophagus. In: Mayer EA, Raybould HE (Eds). *Basic and Clinical Aspects of Chronic Abdominal Pain.* Amsterdam, Elsevier, 1993.

Richter JE, Barish CF, Castell DO. Abnormal sensory perception in patients with esophageal chest pain. *Gastroenterology* 1986; 91:845–852.

Ritchie J. Pain from distension of the pelvic colon by inflating a balloon in the irritable colon syndrome. *Gut* 1973; 14:125–132.

Saeki Y, Atogami F, Takahashi K, Yoshizawa T. Reflex control of autonomic function induced by posture change during the menstrual cycle. *J Auton Nerv Syst* 1997; 66:69–74.

Sato N, Miyake S, Akatsu J, Kumashiro M. Power spectral analysis of heart rate variability in healthy young women during the normal menstrual cycle. *Psychosom Med* 1995; 57:331–335.

Scarinci IC, McDonald-Haile J, Bradley LA, Richter JE. Altered pain perception and psychosocial features among women with gastrointestinal disorders and history of abuse: a preliminary model. *Am J Med* 1994; 97:108–118.

Schmidt PJ, Nieman LK, Grover GN, et al. Lack of effect of induced menses on symptoms in women with premenstrual syndrome. *N Engl J Med* 1991; 324:1174–1179.

Silverman DH, Munakata JA, Ennes H, et al. Regional cerebral activity in normal and pathological perception of visceral pain. *Gastroenterology* 1997; 112:64–72.

Smart HL, Atkinson M. Abnormal vagal function in irritable bowel syndrome. *Lancet* 1987; 2:475–478.

Smith RC, Greenbaum DS, Vancouver JB, et al. Gender differences in manning criteria in the irritable bowel syndrome. *Gastroenterology* 1991; 100(3):591–595.

Svedlund J, Sjodin I, Ottosson J-O, Dotevall G. Controlled study of psychotherapy in irritable bowel syndrome. *Lancet* 1983; 2:589–592.

Talley NJ. Diagnosing an irritable bowel: does sex matter? *Gastroenterology* 1991; 100(3):834–837.

Talley NJ, Fett SL, Zinsmeister AR, Melton III LJ. Gastrointestinal tract symptoms and self-reported abuse: a population-based study. *Gastroenterology* 1994; 107:1040–1049.

Talley NJ, Zinsmeister AR, Melton LJ III. Irritable bowel syndrome in a community: symptom subgroups, risk factors, and health care utilization. *Am J Epidemiol* 1995; 142:76–83.

Talley NJ, Boyce PM, Jones M. Predictors of health care seeking for irritable bowel syndrome: a population based study. *Gut* 1997; 41:394–398.

Talley NJ, Boyce P, Jones M. Identification of distinct upper and lower gastrointestinal symptom groupings in an urban population. *Gut* 1998a; 42:690–695.

Talley NJ, Boyce PM, Jones M. Is the association between irritable bowel syndrome and abuse explained by neuroticism? A population based study. *Gut* 1998b; 42:47–53.

Taub E, Cuevas JL, Cook EW, Crowell M, Whitehead WE. Irritable bowel syndrome defined by factor analysis. Gender and race comparisons. *Dig Dis Sci* 1995; 40:2647–2655.

Thompson WG. Gender difference in irritable bowel syndromes. *Eur J Gastroenterol Hepatol* 1997; 9:299–302.

Thompson WG, Longstreth GF, Drossman DA, et al. Functional bowel disorders and functional abdominal pain. *Gut* 1999; 45:1143–1147.

Toner BB. Cognitive-behavioral treatment of functional somatic symptoms: integrating gender issues. *Cogn Behav Practice* 1994; 1:157–178.

Trimble KC, Farouk R, Pryde A, Douglas S, Heading RC. Heightened visceral sensation in functional gastrointestinal disease is not site-specific. Evidence for a generalized disorder of gut sensitivity. *Dig Dis Sci* 1995; 40:1607–1613.

Unruh AM. Gender variations in clinical pain experience. *Pain* 1996; 65:123–167.

Valentino RJ, Miselis RR, Pavcovich LA. Pontine regulation of pelvic viscera: pharmacological target for pelvic visceral dysfunction. *Trends Pharmacol Sci* 1999; 20:253–260.

Wald A, Van Thiel DH, Hoechstetter L, et al. Gastrointestinal transit: the effect of the menstrual cycle. *Gastroenterology* 1981; 80:1497–1500.

Walker EA, Katon WJ, Jemelka RP, Roy-Byrne PP. Comorbidity of gastrointestinal complaints, depression, and anxiety in the epidemiologic catchment area (ECA) study. *Am J Med* 1992; 92:26S–30S.

Walker EA, Gefand AN, Gelfand MD, Green C, Katon WJ. Chronic pelvic pain and gynecological symptoms in women with irritable bowel syndrome. *J Psychosom Obstet Gynaecol* 1996; 17:39–46.

Walker EA, Gelfand A, Katon WJ, et al. Adult health status of women with histories of childhood abuse and neglect. *Am J Med* 1999; 107:332–339.

Walker LS. Pathways between recurrent abdominal pain and adult functional gastrointestinal disorders. *J Dev Behav Pediatr* 1999; 20:320–322.

Walsh JW, Hasler WL, Nugent CE, Owyang C. Progesterone and estrogen are potential mediators of gastric slow-wave dysrhythmias in nausea of pregnancy. *Am J Physiol* 1996; 33:G506–G514.

Welgan P, Meshkinpour H, Beeler M. The effect of anger on colon motor and myoelectric activity in irritable bowel syndrome. *Gastroenterology* 1988; 94:1150–1156.

Whitehead WE, Winget C, Fedoravicius AS, Wooley S, Blackwell B. Learned illness behavior in patients with irritable bowel syndrome and peptic ulcer. *Dig Dis Sci* 1982; 27:202–208.

Whitehead WE, Bosmajian L, Zonderman AB, Costa PT Jr, Schuster MM. Symptoms of psychological distress associated with irritable bowel syndrome. *Gastroenterology* 1988; 95:709–714.

Whitehead WE, Cheskin LJ, Heller BR, et al. Evidence for exacerbation of irritable bowel syndrome during menses. *Gastroenterology* 1990a; 98:1485–1489.

Whitehead WE, Holtkotter B, Enck P, et al. Tolerance for rectosigmoid distention in irritable bowel syndrome. *Gastroenterology* 1990b; 98(5 Pt 1):1187–1192.

Whitehead WE, Crowell MD, Robinson JC, Heller BR, Schuster MM. Effects of stressful life events on bowel symptoms: subjects with irritable bowel syndrome compared with subjects without bowel dysfunction. *Gut* 1992; 33:825–830.

Whorwell PJ, McCallum M, Creed FH, Roberts CT. Non-colonic features of irritable bowel syndrome. *Gut* 1986; 27:37–40.

Whorwell PJ, Prior A, Colgan SM. Hypnotherapy in severe irritable bowel syndrome: further experience. *Gut* 1987; 28:423–425.

Yasui Y, Saper CB, Cechetto DF. Autonomic responses and efferent pathways from the insular cortex in the rat. *J Comp Neurol* 1991; 303:355–374.

Correspondence to: Bruce D. Naliboff, PhD, CURE, Building 115, Room 223, WLA VA Medical Center, 11301 Wilshire Boulevard, Los Angeles, CA 90073, USA. Tel: 310-268-3242; Fax: 310-784-2864; email: naliboff@ ucla.edu.

Sex, Gender, and Pain, Progress in Pain Research and Management, Vol. 17, edited by R.B. Fillingim, IASP Press, Seattle, © 2000.

17

Female Genital Pain

R. William Stones

Department of Obstetrics and Gynaecology, University of Southampton, Southampton, United Kingdom

Women experience pain as part of normal reproductive life in a manner that has no analogy in men. Menarche is associated with the onset of menstrual cramps, which range in intensity in different individuals. Ovulation may be associated with mittelschmerz (intermenstrual pain). While some women experience almost pain-free childbirth, this is the exception across a range of societies and cultures. These physiological instances of pain call into question our basic concepts of pain, which in terms of the International Association for the Study of Pain's definition (Merskey and Bogduk 1994, p. 210) center on its unpleasantness and close association with at least the perception of actual or potential tissue damage. The closest nonreproductive analogy to the pain associated with female reproductive function might be the pain associated with vigorous physical exercise—for the athlete, muscle pain during a race might indicate the attainment of a training goal rather than something to be avoided.

Women are also subject to a range of pathological conditions and syndromes of genital origin that cause pain (see Table I). Again, many of these conditions have no direct counterpart in men. A complex and comprehensive sociocultural model would be required to explain whether and how individual genital pain syndromes differ in their unpleasantness, their impact on function, and their psychological correlates, and how they differ in comparison to each other, to other types of pain experienced by women, or by sex where there is a male counterpart. Such a model remains elusive.

This chapter provides an overview of important causes of female genital pain, first discussing labor pain and dysmenorrhea, and then focusing on two functional and pathological conditions associated with distress and disability, and setting these within a sociocultural context.

Table I
Main pathological processes associated with chronic pelvic pain in women

Inflammatory, infective
Chronic salpingitis
Inflammatory, noninfective
Endometriosis
Vulvar vestibulitis
Vulvodynia with dermatosis
Mechanical
Uterine retroversion
Adhesions
Functional
Pelvic congestion
Neuropathic
Postsurgical
Dysesthetic vulvodynia
Musculoskeletal
Pelvic floor myalgia
Abdominal and pelvic trigger points
Postural muscle strain

"PHYSIOLOGICAL" PAIN OF GENITAL ORIGIN

PAIN DURING LABOR

Labor pain has been the subject of extensive research, numerous interventions, and extensive and heated debate. Practical issues in experimental work have included the extent to which studies can be controlled for the large number of potential confounding variables, and the method of contemporaneous or recall-based pain assessment. A key contribution to the literature is a study by Waldenström and colleagues (1996). The authors reviewed the literature on pain recall, emphasizing the inconsistent findings from different studies. They highlight the intriguing observation that women's reports of pain relief show only moderate associations with the use of different modalities of analgesia. This finding may be a result of self-selection: for example, women experiencing more severe pain during labor might request more effective analgesia; the authors postulated that women use analgesics to bring pain down to similar levels under different conditions.

In their own investigation of 278 women around the time of childbirth, Waldenström's group (1996) reported that 28% of them experienced labor pain in a positive way, reflecting the generally positive outcome of labor. The descriptors used in pain questionnaire instruments may need to include words such as "happy" as well as the negative terms usually used. Drawing on an early "mastery model" (Humenick 1981) of satisfaction during childbirth, the authors reviewed the changes that have been identified in women's preferences before, during, and after labor, and the wide disparity among individual women in their perceptions and preferences. They concluded that birth attendants should take these differences into account when deciding whether to encourage or discourage the use of analgesia on an individual basis.

DYSMENORRHEA

Traditional clinical teaching divides dysmenorrhea into two subcategories: *primary* or *spasmodic* dysmenorrhea is diagnosed where symptoms have been present since the menarche, where pain starts on the first day of menstruation, and where identifiable pathology is absent. *Secondary* or *congestive* dysmenorrhea occurs at a later stage in menstrual life. Pain may build up before the onset of menstruation; associated menstrual disturbance is common, and specific pathology such as endometriosis is more likely. These clinical categories have been used in experimental studies (Amodei et al. 1987), but they may overlap considerably in clinical practice. For example, in very young women with endometriosis, dysmenorrhea was the most prominent symptom, but it was not necessarily of the congestive type (Punnonen and Nikkanen 1980).

Research studies have used questionnaires to rate pain and a range of other symptoms associated with dysmenorrhea (Moos 1968), and have used pain relief measures developed specifically for drug efficacy studies (Zhang and Li-Wan 1998). Such measures have the advantage of psychometric reliability. It is likely that to some extent the pain of primary dysmenorrhea has a positive element, as discussed above with regard to labor pain. Hypotheses for such positive elements could be conceived in terms of a pain mastery model, or as part of the sociocultural value placed on menstruation as symbolic of female reproductive potency. Surprisingly, the social science literature has not explored these aspects, although the positive side of women's experience of the perimenstrual phase has at least been recognized (Logue and Moos 1988). To complete the biopsychosocial perspective, a twin study has attempted to characterize the genetic contribution to a range of menstrual symptoms, concluding that about half the variance in menstrual pain can be explained by genetic factors (Treloar et al. 1998).

GENITAL PAIN SYNDROMES

Use of the term "genital pain syndromes" indicates a practical problem in the clinical evaluation of women reporting abnormal pain apparently arising from the genital tract. Frequently, establishing a direct link between the symptoms and an identifiable pathological process is problematic. Following a routine history, physical examination, and investigations such as laparoscopy, ultrasound imaging, or microbiological tests, the physician is often unable to reach a positive diagnosis. Furthermore, where pathology is identified, the abnormality may be coincidental rather than causal. Perhaps the best example of this is the visualization of pelvic adhesions at laparoscopy. The first systematic study of this entity compared the findings at laparoscopy in women undergoing investigation for pain or for infertility. The density of pelvic adhesions was similar in the two groups, suggesting that a causal role in pain was unlikely (Rapkin 1986). This reasoning was further substantiated in a randomized trial of surgery for adhesions, where benefit was only achieved where the adhesions were dense, vascularized, or adherent to the bowel (Peters et al. 1992).

The example of adhesions as either a coincidental finding or a cause of pain illustrates a further feature of research and clinical practice in the field: technical developments may allow more precise attribution of cause than was formerly possible. In this instance, the development of pain mapping by laparoscopy under local anesthesia (Palter and Olive 1997) may enable direct determination of whether particular adhesions are responsible for pain, and may permit evaluation of the effects of laparoscopic surgery. The extent to which this technical development will lead to better therapeutic outcomes remains to be established.

Negative laparoscopic investigation in itself was suggested to have some therapeutic value (Baker and Symonds 1992). However, a further retrospective follow-up study did not support this observation (Doyle et al. 1998), and a substantial and carefully designed prospective study, whose results are yet to be reported in full, suggested that "photographic reinforcement" by using laparoscopic images as an aid to postoperative counseling was associated with adverse outcomes (Currie et al. 1995).

"Chronic pelvic pain" covers a range of conditions that are common in the population. The single available population-based study, undertaken in the United States, found that 15% of women had experienced pelvic pain of at least 6 months' duration (Mathias et al. 1996). This chapter will concentrate on two conditions associated with chronic genital pain: endometriosis, widely accepted as an important cause of pain in lay as well as professional domains, and pelvic congestion syndrome, which is less commonly recognized but gives rise to a consistent symptom complex and may represent a good model of stress-related genital pain.

ENDOMETRIOSIS

Definition and pathogenesis. Endometriosis is defined as the presence of endometrial glands and tissue in locations other than the uterine endometrium. Current opinion favors the hypothesis that endometrial tissue shed during menstruation reaches the peritoneal cavity by retrograde flow through the fallopian tubes and, in susceptible individuals, implants at abnormal sites. There are similarities between the behavior of endometriosis, a "benign" condition, and cancers. Malignant ovarian tumors of the endometrioid type have been associated with endometriosis (Vercellini et al. 1993); this type of association could result from cytogenetic abnormalities of the tissue that mirror the progress of normal tissue toward malignancy, as detectable in studies of loss of heterozygosity (Jiang et al. 1996).

Endometriosis may be asymptomatic, or may present with pain, infertility, or both. The causal role of endometriosis in an individual case is by no means always clear. The extent of endometriosis seen at laparoscopy can be scored using the revised American Society for Reproductive Medicine (ASRM) classification (1997), which identifies minimal (I), mild (II), moderate (III), and severe (IV) stages of the disease. However, the score correlates poorly with symptoms. For example, in 160 women with newly diagnosed endometriosis, of whom 75% were nulliparous, the presenting symptoms were infertility (41%), pelvic pain (26%), and a pelvic mass (34%) (Fedele et al. 1990). No statistical relationships were identified between pain symptoms and the stage or localization of endometriotic deposits. The same group investigated a group of infertility patients in more detail and noted more pelvic pain and dyspareunia, but not dysmenorrhea, in those with stages I–II compared to stages III–IV endometriosis (Fedele et al. 1992). In asymptomatic multiparous women, such as those undergoing laparoscopic sterilization, a typical study reported a prevalence of 126/3384 (3.7%) (Sangi-Haghpeykar and Poindexter 1995). In general, the condition is identified in women with a greater exposure to menstruation, such as those who were nulliparous and those who had prolonged or heavy menstrual periods; its frequency increases in relation to age (Parazzini et al. 1995). The oral contraceptive pill is protective.

Endometriosis and pain. At least three mechanisms can be postulated whereby pelvic endometriosis might generate or exacerbate pelvic pain in women. First, an increased quantity of endometrial tissue, even in inappropriate locations, might influence physiological mechanisms associated with pain sensation during normal menstruation. Second, agents released from endometriotic tissue could have direct effects on sensory nerves in the pelvis. Third, the distortion and restriction of normal mobility caused by adhesion formation, especially around the tubes and ovaries, may cause pain through traction and kinking. Deep dyspareunia may also result from the uterus becoming fixed in retroversion by adhesions, or by the formation of tender nodules of active endometriotic tissue.

Laboratory investigation of tissue excised from endometriotic lesions shows that it consists of functional tissue with many similarities to the endometrium. Many agents localized in endometrial tissue have pain-producing properties; these include prostaglandins of the E and F series. Production of the prostacyclin metabolite 6-keto-$PGF_{1\alpha}$ increases in adenomyosis and ovarian endometriosis (Koike et al. 1992). Other locally active agents identified in endometrial tissue include the endothelins, which are synthesized in the glandular and stromal endometrial cells in a cycle-dependent manner (Economos et al. 1992) and act locally to release prostaglandin $F_{2\alpha}$ (Cameron et al. 1991). Endothelins 1, 2, and 3 are algesic in a mouse model (Raffa and Jacoby 1991). Endometriosis is associated with local angiogenesis, which may be mediated by vascular endothelial growth factor (McLaren et al. 1996). Increased vascularity of the tissues would tend to promote the local and regional distribution of algesic agents. It is likely that pain is associated with deep invasion of endometriosis rather than with the surface area of affected peritoneum as reflected in the ASRM score. A careful histological study has suggested that implants penetrating more than 10 mm are strongly associated with pain (Cornillie et al. 1990).

Diagnosis and treatment. Traditionally endometriosis has been a laparoscopic diagnosis on the basis of clinical suspicion. Signs and symptoms are rather nonspecific, given that dysmenorrhea, dyspareunia, and menstrual disturbance are common in women who do not have endometriosis. Severity of dysmenorrhea has some predictive value (Punnonen and Nikkanen 1980). Specific signs on pelvic examination include uterine fixity and the presence of nodularity or induration in the posterior vaginal fornix. Efforts have been made to develop less invasive diagnostic modalities, but none has proved to be sufficiently sensitive and specific. In recent years a cost-utility argument has been advanced in favor of surgical treatment of endometriosis; if laser vaporization or diathermy destruction of endometriotic deposits is performed on the same occasion as diagnostic laparoscopy, the costs of a subsequent admission or of medical treatments are avoided. An evaluation was made of the cost of laser vaporization of endometriotic deposits at the time of laparoscopic diagnosis (Lassey and Garry 1994). Symptomatic improvement of dysmenorrhea was reported in 21/29 (73%), of dyspareunia in 14/17 (82%), and of pelvic pain in 14/25 (56%) of women, with a 19–48-month follow-up. The expense of laparoscopy with laser ablation was £755 (U.K. pounds at 1994 prices), including an allowance for equipment depreciation. Costs were higher for a diagnostic laparoscopy combined with a 6-month course of medroxyprogesterone (£785), danazol (£943), or goserelin (£1327).

More recently researchers have considered the possibility of presumptive treatment with a gonadotropin-releasing hormone (GnRH) agonist prior to laparoscopy, with laparoscopy reserved for nonresponders (Barbieri 1999). This approach has yet to be tested in a prospective series; it would be interesting to know what proportion of women would accept treatment with a potent modulator of hormonal function in the absence of a positive diagnosis. On the other hand, while a definite therapeutic advantage was required to offset the marked metabolic consequences of GnRH agonist therapy, especially bone loss, the use of a GnRH agonist in combination with estrogen "add-back" makes this approach more feasible. It appears that the combined regimen can prevent bone loss, with some diminution in the efficacy of treatment (Gnoth et al. 1999).

The efficacy of medical and surgical treatments for endometriosis has been the subject of a number of studies. Randomized trials of surgical modalities are rare; the only randomized comparison of laser vaporization with diagnostic laparoscopy alone was reported in 1994 (Sutton et al. 1994). Data were compared for 32 women randomized to laser treatment and 31 randomized to a control condition of expectant management. The groups were well matched with regard to age, parity, and stage of endometriosis. The improvement in pain was not significantly different between the groups at 3 months, but became significant in favor of the laser group (20/32 improved) at 6 months compared to controls (7/31 improved). Results in stage I endometriosis were not as good as those in stages II and III, with 6/13 of the laser group reporting improvement at 6 months compared to 4/16 of the controls. This study was the subject of a follow-up study that reported continuing benefit at 1 year in 90% of the 20 women who responded.

With regard to medical treatments, more data from randomized trials are available. In general, the efficacy of medical treatments and duration of benefit are proportional to the degree of ovarian suppression obtained and the duration of therapy. Systematic reviews confirm the benefits of treatment with the combined oral contraceptive pill (Moore et al. 1999) and GnRH agonists (Prentice et al. 1999). Danazol is effective, but is associated with troublesome side effects (Selak et al. 1999). Women's preference for medical or surgical treatment is strongly influenced by aspirations for fertility because hormonal treatments are contraceptive and do not enhance future fertility. The latter characteristic is clearly established from the large number of studies that have attempted, but failed, to show enhanced fertility after hormonal therapy following the initial negative report (Thomas and Cooke 1987). A review and meta-analysis of the results of randomized, controlled trials and cohort studies reporting pregnancies in two or more treatment modalities identified 37 treatment comparisons among 25 studies. The odds ratios (OR) for individual studies comparing ovulation suppression with no treatment ranged from 0.4 to 1.33 with 95% confidence intervals (CI) including unity. The overall OR was 0.85 (95% CI = 0.95–1.22). Data from six randomized, controlled trials comparing ovulation suppression by means of gestrinone, a GnRH analogue, or an oral contraceptive with danazol gave an overall OR for pregnancy of 1.07 (95% CI = 0.71–1.61) (Hughes et al. 1993).

Some evidence indicates improved fertility following laparoscopic surgery: a meta-analysis of five studies gave an overall OR for pregnancy of 2.67 (Hughes et al. 1993). A multicenter Canadian study reported pregnancy outcomes in 341 women randomized to undergo either diagnostic laparoscopy or ablation of endometriosis at the time of diagnosis. Fifty of the 172 women who had ablation of endometriosis carried a pregnancy beyond 20 weeks, compared to 29 of the 169 women who had diagnostic laparoscopy alone. The fecundity rate ratio was 1.9 (95% CI = 1.2–3.1). The comparative cumulative pregnancy probability curves presented in the report of this study appear to show a sustained effect of surgery over the 36-month follow-up period (Marcoux et al. 1997).

PELVIC CONGESTION SYNDROME

Definition and pathogenesis. Pelvic congestion syndrome, previously described as "congestion-fibrosis syndrome" (Taylor 1949b), has more recently been investigated in clinical and radiological studies conducted by Beard and his group in the United Kingdom. Transuterine venography was used to compare the findings in a series of women with pelvic pain with those of women with other pathology and a small number of normal controls. Pelvic venous congestion was characterized both by dilatation of the uterine and ovarian veins and by delayed venous clearance following the injection of contrast medium. Further studies established a relationship between the vascular appearances and symptoms; for example, injection of the vasoconstrictor dihydroergotamine provided symptomatic relief of acute exacerbations of pain (Reginald et al. 1987). The venous response to injection of this agent was also observed using transvaginal ultrasound (Stones et al. 1990).

As with endometriosis, pelvic congestion is essentially a condition of the reproductive years. The relationship between ovarian activity and vascular function may therefore provide a basis for understanding the pathogenesis of this syndrome. The different phases of reproductive life are associated with changes both in size and volume flow in the uterine and ovarian arteries and veins. In pregnancy, although the ovaries are inactive, markedly dilated ovarian veins contribute to the venous drainage of the uterus. Thrombosis of massively dilated ovarian veins causes acute abdominal pain in the puerperium (Savader et al. 1988). Some of the changes in the uterine and ovarian veins may result from fluctuating levels of ovarian steroid hormones. During the normal menstrual cycle the ovarian veins are exposed to 100-fold higher concentrations of estrone and estradiol compared to peripheral plasma (Baird and Fraser 1975). In ovariectomized mice the uterine and ovarian veins, but not the femoral or iliac veins or inferior vena cava, were enlarged in response to estradiol or testosterone administration (Forbes and Kapadia 1976). This finding suggests that uterine and ovarian vessels have a special sensitivity to ovarian steroid hormones. Systemic vascular changes have also been observed during the menstrual cycle: in normal women the peripheral arteriolar vasoconstrictor reflex was attenuated during the luteal phase (Hassan et al. 1990). Women with pelvic congestion exhibited altered vascular responsiveness to posture change (Thomas et al. 1992) and to intravenous calcitonin gene-related peptide (Stones et al. 1992).

Pelvic congestion and pain. Venous congestion may be associated with pelvic pain through direct or indirect mechanisms. Large veins may contribute to pain via the release of endothelial factors stimulating production of nitric oxide, which itself has algesic properties in a human model (Kindgen Milles and Arndt 1996). Experimental evidence is available for the sympathetic innervation of ovarian vessels (Stones et al. 1994) and the localization and release of endothelial agents (Stones et al. 1995, 1996). It is possible that the congestion is a secondary effect of sympathetically mediated vascular perturbation at the arteriolar level, by analogy with cerebral migraine and other types of vascular pain (Burnstock 1996). This hypothesis provides a possible physiological link with stress as a causative or exacerbating factor. However, while some research data support a link between stress and pelvic pain without obvious pathology (Heim et al. 1998), this association has not been investigated systematically in women with pelvic congestion.

Diagnosis and treatment. Beard et al. (1988) investigated the clinical characteristics of women with pelvic pain associated with pelvic congestion. Features most suggestive in the history were a relationship to posture, shifting location of pain, dyspareunia, and postcoital pain. Transuterine venography may be appropriate in a research setting, but ultrasound often permits visualization of dilated pelvic veins in patients. Laparoscopy may not be informative when performed with the operating table tilted head-down.

The approach to treatment includes establishing rapport with the patient and her partner to the extent that a useful discussion of stress factors can occur, leading where appropriate to formal psychological support. Hormonal therapy has been studied in a randomized trial setting, where continuous medroxyprogesterone acetate was effective over a 4-month period (Farquhar et al. 1989). The long-term outcome appeared to be improved in the subgroup randomized to psychotherapy in addition to hormonal therapy. A response to GnRH agonists may be anticipated (Beard and Stones 1999), and occasionally surgery is required (Beard et al. 1991).

PELVIC PAIN IN SOCIOCULTURAL CONTEXT

Because of its link to sexual activity and fertility, the female reproductive apparatus is invested with potent personal, psychosocial, and cultural symbolism. Therefore, it is essential to consider pelvic pain in a sociocultural context. The distress and disability associated with endometriosis and the sometimes serious consequences of treatment have led to the formation of active, vocal, and effective patient support groups, together with manifestations of dissent, as seen on Internet sites such as the "National Lupron Victims Network" (http://www.lupronvictims.com). (Lupron is a proprietary formulation of a GnRH agonist frequently used to treat endometriosis.) The language used in relation to medical and surgical treatments of endometriosis has been identified as a field worthy of study in itself (Shohat 1992). According to Shohat, "in hegemonic endo discourse the video camera renders the interior body accessible, while also transforming the doctor into the author of a videotape of a newly fashioned body. Along with the language of voyeurism and auteurship, one also finds in this discourse a rhetoric of pollution and purity." This thought-provoking contribution places a chronic, painful condition that affects women within its sociocultural context, especially within the wider dynamics of the doctor-patient relationship.

It is interesting and perhaps surprising to note that such issues should have arisen in relation to doctor-patient interactions in a condition involving visible and often causative pathology. Discourse has centered on the dichotomizing of women into those with and without "pathology," with the emphasis on psychological antecedents in the latter group. Pelvic pain has been associated with adverse early experience such as child sexual abuse (Collett et al. 1998), but there appears to be no specific link with mood disturbance; women with pelvic pain but no evidence of gross pathology had similar levels of depressive symptoms to those with endometriosis (Waller and Shaw 1995). Women have certainly been given the message that in the absence of a ready diagnosis their problem is "psychological," and the manner in which this evaluation is conveyed is often experienced negatively (Grace 1995).

In a group of 105 women referred by general practitioners to a hospital gynecology clinic, notable features were the overlap of symptom complexes and diagnoses and the significant proportion of women in whom no diagnosis could be established. Twelve women (11.4%) had endometriosis, 10 women (9.5%) had adhesions, and 15 women (14.2%) had other significant gross pathology. No positive diagnosis could be deduced in 29 women (27.6%). A symptom complex suggestive of irritable bowel syndrome (IBS) was present in 15 women (14.2%), but it overlapped with other diagnoses in 13 women. A symptom complex suggestive of pelvic congestion syndrome was present in 57 women (59.9%), but it overlapped with 7 of 12 diagnoses of endometriosis, with 6 diagnoses of adhesions, and with 8 diagnoses of other gross gynecological pathology. Nine cases shared IBS and pelvic congestion syndrome symptom complexes (Selfe et al. 1998b). Outcome 6 months later was linked in statistical models to the presence or absence of endometriosis, to women's rating of the initial hospital consultation, and to the individual doctor concerned, although not to the doctor's gender or seniority; these findings suggest an interaction between "objective" disease factors and the dynamics of the medical consultation.

Selfe et al. (1998a) examined the underlying attitudes of U.K. gynecologists that might influence some of the negative experiences of women with chronic pelvic pain. A questionnaire, which developed from focus group work, was used to identify five attitudinal constructs. Of these, scores for "sociocultural liberalism" were higher among gynecologists in younger age groups, in women gynecologists, and in those who gave their ethnic origin as Caucasian. Scores for "pathology" were lower among younger gynecologists. This questionnaire item referred to a tendency to view hospital consultations in terms of identifying pathological processes as expressed by the phrase: "The most important aspect of treating chronic pelvic pain is to exclude malignant conditions." It was not possible to link consulting style or outcome with these constructs, but the study indicates how gynecologists function within a sociocultural context, which exerts an influence that may not be fully recognized.

CONCLUSIONS

This discussion of biological and psychosocial factors associated with two common forms of female genital pain highlights the need for inclusive diagnostic and therapeutic models. Pelvic pain is somewhat unusual among sex-related pain conditions in that certain disorders are unique to women with no clear clinical counterpart in men. It is not clear to what extent the phenomenon of "positive" pain experienced in the normal physiological conditions of menstruation and parturition is governed by a biopsychosocial framework that also influences how "nonphysiological" genital pain is experienced. Further interdisciplinary research is required to illuminate these processes and to translate insights arising across the divide between biological and social science into useful strategies for women in pain and their doctors.

REFERENCES

American Society for Reproductive Medicine. Revised ASRM classification of endometriosis. *Fertil Steril* 1997; 67:819.

Amodei N, Nelson RO, Jarret RB, Sigmin S. Psychological treatments of dysmenorrhea: differential effectiveness for spasmodics and congestives. *J Behav Ther Exp Psychiatry* 1987; 18:95–103.

Baird DT, Fraser IS. Concentrations of oestrone and oestradiol in follicular fluid and ovarian venous blood of women. *Clin Endocrinol* 1975; 4:259–266.

Baker PN, Symonds EM. The resolution of chronic pelvic pain after normal laparoscopy findings. *Am J Obstet Gynecol* 1992; 166:835–836.

Barbieri RL. Primary gonadotropin-releasing hormone agonist therapy for suspected endometriosis: a nonsurgical approach to the diagnosis and treatment of chronic pelvic pain (reprinted from *Am J Managed Care* 1997; 3:285–290). *Am J Managed Care* 1999; 5:S291–298.

Beard RW, Highman JH, Pearce S, Reginald PW. Diagnosis of pelvic varicosities in women with chronic pelvic pain. *Lancet* 1984; ii:946–949.

Beard RW, Reginald PW, Wadsworth J. Clinical features of women with chronic lower abdominal pain and pelvic congestion. *Br J Obstet Gynaecol* 1988; 95:153–161.

Beard RW, Kennedy RG, Gangar KF, et al. Bilateral oophorectomy and hysterectomy in the treatment of intractable pelvic pain associated with pelvic congestion. *Br J Obstet Gynaecol* 1991; 98:988–992.

Beard RW, Stones RW, O'Brien PMS (Eds). Chronic pelvic pain: the gynaecologist's perspective. In: *The Yearbook of Obstetrics and Gynaecology,* 7th ed. London: RCOG Press, 1999, pp 76–86.

Burnstock G. A unifying purinergic hypothesis for the initiation of pain. *Lancet* 1996; 347:1604–1605.

Cameron IT, Davenport AP, Brown MJ, Smith SK. Endothelin-1 stimulates prostaglandin F2 alpha release from human endometrium. *Prostaglandins Leukot Essent Fatty Acids* 1991; 42:155–157.

Collett BJ, Cordle CJ, Stewart CR, Jagger C. A comparative study of women with chronic pelvic pain, chronic nonpelvic pain and those with no history of pain attending general practitioners. *Br J Obstet Gynaecol* 1998; 105:87–92.

Cornillie FJ, Oosterlynck D, Lauweryns JM, Koninckx PR. Deeply infiltrating pelvic endometriosis: histology and clinical significance. *Fertil Steril* 1990; 53:978–983.

Currie I, Thornton J, Lillyman J, et al. A randomised trial of photographic reinforcement during postoperative counselling after diagnostic laparoscopy for pelvic pain. *Abstracts of the 27th British Congress of Obstetrics and Gynaecology,* 1995, no. 571.

Doyle DF, Li TC, Richmond MN. The prevalence of continuing chronic pelvic pain following a negative laparoscopy. *J Obstet Gynaecol* 1998; 18:252–255.

Economos K, MacDonald PC, Casey ML. Endothelin-1 gene expression and protein biosynthesis in human endometrium: potential modulator of endometrial blood flow. *J Clin Endocrinol Metab* 1992; 74:14–19.

Farquhar CM, Rogers V, Franks S, et al. A randomized controlled trial of medroxyprogesterone acetate and psychotherapy for the treatment of pelvic congestion. *Br J Obstet Gynaecol* 1989; 96:1153–1162.

Fedele L, Parazzini F, Bianchi S, Arcaini L, Candiani GB. Stage and localization of pelvic endometriosis and pain. *Fertil Steril* 1990; 53:155–158.

Fedele L, Bianchi S, Bocciolone L, di Nola G, Parazzini F. Pain symptoms associated with endometriosis. *Obstet Gynecol* 1992; 79:767–769.

Forbes TR, Kapadia SE. Specific response of ovarian and uterine veins of mice to sex hormones. *Am J Anat* 1976; 147:325–328.

Gnoth C, Godtke K, Freundl G, Godehardt E, Kienle E. Effects of add-back therapy on bone mineral density and pyridinium crosslinks in patients with endometriosis treated with gonadotropin- releasing hormone agonists. *Gynecol Obstet Invest* 1999; 47:37–41.

Grace VM. Problems of communication, diagnosis, and treatment experienced by women using the New Zealand health services for chronic pelvic pain: a quantitative analysis. *Health Care Women Internat* 1995; 16(6):521–535.

Hassan AAK, Carter G, Tooke JE. Postural vasoconstriction during the normal menstrual cycle. *Clin Sci* 1990; 78:39–47.

Heim C, Ehlert U, Hanker JP, Hellhammer DH. Abuse-related posttraumatic stress disorder and alterations of the hypothalamic-pituitary-adrenal axis in women with chronic pelvic pain. *Psychosom Med* 1998; 60:309–318.

Hughes EG, Fedorkow DM, Collins JA. A quantitative overview of controlled trials in endometriosis- associated infertility. *Fertil Steril* 1993; 59:963–970.

Humenick SS. Mastery—the key to childbirth satisfaction—a review. *Birth Family J* 1981; 8:79–83.

Jiang X, Hitchcock A, Bryan EJ, et al. Microsatellite analysis of endometriosis reveals loss of heterozygosity at candidate ovarian tumor suppressor gene loci. *Cancer Res* 1996; 56:3534–3539.

Kindgen Milles D, Arndt JO. Nitric oxide as a chemical link in the generation of pain from veins in humans. *Pain* 1996; 64:139–142.

Koike H, Egawa H, Ohtsuka T, et al. Correlation between dysmenorrheic severity and prostaglandin production in women with endometriosis. *Prostaglandins Leukot Essent Fatty Acids* 1992; 46:133–137.

Lassey AT, Garry R. Simultaneous diagnosis and treatment of early stage endometriosis. *Gynaecol Endosc* 1994; 3:97–99.

Logue CM, Moos RH. Positive perimenstrual changes—toward a new perspective on the menstrual-cycle. *J Psychosom Res* 1988; 32:31–40.

Marcoux S, Maheux R, Berube S, et al. Laparoscopic surgery in infertile, women with minimal or mild endometriosis. *N Engl J Med* 1997; 337:217–222.

Mathias SD, Kuppermann M, Liberman RF, Lipschutz RC, Steege JF. Chronic pelvic pain: prevalence, health-related quality of life, and economic correlates. *Obstet Gynecol* 1996; 87:321–327.

McLaren J, Prentice A, Charnock-Jones DS, et al. Vascular endothelial growth factor is produced by peritoneal fluid macrophages in endometriosis and is regulated by ovarian steroids. *J Clin Invest* 1996; 98:482–489.

Merskey H, Bogduk N. *Classification of Chronic Pain,* 2nd ed. Seattle: IASP Press, 1994.

Moore J, Kennedy S, Prentice A. Modern combined oral contraceptives for pain associated with endometriosis. *The Cochrane Library* 1999, Update Software, Oxford (updated quarterly).

Moos RH. The development of a menstrual distress questionnaire. *Psychosom Med* 1968; 30:853–867.

Palter SF, Olive DL. Office microlaparoscopy under local anesthesia for chronic pelvic pain. *J Am Assoc Gynecol Laparosc* 1997; 3:359–364.

Parazzini F, Ferraroni M, Fedele L, Bocciolone L, et al. Pelvic endometriosis: reproductive and menstrual risk factors at different stages in Lombardy, northern Italy. *J Epidemiol Community Health* 1995; 49:61–64.

Peters AAW, Trimbos-Kemper GCM, Admiraal C, Trimbos JB. A randomized clinical trial on the benefit of adhesiolysis in patients with intraperitoneal adhesions and chronic pelvic pain. *Br J Obstet Gynaecol* 1992; 99:59–62.

Prentice A, Deary AJ, Goldbeck WS, Farquhar C, Smith SK. Gonadotrophin-releasing hormone analogues for pain associated with endometriosis. *The Cochrane Library,* Oxford: Update Software, 1999 (updated quarterly).

Punnonen RH, Nikkanen VP. Endometriosis in young women. *Infertility* 1980; 3:1–10.

Raffa RB, Jacoby HI. Endothelin-I, -2 and -3 directly and big-endothelin-1 indirectly elicit an abdominal constriction response in mice. *Life Sci* 1991; 48:PL85–90.

Rapkin AJ. Adhesions and pelvic pain: a retrospective study. *Obstet Gynecol* 1986; 68:13–15.

Reginald PW, Beard RW, Kooner JS, et al. Intravenous dihydroergotamine to relieve pelvic congestion with pain in young women. *Lancet* 1987; ii:352–353.

Sangi-Haghpeykar H, Poindexter AN III. Epidemiology of endometriosis among parous women. *Obstet Gynecol* 1995; 85:983–992.

Savader SJ, Otero RR, Savader BL. Puerperal ovarian vein thrombosis: evaluation with CT, US, and MR imaging. *Radiology* 1988; 167:637–639.

Selak V, Farquhar C, Prentice A, Singla A. Danazol for pelvic pain associated with endometriosis. *The Cochrane Library* 1999, Oxford: Update Software (updated quarterly).

Selfe SA, van Vugt M, Stones RW. Chronic gynaecological pain: an exploration of medical attitudes. *Pain* 1998a; 77:215–225.

Selfe SA, Matthews Z, Stones RW. Factors influencing outcome in consultations for chronic pelvic pain. *J Womens Health* 1998b; 7:1041–1048.

Shohat E. 'Lasers for Ladies': endo discourse and the inscriptions of science. *Camera Obscura* 1992; 57–90.

Stones RW, Rae T, Rogers V, Fry R, Beard RW. Pelvic congestion in women: evaluation with transvaginal ultrasound and observation of venous pharmacology. *Br J Radiol* 1990; 63:710–711.

Stones RW, Thomas DC, Beard RW. Suprasensitivity to calcitonin gene-related peptide but not vasoactive intestinal peptide in women with chronic pelvic pain. *Clin Autonom Res* 1992; 2:343–348.

Stones RW, Beard RW, Burnstock G. Pharmacology of the human ovarian vein: responses to putative neurotransmitters and endothelin-1. *Br J Obstet Gynaecol* 1994; 101:701–706.

Stones RW, Loesch A, Beard RW, Burnstock G. Substance P: endothelial localization and pharmacology in the human ovarian vein. *Obstet Gynecol* 1995; 85:273–278.

Stones RW, Vials A, Milner P, Beard RW, Burnstock G. Release of vasoactive agents from the isolated perfused human ovary. *Eur J Obstet Gynecol* 1996; 67:191–196.

Sutton JG, Ewen SP, Whitelaw N, Haines P. Prospective, randomized, double-blind, controlled trial of laser laparoscopy in the treatment of pelvic pain associated with minimal, mild and moderate endometriosis. *Fertil Steril* 1994; 62:696–700.

Taylor HC. Vascular congestion and hyperaemia: Part 1. Physiologic basis and history of the concept. *Am J Obstet Gynecol* 1949a; 57:211–230.

Taylor HC. Vascular congestion and hyperaemia: Part II. The clinical aspects of the congestion-fibrosis syndrome. *Am J Obstet Gynecol* 1949b; 57:637–653.

Taylor HC. Vascular congestion and hyperaemia: Part III. Etiology and therapy. *Am J Obstet Gynecol* 1949c; 57:654–668.

Thomas DC, Stones RW, Farquhar CM, Beard RW. Measurement of pelvic blood flow changes in response to posture in normal subjects and in women with pelvic pain owing to congestion by using a thermal technique. *Clin Sci* 1992; 83:55–58.

Thomas EJ, Cooke ID. Successful treatment of asymptomatic endometriosis: does it benefit infertile women? *BMJ* 1987; 294:1117–1119.

Treloar SA, Martin NG, Heath AC. Longitudinal genetic analysis of menstrual flow, pain, and limitation in a sample of Australian twins. *Behav Genet* 1998; 28:107–116.

Vercellini P, Parazzini F, Bolis G, et al. Endometriosis and ovarian cancer. *Am J Obstet Gynecol* 1993; 169:181–182.

Waldenström U, Bergman V, Vasell G. The complexity of labor pain: experiences of 278 women. *J Psychosom Obstet Gynecol* 1996; 215–228.

Waller KG, Shaw RW. Endometriosis, pelvic pain, and psychological functioning. *Fertil Steril* 1995; 63:796–800.

Zhang WY, Li-Wan PA. Efficacy of minor analgesics in primary dysmenorrhoea: a systematic review. *Br J Obstet Gynaecol* 1998; 105:780–789.

Correspondence to: R. William Stones, MD, Level F (815), Princess Anne Hospital, Southampton, SO16 5YA, United Kingdom. Tel: 44-2380-796033; Fax: 44-2380-786933; email: rws1@soton.sc.uk.

Part IV

Conclusions

Sex, Gender, and Pain, Progress in Pain Research and Management, Vol. 17, edited by R.B. Fillingim, IASP Press, Seattle, © 2000.

18

Female Pain Versus Male Pain?

Karen J. Berkley

Program in Neuroscience, Florida State University, Tallahassee, Florida, USA

This extraordinary collection of scholarly chapters on sex-gender variations in pain addresses a difficult set of questions. What are the variations—in both appearance and mechanisms? Can variations observed in the clinic inform and improve basic research? Can variations uncovered by basic research inform and improve clinical practice? Is the approach even warranted?

WHAT ARE THE VARIATIONS?

It is evident from Chapter 2 by Aloisi that sex differences appear in virtually every sensory system, with females generally appearing "more sensitive" than males. Thus it is not surprising that the same generality appears to hold for nociceptive stimuli. Added to the greater female sensitivity is the higher female prevalence of many painful disorders such as the four discussed here—headache (Chapter 13), fibromyalgia (Chapter 14), temporomandibular disorders (Chapter 15), and irritable bowel syndrome (Chapter 16). But what also emerges—from every chapter—is frustration with applying to individuals the generality of a greater female vulnerability for pain, because exceptions abound. Both in humans and in laboratory animals, patterns of sex-related difference in pain change with age, with testing paradigm, with type or location of pain, with symptomatology, with subject demographics, with reproductive status, with genetic profile, with treatment utilization behavior, with analgesic, with responses to treatment, and so forth.

Thus, we are faced with the problem of dealing with what may be two separate issues: factors that underlie what appears to be a general lifelong greater female vulnerability for pain versus sex-gender factors that contribute to individual and circumstantial variations in pain. It is perhaps in addressing the latter issue that we are beginning to find answers and a meaningful approach.

FROM THE CLINIC

At least three issues recur in the chapters that review clinical issues of symptom presentation (i.e., pain) and therapy. These issues include reproductive status and hormones, coexistence of clinical conditions, and sociocultural influences, including patient-doctor relationships.

Reproductive status and hormones. One obvious set of differences between females and males is reproductive status; these differences begin at conception and continue throughout life. Thus it is not surprising that much of the discussion in the clinical chapters addresses how reproductive conditions and their sex differences might contribute to individual variability in both symptom presentation and response to therapy. The answers remain unclear. As pointed out by Fillingim and Ness in Chapter 10, part of the problem involves technical or strategic issues. For example, the definitions of different reproductive conditions can vary widely across studies. Statistical approaches necessary to demonstrate cyclicity or entrainment such as cosine analysis are prohibitive for most clinical studies. Accurate measurements of hormones are neither simple nor inexpensive.

Even more problematic are assessments and conceptualizations of *how* reproductive condition might affect pain in the clinical setting. Frustration with this problem is almost palpable across chapters. Is it hormones? If so, is it current hormone milieu, or past history of hormone milieu (i.e., acute increases or decreases, long-term high or low levels, hormonal conditions during fetal development), or some combination? Which hormones (or combinations of hormones) are most relevant? What is the significance of variations associated with endogenous hormone changes versus exogenous hormone manipulations? If not hormones, or if in addition to hormones, is it simply some aspect of chronobiology such as differences in the age of onset of puberty, the existence of cyclical changes and pregnancy in females but not males, or differences in characteristics of reproductive senescence (i.e., menopause versus the longer andropause). Could it also be, as pointed out by Stones in Chapter 17 and by Komisaruk and Whipple in Chapter 7, that contributions to variance involve the meaning or significance of reproductive status (in that for females certain reproductive-related events such as childbirth, menses, and copulation involve noxious events that also have positive valence)? One could argue, often from ignorance, because most of the clinical studies have focused on menstrual variations, for the relevance of each one of these factors. Here, then, is a clarion call for future basic researchers: find a way to understand how the complex interactions of these factors might affect pain symptomatology, perhaps differently, in different clinical circumstances.

Coexistence of clinical conditions. While most authors comment on the coexistence of "their" particular disorder with other clinical disorders, some studies are beginning to find evidence that such coexistence may be greater in females than males. Thus, from LeResche (Chapter 12), we learn that, for everyday pains, females report more types of pain but not more overall pain than males. From Naliboff, Heitkemper, Chang, and Mayer (Chapter 16), we hear of a greater female co-occurrence of irritable bowel syndrome with urinary dysfunction, fibromyalgia, and chronic pelvic pain. From Holroyd and Lipchik (Chapter 13), we hear of the higher female co-occurrence of pericranial tenderness with tension-type headache.

Some of this greater co-occurrence may be due to disorders associated with reproductive organs (less common in men). Thus, from Giamberardino (Chapter 8), we hear how dysmenorrhea influences pain crises arising from a ureteral calculosis. From Fillingim and Maixner (Chapter 15), we learn that temporomandibular disorder coexists not only with fibromyalgia, irritable bowel syndrome, and depression, but also with premenstrual syndrome. And from Bradley and Alarcón (Chapter 14), we hear of the coexistence of fibromyalgia not only with migraine and tension headaches, irritable bowel syndrome, urinary frequency, paresthesias or dysesthesias, photosensitivity, and Raynaud's phenomenon, but also with dysmenorrhea.

This information raises a general, as yet poorly studied, set of issues concerning how the presence or past history of one pathophysiological condition influences either signs and symptoms arising from another condition or the probability that another condition might arise in the future. Thus, not only do we have yet another issue ripe for basic researchers to examine, but the delightful possibility that some of the answers might be found in assessing sex-gender factors.

Sociocultural factors, including patient-doctor relationships. Most of the chapters that deal specifically with clinical issues comment on the greater female prevalence of treatment-seeking (i.e., the female-male ratio of the disorder in the general population is lower than that in the clinical population). However, Holroyd and Lipchik (Chapter 13) describe studies showing sex differences in the reasons individuals seek health care for their headaches (severity of symptoms is a more likely provocation in females than males) as well as differences in the diagnosis and treatment advice they receive (females are more likely to receive a headache diagnosis and possibly more drugs), while Stones (Chapter 17) describes the initiation of studies designed to assess how the belief systems of the doctor can affect diagnosis and patient satisfaction. Chapter 4 by Robinson, Riley, and Myers focuses on this issue, going much further to show the enormous impact of sociocultural factors on pain behaviors of all types (both experimental and clinical). The authors end this enlightening chapter with a call for all research efforts on sex-related or sex-correlated differences in pain to incorporate the complex interacting variables of physiology, psychology, and sociocultural factors into experimental design and interpretation. This call is echoed by Naliboff and colleagues (Chapter 16), by Bradley and Alarcón (Chapter 14), and by Rollman, Lautenbacher, and Jones (Chapter 9), with their descriptions of how improvements in outcome are likely to come from approaches that adopt a biobehavioral model. Again, we have another enormous challenge for basic researchers.

FROM BASIC RESEARCH

At least two broad themes are common among the chapters that review basic research. The first relates to reproductive status, hormones, and opioid analgesics, and the second concerns human psychophysical evaluations and psychosocial issues.

Reproductive status, hormones, and analgesics. While chapters that concern themselves with basic research in humans reveal the potent influence that reproductive status, particularly the ovarian cycle, appears to have on pain measures (see Chapter 10), the nature of that influence remains unclear. However, experimental manipulations of hormones and analgesics, mainly in rodent studies, are beginning to yield important clues. What is emerging from this work, as detailed in Chapters 2, 3, 5, and 6, is the realization that there are qualitative differences between males and females in the mechanisms by which nociceptive behaviors are modulated. The differences seem to lie in how sex steroid hormones exert their effects. Thus, stress gives rise to a non-opioid, NMDA-mediated analgesic effect that is present primarily in males but also in some females—those that have been ovariectomized or neonatally exposed to testosterone. Stress also gives rise to an estrogen-dependent, non-opioid, non-NMDA-mediated analgesia that is present only in intact females; its mechanisms are not yet known. Furthermore, the hormonal milieu of pregnancy creates an antinociception that involves δ- and κ-, but not μ-opioid systems. Such an analgesia, when created artificially by hormone treatments in gonadectomized rats, acts synergistically in females but additively in males. And finally, estrogen can influence cardiovascular responses to injury (e.g., by promoting vasodilatory or spasmodic effects) as well as neuronal responses to injury (e.g., gene expression of trkA), thereby influencing nociception differently in females and males.

Human psychophysics and psychosocial issues. Several chapters review studies in humans on the relationship between the intensity of the stimulus and its perception. Most studies so far have used cutaneous stimuli, but studies with visceral or muscle stimulation are now underway (see Chapters 8 and 13–16). Although most psychophysical studies conducted in healthy individuals still show that women have lower thresholds or tolerance than men, what is becoming more and more and more evident as the literature grows is that even seemingly minor manipulations of the testing situation, testing protocol, incentive for reporting, subject expectation, or subject demographics significantly influence the presence or direction of sex differences in interesting ways that defy simple unifying explanations (as reviewed in Chapters 4, 9, and 10). This situation makes it more complicated to understand how a painful disorder might influence an individual's pain in general (e.g., see Chapter 15). While this situation might make some basic scientists consider moving to another field, it also encourages us to develop a more constructive framework from which to move forward, perhaps one that incorporates a biobehavioral approach, as discussed below.

CLINICAL ↔ BASIC RESEARCH

All chapters, regardless of focus, deal to some extent with both clinical findings and basic research, revealing considerable gaps, as illustrated by comparing the two sections above. But this gap is highlighted most directly in the interesting and provocative contribution by Miaskowski, Gear, and Levine (Chapter 11). This chapter presents a table of results from rodent studies that appears to demonstrate the greater efficacy of μ-opioid analgesics in males, and another table of results from human studies that appears to indicate just the opposite—a greater efficacy of μ-opioid analgesics in women. Also described is a series of studies conducted by this group that provides convincing evidence for the greater efficacy of κ-opioid analgesics in women. These two sets of findings provide two excellent examples for considering how clinical findings and basic research on sex-related differences can inform and advance each other.

Sex-related differences in efficacy of μ-opioid analgesics. Several chapters pointed out the consistency of rodent studies in demonstrating a greater efficacy of μ opioids in males, as measured by effects on the rodents' responses to nociceptive stimuli. For humans, however, as pointed out by Miaskowski and colleagues, the effects have been measured mainly by how much μ-opioid medication females and males consume postsurgically. Males in most studies consume more μ opioids than females to achieve (when measured) comparable pain reduction. The question then arises as to whether the greater postsurgical consumption of μ-opioid medications by men indicates its *lesser* efficacy in men.

One possible way to interpret the finding of greater μ-opioid usage by males is to consider results of other studies demonstrating that women and men use different strategies to reduce pain. As discussed at length by Robinson and colleagues (Chapter 4), women bring a greater variety of coping strategies to bear on their pains then do men; that is, women make greater use than men of what might be called *self-polytherapy* (see Berkley and Holdcroft 1999). Is it possible, then, that men use more μ opioids because they actually work *better* for them, and that women use less μ opioids but engage in other forms of positive coping strategies to make up the difference? This is an example of how basic and clinical research can inform each other and give rise to constructive hypotheses to be tested, and then possibly applied. Is it in fact the case that postoperatively women engage in more coping mechanisms than do men? If so, could opioid usage be reduced in men if they were encouraged and educated on how to engage in additional constructive coping mechanisms?

Sex-related differences in efficacy of κ-opioid analgesics. What might explain the greater efficacy of κ-opioid analgesics in females? For that, we turn to studies discussed by Gintzler and Liu (Chapter 6), and by Sternberg and Wachterman (Chapter 5), which demonstrate a similar finding in rodents. Relevant to the mechanisms of this sex difference are the surprising new findings by Gintzler's group that pregnancy levels of a *combination* of estradiol and progesterone delivered to gonadectomized rats can elicit an antinociception in males (in which the hormone treatment is clearly pharmacological rather than physiological) as profound as that produced in females. Importantly, it appears that the analgesia revealed in females results from a synergistic combination of spinal κ- and δ-opioid and α_2-noradrenergic, but not μ-opioid pathways, whereas the analgesia revealed in males results from independent additive contributions of spinal κ- and μ-opioid, but neither δ-opioid nor α_2-noradrenergic pathways. What may be masked by this pharmacological hormone manipulation in males, however, is a contribution from their non-opioid, NMDA-mediated antinociceptive system, as described by Sternberg and Wachterman (Chapter 5). This complicated set of findings further demonstrates profound sex differences in the neurochemical mechanisms of nociceptive modulation, some of which depend on hormonal milieu.

These data help to explain some of the clinical findings and suggest directions for future clinical studies. For example, studies could be conducted to address whether and how the delivery of exogenous hormones changes the effectiveness of κ opioids in females (e.g., postmenopausal hormone replacement therapy or oral contraceptive use). Others could address whether κ opioids become more effective in men when they receive hormone therapy for prostate cancer. Still others could examine whether analgesia would be improved in men if they were given a combination of κ and μ opioids. Results from such clinical studies could then drive further basic research.

FOR THE FUTURE: A DEVELOPMENTAL LIFESPAN PERSPECTIVE

The complexity of the answers to questions addressed in this book might lead many to concede that it is simplistic and naive to conclude that pain differs in females and males. But if one asks whether anything of value is being revealed, in mechanisms of pain or potential therapies by seeking sex-related variation in pain, the answer—as can be seen from the examples above—is clearly a resounding *yes*. Even when no sex differences emerge, simply asking the question can reveal mechanisms and approaches to therapy that might otherwise not have been considered. Nevertheless, because the field is becoming so immense, with virtually everyone acknowledging that there are no easy answers, it seems we could benefit by enlisting a framework from which to move ahead.

Clues abound within the chapters here. First, we have Mogil's elegant contribution (Chapter 3) in which he describes his own and others' astonishing findings on the interactions of sex differences in nociceptive sensitivity and (even more strikingly) in mechanisms of analgesia with genotype. Using specific experimental tests carried out under well-controlled experimental circumstances on a large number of inbred strains of rodents, these studies provide clear evidence that the existence and direction of sex differences under those circumstances depends upon *genotype*. Additionally, these observations herald the huge potential for individual differences in *phenotype* that would emerge as these genotypic influences are further influenced by individual differences in environmental circumstances (e.g., Crabbe et al. 1999) that accrue as life moves on. Thus, consider the work described by Sternberg and Wachterman (Chapter 5) showing that *prenatal* stress of the mother influences analgesic efficacy and nociceptive behaviors in her offspring when they become adults, sometimes acting differently in females and males. Consider also LeResche's contribution (Chapter 12), where we learn how patterns of pain in humans, including sex differences, change across the adult lifespan, sometimes dramatically.

Further clues come from observations in several chapters on how illness can affect sex-related differences. In other words, sex-correlated patterns in pain found in healthy individuals are likely to differ when those same individuals develop pathophysiology or experience stress, the changes depending on the type of pathophysiology or stress. A related set of observations comes from brain-imaging studies (reviewed by Ingvar and Hsieh 1999), demonstrating that (a) *many* different and unexpected areas (such as premotor cortex and cerebellum) alter their activity when an individual is experiencing pain, (b) activation patterns differ considerably when pain associated with clinical conditions is compared with pain derived from the delivery of noxious stimuli to healthy people (see Chapter 14), and, most importantly, (c) patterns of activation differ across individuals (e.g., Gelnar et al. 1999; Davis et al. 1998). How these patterns differ by sex is only just beginning to be explored (Silverman et al. 1997; Becerra et al. 1998; Paulson et al. 1998).

Taken together, such observations call our attention to the fact that the experience of pain is a dynamic entity that develops and changes throughout life. Therefore, one constructive way to frame emerging information on how sex and gender contribute to individual and circumstantial variations in pain may be a developmental systems perspective. Such a perspective is clearly articulated in two recent books (Bateson and Martin 1999; Fausto-Sterling 2000). Here, sex and gender characteristics would be only one set of many factors that change continually over the lifespan and influence how *pain develops and changes in each individual* as that individual moves through her or his own unique life's circumstances. Such a framework encourages us to look back onto an individual's history in order to understand how pain behaviors and potential pain mechanisms operate at the moment of their assessment, and how they might change in the future with the deliberate introduction of therapy directed at that individual.

REFERENCES

Bateson P, Martin P. *Design for a Life*. London: Jonathan Cape, 1999.

Becerra L, Comite A, Breiter H, Gonzalez RG, Borsook D. Differential CNS activation following a noxious thermal stimulus in men and women: an fMRI study. *Soc Neurosci Abstracts* 1998; 24:1136.

Berkley KJ, Holdcroft A. Sex and gender differences in pain. In: Wall PD, Melzack R (Eds). *Textbook of Pain*, 4th ed. Edinburgh: Churchill Livingstone, 1999, pp 951–965.

Crabbe JC, Wahlsten D, Dudek BC. Genetics of mouse behavior: interactions with laboratory environment. *Science* 1999; 284:1670–1672.

Davis KD, Kwan CL, Crawley AP, Mikulis DJ. Functional MRI study of thalamic and cortical activations evoked by cutaneous heat, cold, and tactile stimuli. *J Neurophysiol* 1998; 80:1533–1546.

Fausto-Sterling A. *Sexing the Body*. New York: Basic Books, 2000.

Gelnar PA, Krauss BR, Sheehe PR, Szeverenyi NM, Apkarian AV. A comparative fMRI study of cortical representations for thermal painful, vibrotactile, and motor performance tasks. *Neuroimage* 1999; 10:460–482.

Ingvar M, Hsieh J-C. The image of pain. In: Wall PD, Melzack R (Eds). *Textbook of Pain*, 4th ed. Edinburgh: Churchill Livingstone, 1999, pp 215–233.

Paulson PE, Minoshima S, Morrow TJ, Casey KL. Gender differences in pain perception and patterns of cerebral activation during noxious heat stimulation in humans. *Pain* 1998; 76:223–229.

Silverman DHS, Munakata J, Hoh C, Mandelkern E, Mayer EA. Gender differences in regional cerebral activity associated with visceral stimuli. *Soc Neurosci Abstracts* 1997; 23:1955.

Correspondence to: Karen J. Berkley, PhD, Program in Neuroscience, Florida State University, Tallahassee, FL 32306-1270, USA. Tel: 850-644-5741; Fax: 850-644-9874; email: kberkley@psy.fsu.edu.

Index

Locators in *italic* refer to figures.
Locators followed by t refer to tables.

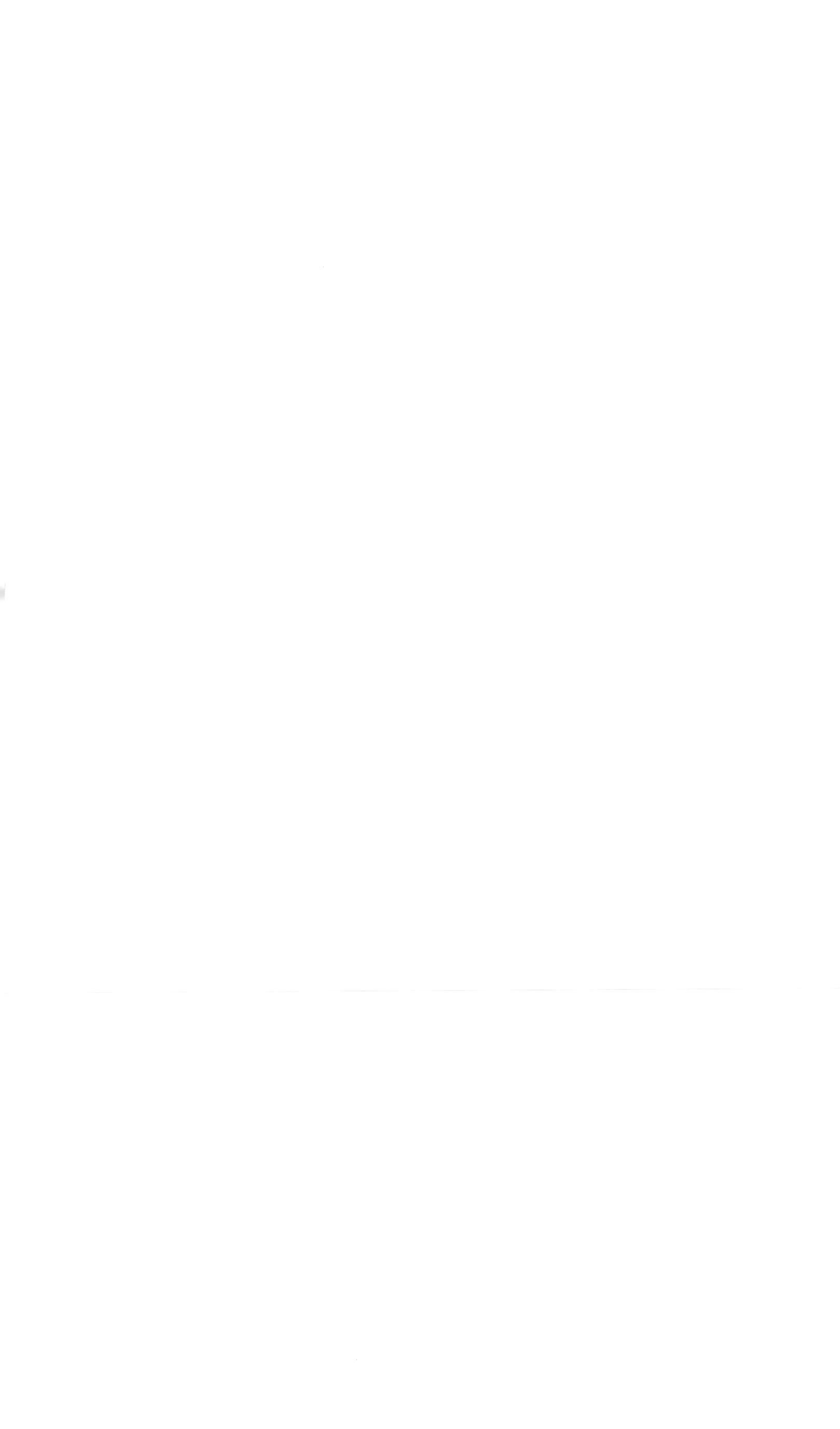